thi...

help

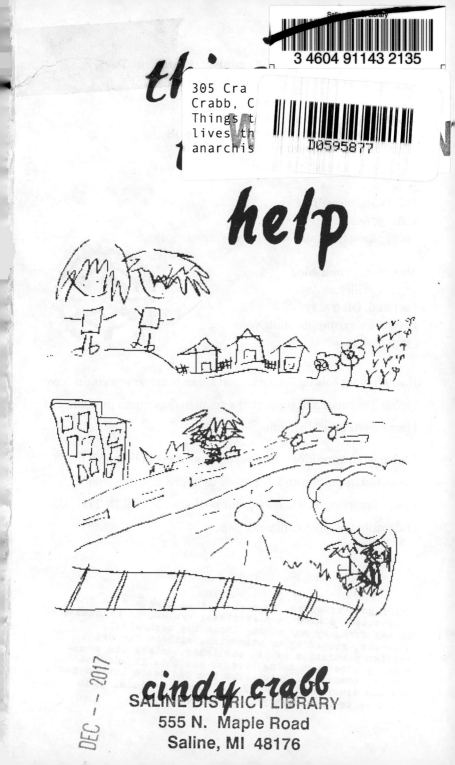

cindy crabb

Things That Help

Healing Our Lives Through Feminism, Anarchism, Punk, & Adventure

© Cindy Crabb, 2011, 2018
This Edition © Microcosm Publishing, 2018

Originally published as *The Encyclopedia of Doris*, 2011

This is Microcosm #204
ISBN 978-1-62106-864-8
This edition first published December 12, 2017

Microcosm Publishing
2752 N Williams Ave.
Portland, OR 97227
www.microcosmpublishing.com
(503) 799-2698

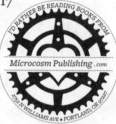

Global labor conditions are bad, and our roots in industrial Cleveland in the 70s and 80s made us appreciate the need to treat workers right. Therefore, our books are MADE IN THE USA and printed on post-consumer paper.

MICROCOSM · PUBLISHING

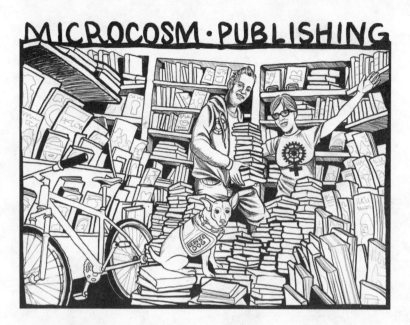

Microcosm Publishing is Portland's most diversified publishing house and distributor with a focus on the colorful, authentic, and empowering. Our books and zines have put your power in your hands since 1996, equipping readers to make positive changes in their lives and in the world around them. Microcosm emphasizes skill-building, showing hidden histories, and fostering creativity through challenging conventional publishing wisdom with books and bookettes about DIY skills, food, bicycling, gender, self-care, and social justice. What was once a distro and record label was started by Joe Biel in his bedroom and has become among the oldest independent publishing houses in Portland, OR. We are a politically moderate, centrist publisher in a world that has inched to the right for the past 80 years.

things
that
help

Healing Our
Lives Through
Feminism,
Anarchism, Punk,
& Adventure

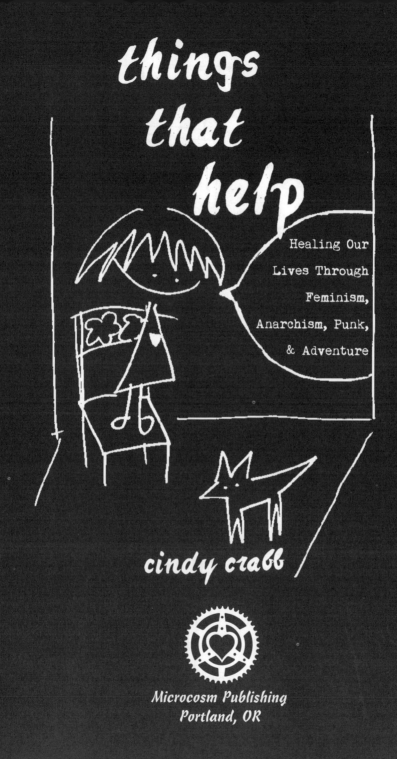

cindy crabb

Microcosm Publishing
Portland, OR

Table of Contents

more contents

PUBLISHER'S NOTE:

We believe in and support Cindy
Crabb's work because of its capacity
to have a positive impact and help
people; especially now.

a small start

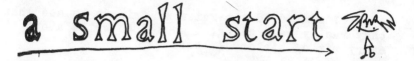

Once upon a time there was no stable home. I moved around a lot. I tried to pare down my possessions to fit into two shopping carts, but I tended to gather things quickly; a little dragon stuffed animal found sitting on top of a recycling bin, bus passes with still a little bit of money on them, a gadget to turn any faucet into a personal drinking fountain (I found that at the Ashby flea).

I liked to make wherever I lived beautiful. I liked to build shelves, make secret spaces, and cover the walls with flyers and found art. I liked to make little boxes with little surprises inside. I liked for my room to look chaotic, and only I could know where every single thing was, where it all belonged. But when I was moving around so much, it was hard to always pack and unpack and find out where each precious thing went. It took too much time, too much thought. I ended up just putting everything in piles, alphabetically.

I read a ton those days. I walked around a lot and tried to figure out how people lived. I looked for projects that could make a life fulfilling. I met and fell in love with people who were living on various edges. I gathered everything to me. I wanted to know it all. I wanted to experience it all. I wanted to remember it all. My body couldn't contain it.

I wrote because I loved writing, and because I wanted to break down the secrets and barriers of our cultures and worlds. I wanted realness in my life, and I wanted to push myself to find the real inside me. I wanted a politic of curiosity and exploration instead of defensive debate. I wanted celebration of the ways we protected ourselves

and I wanted to draw out anything beautiful I could find.

I wanted to interview my friends to see what they really were doing. I wanted to write about every bit of history I learned.

It was too much to keep track of, so I decided to alphabetize. My zine, Doris, came out about twice a year (zines are little self-published, usually non-commercial, mostly self-distributed magazines). I figured I'd dedicate each issue to three letters, and in nine years I'd have an encyclopedia! Which is what you hold in your hands now!

There were years when I stuck well to the task, and years where I wrote about whatever was on my mind and just found titles to fit them into the proper letter. There were a lot of subjects I didn't get to. Some of these I managed to cram in to the new 26 pages, one for each letter, I wrote just for this book. There are also a lot of interviews and articles and stories that never appeared in Doris, but were written for other zines or for Maximum Rock and Roll, Slug and Lettuce, or Punk Planet.

I want to thank Caty Crabb and everyone who ever helped me with Doris or with my life. Everyone who writes zines that are made with thought and care. my bands, my friends, my horses, my readers, and everyone who is working to create a world worth living in. everyone who's trying to figure out what makes sense at all. everyone who's trying to find a reason not to kill themselves. everyone who dances or wishes they would dance. everyone who screams or wishes they would scream. everyone who wonders who they could be if they could get rid of all the bullshit all around us. thanks.

a is for...

apple crisp *my mom's*

6-7 granny smith apples

1/2 cup butter
1 cup sugar
3/4 cup flour
1 teaspoon cinnamon

cut up apples really thin.
put 1/2 the apples in a
square pan and sprinkle with
a little sugar and cinnamon.
put on the rest of the apples.

It will really fill up the
pan and if you don't cut them
thin they won't fit.

preheat oven to 350
mix together all the
ingredients (aside
from the apples)
then sprinkle them
on top of the apples
bake for 1 hour.

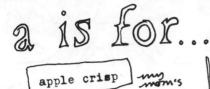

AUDRE LORDE
black lesbian poet theorist

AUDRE LORDES WORDS MADE
ME BELIEVE IN MYSELF and
IN OUR ABILITY TO CHANGE
THE WORLD FUNDAMENTALLY +
IN THE IMPORTANCE OF POETRY
and FEELING and BODY IN
THE FIGHT FOR FREEDOM.

*"What are the words you do not have?
What do you need to say? what are the
tyrannies you swallow day by day and
attempt to make your own, until you will
sicken and die of them, still in silence?"*
                - The Transformation of Silence
                     into Language and Action

favorite books by Audre Lorde:
Sister Outsider: Essays and Speeches
Zami: A New Spelling of My Name

Abiku

Jane said "Will you play with us? I like to play
with other girls who scream." and man could she
scream. all dressed up in a metallic cape and hood,
and Josh too, covered head to toe. there was a keytar,
a headset microphone. so loud it overtook you.
electronicapunk. she sang right up to us. and after
the show they are the nicest people. they offered
to come help me redo the electricity in my house.
they had just bought a keyboard from a guy who
turned out to be Captain Planet. They are in love
with the hotdog shop where Miguel works at and
they eat a billion tofu dogs. we become instant
                                    friends.

alligators

actuporalhistory.org

(13)

anna

her, not me!

He called her the woman who would bear his
children, she called me his wife and kids. I
was like that, kids and wife, underfoot,
around too much, in the way, but also one of
the only solid things he had.

I would wake up in the morning and skate down to
his house, bring him coffee and try to get him
out of bed. and I'd wait, wondering, and nervous,
hoping that eventually he would let me in.

I had decided that I would become his best
friend. It was obvious that we should be, that
he needed me as much as I wanted him and I knew
that it would take a long time for him to see it,
but in the meantime I was going to force my way in.
In the meantime I was gonna do exactly what I felt
like doing, even if it would bug the shit
out of him. like "wake up, wake up, walk
around with me!" and when he tried to leave
town, I stole a car and followed.

Anna was the woman who would bear his
children, turkey baster style, sure, that's
what they said; But she was the one the
songs were written for, she was the one
thanked first in the magazines, she was the
once upon a time a punk rock bombshell, she
could sing her guts out, she wrote too, and
she had a girlfriend.

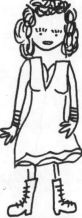

I wanted all those things, but especially just
to have a girlfriend for once and be solid in
it and sure of myself.

I wanted to be jealous of Anna but I had
never really felt that way.

At least not in the way I'd
seen it in boys I'd been with who said

non monogamy was what they
wanted also - no possession. I thought it would
be pretty easy, that it was the thing that made
the most sense. I tried to learn what was going

on inside of me. what was want and what was habit
and what was me trying to get something else
all together, trying to prove something, good or
bad. I tried to stop judging myself so much. Tried
to hold my ground. Tried this supposedly easy going
thing, non monogamy.

The people I was involved with would change so
quickly. They would get that crazy jealous, hurt
look in their eyes, and they'd ask "Where were
you? Oh, with that dude", so full of condescension
and hate. There was a part of them wanting to keep
me and a part of me wanting to be kept. And a part
of me thinking I was stupid and bad for sleeping
around.   But I knew in my mind and I had to say
outloud - I am not an owned thing. It is my body.
Mine.   I said it until I believed it and I didn't
need to prove it. I got sick of smoothing over

feelings, trying to explain; sick of the whole
mess of it, and all the time wasted.

But Anna Joy, I wanted to feel jealous of
her. I wanted to feel a strong, irrational feeling
like that.   mostly I wanted to pretend. I
thought it would be funny. I wanted to walk up
to her, hands on my thin waist, small hips, look
her mean and tough in the eyes, right in the eyes,
and say

Hi, I'm the wife and kids

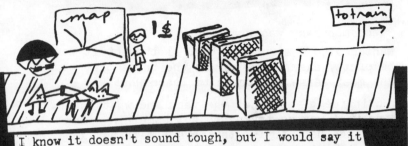

I know it doesn't sound tough, but I would say it so tough, and she would open her mouth in surprise, so nicely, and with that, we would make friends.

So with this in mind, I went to see her read. Alone with my wig, my dark glasses, my dog. I crossed the Bay in the subway, on the train, faking blind. I walked to the Bearded Lady and I sat in the back. All the chairs filled up, and everybody, all of them, comfortable and knowing. I sat in the back, waiting.

People read, and then she did. They said her name and she stood up, in her antique dress, her full long hair, and this feels like a weird word to use, but I will, she was voluptuous. She was something I could never be.

She started reading in this voice, a lower range than seemed possible, a sexy swallowing voice, like she was in a booth, you know. She was in the booth and all of us behind the curtain on the other side of the window, putting in quarters to see her read. It scared me. Before she had come on, the m.c. had said, "When I first met Anna she wore blue jeans and a tool belt". Everyone whistled and hooted and said her name, and then again when she was done, and hugs all around, except for me, sitting alone.

They had it all; raised voices and art and closeness. Lives interesting to look at, lives lived together. And I couldn't force my way in. Didn't want to fake jealousy. didn't want to fake that I was interesting - not that I was pulling anything off anyway. not that I was tricking anyone but myself. My fake world. my fake strength. fake life. I wanted to be inside already, in their languages, in their embraces, and not this. I wanted to be something, but not this nervous girl, in the back row, biting her nails, as always, unsure.

ANARCHY

I hardly ever talk about my beliefs because I really don't like having to defend them, and for the most part, anarchism just seems like common sense. It's about being a good person and believing that the world would be much better off if we got rid of all forms of domination and oppression and if we had the power to decide how we wanted to live our lives.

It seems like such common sense, but I know that reading about anarchism and hashing out ideas really made a giant difference in how I understood the world and saw possibility in it.

When I first read about anarchism, I was so excited. I was excited about people really committing themselves to figuring out how to build community, how to work together and make decisions together in ways that weren't all fucked up. I liked thinking about what an anarchist society would look like; the particulars of it. Like how would our basic needs be met, and what would we produce beyond just the basics? How would we build accountable, democratic structures and federations?

It was inspiring to read about how people had organized themselves in the past - like during the general strikes in Seattle and SanFrancisco in the 1930's.

There was a huge history of resistance that I had never known about, and tons of important, amazing things going on right now, in other countries, that we were kept ignorent about. There were other people who believed that having hope in this hopeless world was not a stupid, naive thing. It was not something I should try to grow out of.

I wanted to see the streets torn up and gardens planted in their place.

I wanted to walk through this world without the fear of rape and nothing but the most fundamental change could ever ensure this.

I wanted to learn so many things. I wanted everything to be different; the very heart of everything; how we see ourselves and eachother and our place in the world.

There are so many things I think are important like figuring out how you want to live, and taking steps to get there

I think it's important for people to push their brains in ways it doesn't normally get pushed, and to think deeply.

When I first started reading about anarchism, a lot of the books were way over my head. I didn't have the vocabulary or language to understand them. I tried to plow through them, hoping it would sink in, but what taught me the most were these lectures I'd go to by

Murray Bookchin. I loved that man. He was so sweet and funny. He would crack jokes all the time that no one seemed to get. They were either too busy taking down every word that he said, or fuming, trying to prove that he was not 100% right.

He had the speaking style of an ex*Marxist who came of age standing on soap boxes on street corners, debating whole crowds of opinionated people who knew their history and their economic theory. He spoke with the utmost confidence, and I knew he wasn't 100% right, no one is. But he had a lot to teach and we had a lot to learn.

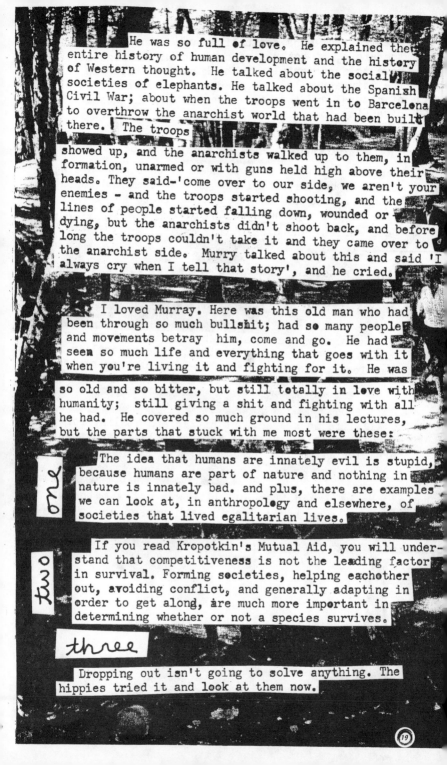

He was so full of love. He explained the entire history of human development and the history of Western thought. He talked about the social societies of elephants. He talked about the Spanish Civil War; about when the troops went in to Barcelona to overthrow the anarchist world that had been built there. The troops

showed up, and the anarchists walked up to them, in formation, unarmed or with guns held high above their heads. They said-'come over to our side, we aren't your enemies - and the troops started shooting, and the lines of people started falling down, wounded or dying, but the anarchists didn't shoot back, and before long the troops couldn't take it and they came over to the anarchist side. Murry talked about this and said 'I always cry when I tell that story', and he cried.

I loved Murray. Here was this old man who had been through so much bullshit; had so many people and movements betray him, come and go. He had seen so much life and everything that goes with it when you're living it and fighting for it. He was

so old and so bitter, but still totally in love with humanity; still giving a shit and fighting with all he had. He covered so much ground in his lectures, but the parts that stuck with me most were these:

one

The idea that humans are innately evil is stupid, because humans are part of nature and nothing in nature is innately bad. and plus, there are examples we can look at, in anthropology and elsewhere, of societies that lived egalitarian lives.

two

If you read Kropotkin's Mutual Aid, you will understand that competitiveness is not the leading factor in survival. Forming societies, helping eachother out, avoiding conflict, and generally adapting in order to get along, are much more important in determining whether or not a species survives.

three

Dropping out isn't going to solve anything. The hippies tried it and look at them now.

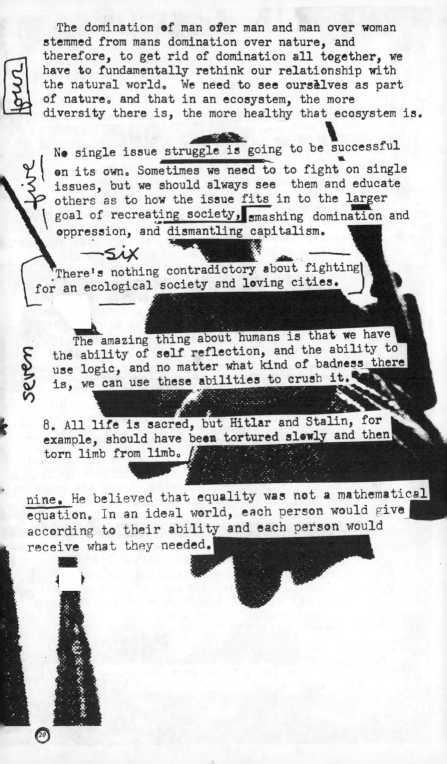

The domination of man over man and man over woman stemmed from mans domination over nature, and therefore, to get rid of domination all together, we have to fundamentally rethink our relationship with the natural world. We need to see ourselves as part of nature. and that in an ecosystem, the more diversity there is, the more healthy that ecosystem is.

four

No single issue struggle is going to be successful on its own. Sometimes we need to to fight on single issues, but we should always see them and educate others as to how the issue fits in to the larger goal of recreating society, smashing domination and oppression, and dismantling capitalism.

five

— six —

There's nothing contradictory about fighting for an ecological society and loving cities.

The amazing thing about humans is that we have the ability of self reflection, and the ability to use logic, and no matter what kind of badness there is, we can use these abilities to crush it.

seven

8. All life is sacred, but Hitlar and Stalin, for example, should have been tortured slowly and then torn limb from limb.

nine. He believed that equality was not a mathematical equation. In an ideal world, each person would give according to their ability and each person would receive what they needed.

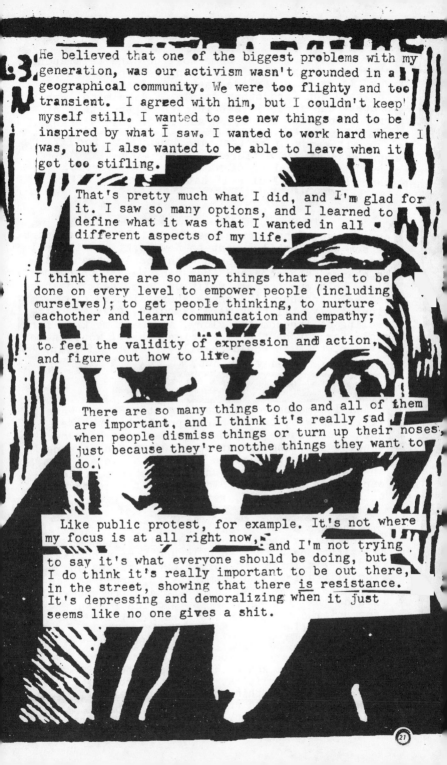

He believed that one of the biggest problems with my generation, was our activism wasn't grounded in a geographical community. We were too flighty and too transient. I agreed with him, but I couldn't keep myself still. I wanted to see new things and to be inspired by what I saw. I wanted to work hard where I was, but I also wanted to be able to leave when it got too stifling.

That's pretty much what I did, and I'm glad for it. I saw so many options, and I learned to define what it was that I wanted in all different aspects of my life.

I think there are so many things that need to be done on every level to empower people (including ourselves); to get people thinking, to nurture eachother and learn communication and empathy; to feel the validity of expression and action, and figure out how to live.

There are so many things to do and all of them are important, and I think it's really sad when people dismiss things or turn up their noses just because they're notthe things they want to do.

Like public protest, for example. It's not where my focus is at all right now, and I'm not trying to say it's what everyone should be doing, but I do think it's really important to be out there, in the street, showing that there is resistance. It's depressing and demoralizing when it just seems like no one gives a shit.

Protest can make us come together and talk about strategies - what we're wanting to accomplish and why. It creates a place where people who are isolated can find other people of like mind. Public protest can force issues into the open, start a process of mass education and force policy change.

I think all kinds of protest are important, for different reasons, at different times. Like I remember the pure feeling of watching cops retreat, when I was 18 and full of self hate and unsure of every move. I had never really felt like I was part of something until I went to New York, and there I was, in black, arms linked with mostly strangers. We charged the cops and they ran. We set things on fire, held one corner, split up, came back together and held another. And those short minutes of winning, even if they were symbolic, gave me this feeling of freedom and glory, and made me know for real, for may be the first time, that I would never give up, that it would be silly and unsatisfying to choose the easy way out.

And I remember once standing at a Roe vs Wade vigil. It was, on one hand, pretty boring. We just stood there, trying hopelessly to keep our candles lit, and one group of women sung a song. But it was amazing to me anyway, to see all these people from my town, all ages and styles; especially to see the old women. It made me want to rededicate myself, refocus.

There's a lot to say about protest. There's a lot to say about everything: like counter institutions - free schools and home schools and free clinics and worker owned co-ops and tool libraries, and community supported agriculture farms. We need to create a different world inside the one we live in, provide for our communities and learn the hard skills of working collectively.

It's important to learn about the world and learn to think deeply. And I think people should be involved in local politics, like school boards and city council (but nothing higher than that), and that we should try and create a really direct, accountable democracy and active citizenship.

Like, in vermont when I lived there, they had once a year town meetings, where everyone in the whole state had the day off and real town meetings were held. decisions made at them were binding. There was one town near mine, where a Walmart was may be going to get put in, but at the town meeting, they not only vetoed the Walmart, they also decided to have a one year moratorium on growth, and in that year they would meet and figure out how and in what ways they wanted their town to develop.

There is so much of this kind of stuff - whole realms of things I could never handle, but I think are important all the same.

And I think it's important to drink in the street, say fuck you to everything expept me and mine. And I think we need to make music, and create a culture that dances and feels; a culture that looks good and crazy, that's full of weird plans and possibilities. And we need to learn to be good enough friends that we can talk about what we feel and think, the held in secrets, the stuff af daily life, the ideas and dreams and all the rediculous shit.

We need to try things out, push ourselves sometimes, and sometimes to just break down. We can create a new ethics, try things, experience things and change.

Britanica World Language Dictionary:

anarchism: the theory that all forms of government are incompatible with individual and social liberty and should be abolished

Philosophic Anarchism: The advocacy of voluntary cooperation and mutual aid as a substitute for the coercive power of the state.

b is for 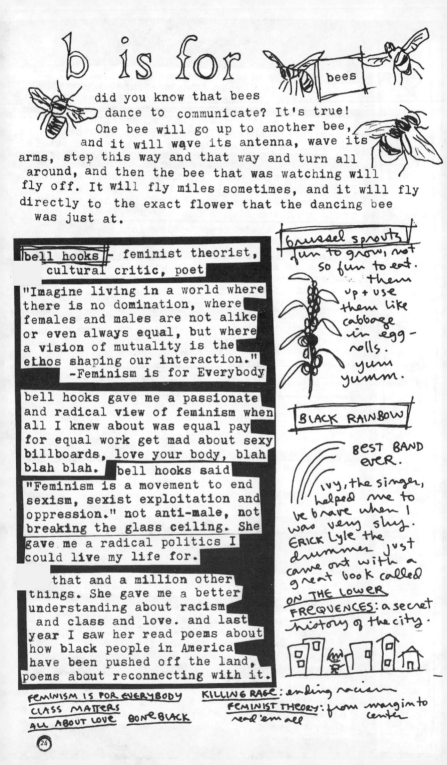 bees

did you know that bees dance to communicate? It's true! One bee will go up to another bee, and it will wave its antenna, wave its arms, step this way and that way and turn all around, and then the bee that was watching will fly off. It will fly miles sometimes, and it will fly directly to the exact flower that the dancing bee was just at.

bell hooks - feminist theorist, cultural critic, poet

"Imagine living in a world where there is no domination, where females and males are not alike or even always equal, but where a vision of mutuality is the ethos shaping our interaction."
       -Feminism is for Everybody

bell hooks gave me a passionate and radical view of feminism when all I knew about was equal pay for equal work get mad about sexy billboards, love your body, blah blah blah. bell hooks said "Feminism is a movement to end sexism, sexist exploitation and oppression." not anti-male, not breaking the glass ceiling. She gave me a radical politics I could live my life for.

that and a million other things. She gave me a better understanding about racism and class and love. and last year I saw her read poems about how black people in America have been pushed off the land, poems about reconnecting with it.

brussel sprouts fun to grow, not so fun to eat. them up + use them like cabbage in egg-rolls. yum yumm.

BLACK RAINBOW

BEST BAND EVER.
Ivy, the singer, helped me to be brave when I was very shy. ERICK Lyle the drummer just came out with a great book called ON THE LOWER FREQUENCES: a secret history of the city.

FEMINISM IS FOR EVERYBODY
CLASS MATTERS
ALL ABOUT LOVE   BONE BLACK

KILLING RAGE: ending racism
FEMINIST THEORY: from margin to center
read 'em all

boats

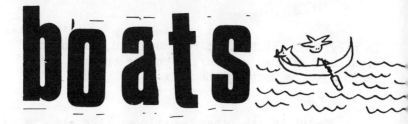

These two started down the river on a pontoon boat,
down the Mississippi, up the Ohio to the Tenessee.
I think what they did was they opened up each

pontoon and filled them with capped plastic pop
bottles, and then sealed the pontoons up and clamped
them down to dry. The pop bottles held air and
hopefully would keep the boat from sinking if the
pontoons leaked, which they did. They also cut holes
in the top so they could pump water out if they
needed to.

I ask the regular questions. How far did you get?
Was it just the two of you? Did you get in trouble
much? and he tells me the anwsers. They wanted lots
and lots of people to come with them, and bring
other boats, but it's funny how everyone talks and

wants, but in the end they are tied to something and
have reasons to stay. There were three people on
the boat, but the other person (I forget what name
he told me), broke her collar bone.   They made it
to Dubque, in this terrible boat wrecking weather,
they got to the marina, tied it up, got drunk,
fell asleep, and woke up with the boat at a sharp
angle, part way sunk. Then they got a house boat,
the one that they have now.

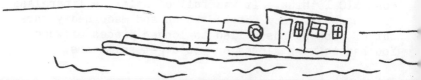

And they haven't gotten
in very much trouble. Not too much bad, except the
wind pushing them upriver, when the current was
suppose to be drawing them down.

I want to ask other questions. Like what is on
the river in the places we don't see? and What
does it feel like, how does it feel in your heart
and in your body, to float into a city,
to enter it that way?

Once, this last spring, my roommates brought a
boat back, they got it free from the I Wanna, or it
cost $10 I think. It was full of holes, a fiberglass
fishing boat. They patched it up and made heavy oars
out of wood boards nailed to longer pieces of wood.
You had to wear gloves or you'd get splinters.

I went in the boat on the first test run. I
didn't think it would hold three people and a dog,
but it did. I navigated. I said "give me the oars,
fuck, there's a rock, give me the oars, you guys
don't know how to steer!" When we got to the part
of the river that is waist high, not just knee deep,
we let go, we floated I can not explain the feeling,

even there, on the take it for granted, stupid and
poluted river across the street. It is something
in my lungs and chest. Something in my head and
eyes that quiets. On the water, so much changes.

I got obsessed with boats again after that and
talked about it - how can it be that they work?
Can you just stick anything together and get on it
and go? I mean, not anything, but you know what I mean.

I started talking about boats,
about things that are so amazing that we usually
forget are spectacular at all. Nora told me she
made a boat out of cardboard and duct tape. It didn't
last long, but it worked for a few minutes, carried
three.

Then she told me about a girl she knew who
took those big Mary Poppins black umbrellas, six
of them, wired them together and built a small
platform on top and she would sit there. It worked.
This is what I want. An umbrella boat.

i believe

I started writing a zine because I believed in the power
of telling secrets. I believed that so much of our lives
were closed up and hidden - the sweet things and the
scar y things and the small beautiful things and the
ways we learned to survive.

I believed in fundamental social change. I wanted to
live in a world without rape, and to create that world
we had to chang e everything - the whole basis of our
society. I wanted to live in a world where we were humans
and not just consumers, where our voices mattered, where
we learned together instead of just arguing.

I wrote a zine because I felt like the public face of
feminism had been watered down and I wanted to change
that. I believed in the quote "What would happen if one
woman told the truth about her life? The whole world
would explode."

I wanted the world to explode. I wanted our truths to be
told.

I had been working on a radical, ecological newsletter and
been involved in anarchism organizing, and I loved theory
but I hated the absolutes, and there was some heart part
that was missing. I hated how I felt like I had to know
for sure what I thought and be able to defend it with facts
and figures and dates. I wanted the process of coming to
ideas to be spoken, not just the end product.

I wrote a zine because I felt alone. I rode the bus and I
watched people and they looked like they felt alone too.
and I thought, 'what if I handed them a small packet of
secrets? Would it open them up a little? Whould they tell
someone a secret too? "

It seemed like there were rules about what was acceptable
t o talk about, and I wanted to be accepted, but I felt so
limited. I want ed to know about peoples childhoods and
their families. I wanted to hear peoples coming out stories,
the complexities of them. I wanted to know what people
felt passionate about but didn't talk about. I wanted to
hear small stories of what gave people courage and strength.
I wanted to remember, each day, to notice something that
made me feel. I wanted to remember to live fully. I
wanted funny stories and hurt stories, so these are the
things I told.

also, I wanted to make sure I kept challenging myself to
research things I was interested in. I would pick a
subject, read about it, talk with people about it, write.

and the feel of scissors, gluestick, paper

Now I am 40, and I still write the zine, still for the
same reasons, and more. I think it is essential that as
women grow older we stay connected to the generations
coming up. We need to rethink our assumptions, reexamine
our ideas, and be the role models most of us didn't have.
I know at least I didn't have many, and the older women
that did stick around, they meant so much to me. They were
proof that you didn't have to give up. I needed older
women to talk to and learn from and to show me that it

was possible to live fully and not be destroyed - that
you can keep your heart open and keep working for

complete fundamental social change, and this work will
sometimes, a lot of times, be difficult, but it will
nourish you. It will feed you. You can tell me your
secrets, the ones you've packed away. It is possible to
feel alive, heart beat to heart beat alive. this is
what I believe. this is my truth. write.

BOOGERS

T.H.O.R. Detective Agency
P.O. Box 954
Bloomington, IN 47402.

CASE: HOW CAN SO MUCH SNOT GET INsIDE A PERSON.
CLIENT: Cindy Ovenrack 309 N. 6th ave. pensacola, FL

Mucus comes from mucus membranes which are in your
nose, sinuses. throat, stomach, lungs, bladder, etc. They
make a fresh batch of snot on a regular schedule of every
twenty minutes. On a normal day this amounts to a quart a
day.   The mucous is made from several different things
suspended in water. The mucin is what makes mucus slimy
and is aslso found in bile, slobber, te ndons, and cartilage.
Leukocytes are white blood cells., which kill the bacteria.
also there is some inorganic salts and some epithelial cells.
those are just little pieces of the inside of your body.

so the mucus membranes are the workhorsses responsible for
cooking all this shit up. normally the cilia which are little
moving hairs shuffle the used up mucus into your throat and
down the tubes to where the stomach acid can denature it(kill kill
kill) your lungs shuffle it up and down. the mucus catches 90%
of anything bigger than 2 microns i guess.

When you are sick with a cold, flu, or other infection
snot production increases wildly. you   could be making
a gallon of snot a day or more. the mucus membranes might also
get infected ~~wxxxxy~~ ~~leaves~~ ~~xIii~~ and swollen which leaves little room
for breathing. so you have to blow it out or cough it out if cilia
are overloaded.
The AMA has a recommended nose blowing strategy which i think
isnt very cool. 1. Hold one nostril shut. 2. Gently blow
into snotrag. 3. repeat 1 and 2 with
other nostril. When your nose gets runny and
puffy that is caused by histamines which
is a way of loosening up cells so antibodies
can get up in them faster. Also your nose when
sneezing releases up to 100,000 droplets of snot
~~Dxxfiiii~~ So always use a snotrag. one book
recomended pressure to your septum with a finger
to stop sneezes in emergencies. havent tested it WORKS!
~~it out yet~~, but its good to know for myself because
my sneezes get me into trouble sometimes.

this information came from the librarry, mostly
from a couple of ch lderens books and a medical
dictionary. If you need more detail let me know.
If you think it's fair we'll TRADE for the FOOD WE ATE
At yOUR HOUSE.

I HAVE lots MORE WORK TO DO ~~on~~ ON
MY MISSINGPERSONS CASES + Stuff.

THANKS FOR   THE BUSINESS.

YOU STILL HAVE SOME CREDIT
IF YOU NEED IT. ~~so~~ ItWAS FUN. ♡ SAM.

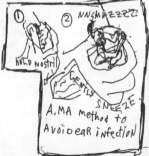

A.MA method to
AVOiD eAR infection

book reviews

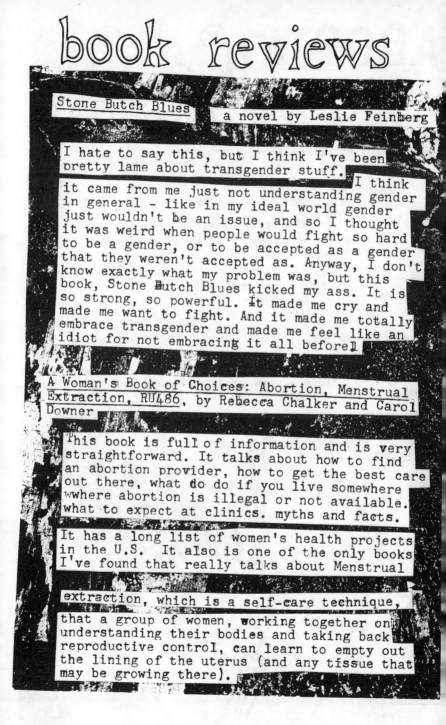

Stone Butch Blues
a novel by Leslie Feinberg

I hate to say this, but I think I've been pretty lame about transgender stuff.
I think it came from me just not understanding gender in general - like in my ideal world gender just wouldn't be an issue, and so I thought it was weird when people would fight so hard to be a gender, or to be accepted as a gender that they weren't accepted as. Anyway, I don't know exactly what my problem was, but this book, Stone Butch Blues kicked my ass. It is so strong, so powerful. It made me cry and made me want to fight. And it made me totally embrace transgender and made me feel like an idiot for not embracing it all before!

A Woman's Book of Choices: Abortion, Menstrual Extraction, RU486, by Rebecca Chalker and Carol Downer

This book is full of information and is very straightforward. It talks about how to find an abortion provider, how to get the best care out there, what to do if you live somewhere where abortion is illegal or not available. what to expect at clinics. myths and facts.

It has a long list of women's health projects in the U.S. It also is one of the only books I've found that really talks about Menstrual

extraction, which is a self-care technique,

that a group of women, working together on understanding their bodies and taking back reproductive control, can learn to empty out the lining of the uterus (and any tissue that may be growing there).

ABORTION

IT IS CRAZY TO ME HOW TABOO A SUBJECT ABORTION IS. SO MANY PEOPLE HAVE HAD THEM, AND SO MANY PEOPLE PROBABLY NEED OR WANT TO TALK ABOUT THEM, BUT THERE IS SUCH A SILENCE AROUND IT. SUCH FEAR AND JUDGEMENT AND DEFENSIVENESS. I WANT TO TALK ABOUT MINE.

I WANT TO HEAR OTHER PEOPLE'S STORIES. I WANT TO CHANGE THE WHOLE WAY THE THING IS SEEN AND FELT AND I WANT TO CHANGE THE WHOLE WAY THE PROCEDURE IS USUALLY DONE. I WANT ABORTION TO BE OURS. FOR IT TO BE DONE WITH WOMEN WHO CARE ABOUT US, IN SPACES WE FEEL SAFE AND COMFORTABLE IN.

FOR US TO HAVE THE SUPPORT WE NEED TO FEEL WHAT WE FEEL SURROUNDING ABORTION AND DURING IT; AND FOR US TO TALK AND FIND WAYS THAT FEEL RIGHT FOR US. I WANT US TO CREATE OUR OWN DEFINITIONS AND INTERPRETATIONS OF WHAT IS GOING ON IN OUR BODIES.

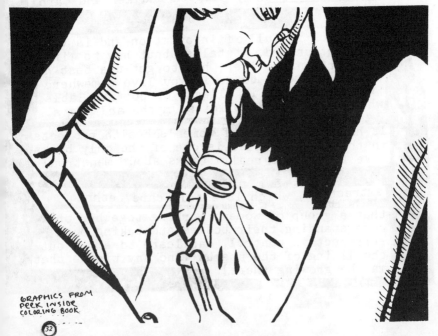

GRAPHICS FROM
PEEK INSIDE
COLORING BOOK

I WANT TO TALK ABOUT ABORTION A LOT, BUT WHEN IT COMES
DOWN TO IT, I NEVER REALLY DO. I'M PROTECTIVE OF MY
EXPERIENCE. THERE IS SO MUCH OF THE WORLD JUDGING
AGAINST ME, THAT I DON'T WANT TO RISK SEEING THAT
JUDGEMENT IN FRIENDS EYES.

WE HAVE BEEN KEPT QUIET. WE HAVE HAD OUR HISTORIES
HIDDEN FROM US, CONTROL OF OUR BODIES AND OUR HEALTH
CARE SYSTEMATICALLY STOLEN FROM US. WE HAVE NOT BEEN
THE ONES CREATING THE WAYS IN WHICH ABORTION IS
TALKED ABOUT PUBLICLY, OR THE LANGUAGE IT IS TALKED
ABOUT IN.

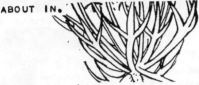

my questions are really different than
the ones people talk about. I don't care
about when "life" begins or when is a
fetus viable. I have different questions
altogether. like even if we define what
is growing inside of us as potential life,
what makes that sacred?

and if we do
see it as sacred, why aren't there a
million ways to honor it, and our decision
not to let it continue to grow.

why is that
particular potential seen in a moral
glare, and why isn't it more of a
moral imperative to create a culture
where women have networks of care and
support, and full reproductive freedom

AND BY REPRODUCTIVE FREEDOM I MEAN FULL
ECONOMIC FREEDOM, THE TIME AND SPACE TO EXPLORE WHAT IT
IS WE WANT IN OUR LIVES, KNOWLEDGE OF OUR BODIES,
ACCEPTANCE AND LOVE OF OUR BODIES, THE DESTRUCTION OF
HETEROSEXISM, SUPPORTIVE RELATIONSHIPS, GOOD SEX, ACCESS
TO SAFE AND AFFORDABLE ABORTIONS, FREE PRENATAL CARE,
GOOD CHILD CARE, AND CONTRICEPTION THAT WORKS AND DOESN T
SUCK.

and a million other things

I want to talk about so much: like where the
guilt and sadness comes from.

I want to talk about the feeling of
body = enemy. I want to talk about
abortion feeling empowering. I want
to talk about isolation + fear. I
want to talk about history and other
cultures ways of seeing abortion. I
want to talk about science and the
representation of the fetus.
so much. save it all for another
time. Here is what I'm going to
talk about here:

ABORTION IN AMERICA
in the 1800's (simplified)

In the U.S., in the 1800's, there were very few
schools of medicine. There was no body of Western
science to be trained in, and so the schools
mainly taught "heroic" measures, such as massive
bleedings, prescription of mass amounts of
laxitives, or opium. The doctors trained in these
schools were called "regulars". It was important
to upper class people to feel like they were
being treated by men of their same class, and so
the regular doctors were given this social standing.

In the early 1800's, when a woman stopped
menstruating, she was not considered to be pregnant
until she could feel the fetus moving inside of
her. Before this movement (which was called
quickening), she was thought of as having blocked
menses.

Even if she felt like something was growing inside of her, it was not considered to be necessarily a potential child. It could be anything, and it was considered perfectly normal and right for a woman to do whatever she could to expell the burden blocking her menses, if she so chose. This view was so common that even religious newspapers carried advertisements of people who would help restore your menses.

there were a lot of medical practitioners other than the regulars. There were the Eclectics, who had their own schools and newspapers and were trained in preventative care and mild herbal cures. There were midwives and general town healers (and some quacks). The regular doctors didn't want to be associated with these folks. They wanted full control of medical practices and knowledge, so they talked to their friends in the legislature and got medical licensing laws passed.

At first, these laws had no popular support, and they spurred a huge popular health movement. This movement was inseparable from feminist and class struggles.

The popular health movement said that doctoring should not be a paid occupation. They believed people should be taught about self-care, that women should learn about their bodies. Around this time, there began to be a lot more literature available to women about their bodies, and there was a general interest in family limitation. It was openly advocated that women shouldn't have to have more kids than they wanted, and that excessive childbearing was sending women to the grave, and also impeding their health and happiness. There was a lot of public discussion about contraception (most of what was available didn't work very well) and about instruments for abortion. Even Parke Davis Co. sold a DIY abortion kit called "Utero Vaginal Syringe" through the mail.

It is estimated that the rate of abortion rose from I in every 25-30 births to I in every 5-6 births. And for the first time, it became apparent that white, married, protestant, middle class women were having abortions.

All this caused a lot of problems for the "regular" doctors. First of all, the regulars were losing clients because the regulars didn't believe in abortion, at any stage (they had all signed the Hippocratic Cath. Hippocrates, a Greek physician from around 400BC, was against abortion. He held a minority view for his time. Both Plato and Aristotle thought it was fine).

Another big problem the regulars had, was they were white supremists, and they were afraid that if white women started limiting their family sizes, and immigration into the U.S. continued, it wouldn't be long before whites were in the minority. They were also scared that women were starting to get funny ideas about their place in society. They wanted to keep women in their place - as housekeepers and child raisers.

So, basically, the regular doctors were racist sexist, money hungry, status and power seeking fucks, and they were friends with the rich guys who tended to get into political office, and the rich guys who owned newspapers. The doctors went around, trying to use all their influence to turn public opinion against abortion. It was a long and hard struggle for them.

The first laws against abortion that were passed - were parts of general public health laws, meant to protect women from bad doctors.

They said it was against the law for a
pregnant woman to take

herbs or undergo medical procedures to induce
miscarriage, but they were really only used to
prosecute doctors who botched abortions.

It's pretty amazing to me that even with these
first few laws, causing miscarriage before
quickening was not considered against the law.
It also was not considered against the law to

perform an abortion if the womans life or health
were in danger. These things didn't even have to
be written into the law - they were just common
understanding.

These laws didn't satisfy the regular
doctors in the least. They started pushing
newspapers to print sensationalized stories
about abortions gone wrong, and they pushed
for laws to be passed that were against the
right of abortion providers to advertise. They
formed the American Medical Association, and
made a long, concerted effort to control and
professionalize medicine; to be the only ones
dictating how it is alowed to be practiced and
how it is talked about and seen. And slowly but
surely, the fuckers won.

but they won't win forever

SOURCES
and
RESOURCES

ABORTION IN AMERICA - JAMES MOHR
WITCHES, MIDWIVES and NURSES - EHRENREICH + ENGLISH
UNDIVIDED RIGHTS: WOMEN OF COLOR ORGANIZE FOR REPRODUCTIVE
JUSTICE - SILLMAN, FRIED, ROSS, GUTIÉRREZ
A WOMAN'S BOOK OF CHOICES - CHALKER + DOWNER
EXPERIENCING ABORTION - KUSHNER
ABORTION WARS - SOLINGER
TARGETS OF HATRED - BAIRD-WINDLE + J. BADER
CONTRACEPTION + ABORTION IN 19TH CENTURY AMERICA
- BRODIE

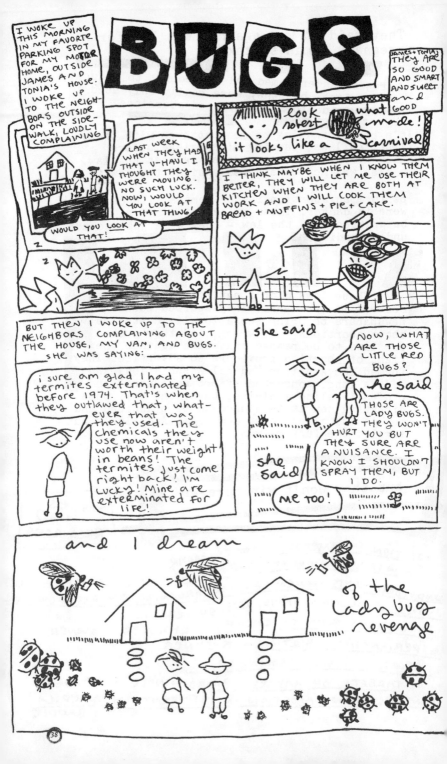

c is for

Chocolate Cake with PeanutButter Frosting

from Raggedy Anarchy's cookbook

in a big bowl, mix
3 c flour
2 c sugar
2/3 c cocoa
2 tsp baking soda
1 tsp salt

in another bowl, mix
2 c cold water
1/2 c plus 2 Tbs Veg oil
2 tsp vanilla
2 Tbs lemon juice or vinegar

add wet ingredients to dry. mix. pour into two 8 or 9 inch round pans, lightly greased and floured. bake at 350° for 25 minutes - half hour. cool for 10 min then take out of the pan to cool the rest of the way

frosting. electric mixers help.
butter must be room temp!

2 c powdered sugar
1/2 c peanut butter
2 T shortning
3 T water or milk.
mix until smooth.
add extra liquid a
teaspoon at a time
if needed.

The Catalyst Project

"...I see no hope of building a successful movement for social justice in this country without the anti-racist training of white activists that will permit us all to come together as equals in the struggle"
- Elizabeth 'Betita' Martinez
Institute for MultiRacial Justice

The Catalyst Project is a really great organization and they do a four month anti-racism training program. Most people I know who have gone to this have been doing activist or community work for a long time, but a while ago someone asked me about growing up and what do you do now that kickball and protests aren't fulfilling and I told them to go to this training. It is run by mostly white women and queers, and they have a multiracial advisory board. They do really thoughtful, serious, amazing work.
"participants in this program will: learn about white supremacy and other systems of oppression and privilege in a holistic, collective liberation framework; develop an understanding of white supremacy in relation to patriarchy, capitalism, heterosexism, imperialism, anti-Jewish oppression, and the gender binary system; learn about histories of racial justice struggles; and develop organizing skills..."
www.collectiveliberation.org

HEY CLAIRE WHATS GOOD THAT STARTS WITH A C?

CHAMPAGNE, CICADAS, CYPRUS TREES. OH! I KNOW! CAPIBARAS!

WHATS A CAPIBARA?

UNSURE OF SPELLING

IT'S A BIG GIANT AMAZONIAN RODENT PIG/RAT WITH WEBBED FEET. GIANT! LIVES IN WATER!

39

Caty's farm

Me: *I thought first we could describe the farm and the land you're on.*

Caty: The property I'm on is about 80 acres, with a creek running along one side and a mountain on the other. We farm about 3 acres.

And you grow… **Caty:** Mostly annual vegetables. (*there is a big tomato hoop-house and grow lots of peppers and lettuce, spinach, squash, beans, flowers, garlic, potatoes, etc.*) We have an orchard, but they're mostly young trees, and we have berries, but we don't sell those.

What's the goal of the farm? **Caty:** My goal is to be able to farm. To make a living off farming. And I've been able to do that. But I have a lot of things I'd like to come out of it. It's confusing and hard to talk about. Sometimes I think building community may be the only real way to change the world. I'm not convinced of this, but maybe. And I think farming can play a role in building community.

How? By making people more aware of food politics? Where things come from? Natural cycles?

Caty: Yeah, I don't know. I think maybe it feels better for people to buy their food directly from the farmer. It makes them feel connected. And that feeling of connection can get people questioning all kinds of things. I have a lot of conversations with customers about the commercialization of it all.

Of food?
Caty: Yes, food. And the commercialization of life in general. But kind of I don't think it makes much of a difference. Part of me does, part of me doesn't.

What was it like, going to market, when you first started your farm? Did people think you were weird?

Caty: I felt weird at first. I tried to grow my mohawk out. I'd comb my hair and wear a baseball hat or something to cover up the fact that, basically, I have a mohawk. I'd try not to wear too weird of clothes. But really, people were pretty nice from the start. Some of the old-timers pretty much just one, was rude to me in the beginning, but most people were accepting and could tell that I was a dedicated farmer. And now, even the guy who was rude to me at first, comes around and asks my advice.

Do you sell at other places than the tailgate market?

Caty: We have 3 tailgate markets a week. We also sell quiet a lot to Earth Fair and a little bit to the co-op, and a little bit to the local wholesaler.

Is it just the two of you? Caty: It's me and Joey, my farming partner. We split all the work and split the profits. And then, this year, we'll have two apprentices. One for 8 months and one for just 3 of the busiest months. And we have various volunteers, friends and family.

I had a couple questions about things that seem weird to me, but probably don't seem weird to you at all. Like the pond. How did it get made and how does it work?

Caty: I'm not sure. I wasn't here when the pond was made, and I'm not sure exactly how it was done. I assume he had someone come with some kind of machine, big earth moving digger machine, to dig the pond in the first place. And I assume he put in a pond liner and more soil back into it and stuff. There's a 4 inch PVC pipe that comes from quite a bit uphill in the creek, that runs underground to the pond. That's where the water comes from. And there's another outtake that's high up on the bank on the other side, so water is continuously flowing through it.

And when you want to use irrigation?
Caty: Then there's a gate valve and another pipe that comes out of the pond and the gate valve you can turn on and off. The pond is uphill from the farm, so all the pressure is gravity.

And the sprinklers just spin.... Caty: Just from that pressure. It's the same thing in my house.

Oh, yeah. That's how you get the water upstairs? Caty: That's why I don't have much pressure up there.

So at your house you have solar, get water from the creek, and compost your toilet. How is that? Caty: It's nice. All of it.

Isn't it gross? Caty: Which part? The composting toilet are you talking about? *Yeah.*

Caty: Oh, it's fine. I guess sometimes it's a little gross, but not really. You just shit in a bucket and put the sawdust on. I have a toilet seat over the bucket. And then when it's full, I bring the bucket somewhere else and compost it. It would be nicer if it was closer, but the outhouse was already built when I got here, and it was close to the creek, and I don't want the compost to be close to the creek. That would be really messed up.

It's kind of nice if I wait until two bucket are full before I compost it, because then if one bucket has been sitting around awhile that's full, it already starts composting, so you don't see the big turds anymore and it doesn't smell as much.

So then I just dump them on the compost (a separate one from the food compost, of course), and I have a bucket of water up there. I rinse it out with water. It's really not bad. And it just feels good to deal with your shit. You know, to actually have to deal with your shit, very literally.

Are you trying to be self-sustainable?

Caty: No, but it ends up I'm moving more toward being that way. I never will be completely, and it's not a goal of mine. I don't feel like I'm changing the world through it. I don't think one person not doing something, like not buying from the power company, is going to change much. And I don't want to just change my life. I guess doing activism and education around those issues, like what's wrong with power companies, is more worthwhile than just not using power. But when I was doing activism, I didn't feel like I was being very effective either. So I'm trying to do something that's not bad, that keeps me sane and happy, while I try to figure things out, like how to confront the system and change the whole world.

I just hate going to the grocery store. I hate grocery stores. And I hate getting bills and having to divide them up with roommates and get money orders and pay the bills. It just feels so much better to not have to do that stuff.

      I've always been really practical. And when I first started farming, I didn't do a lot of the more idealistic things, even thought I wanted them. Mostly I just wanted to get my farm off the ground. Over time, I've been able to start preserving more of my food. I've hooked up solar and get water from the creek. It makes me feel better inside, so I work to get those things. Plus it's the cheapest, most practical way to do it. You can't even get power out here.

You can't?

Caty: Well, I could, but I'd have to get poles put in, power lines, and who wants all that?

What were your reasons, originally, for wanting to get into farming. Maybe the short version. I'm curious about the politics around it and how the politics have changed.

Caty: I didn't really know I was interested in farming at all, really. Originally I went to the Institute For Social Ecology for other reasons, and took that class (Bioregional Agriculture) because I was somewhat interested in it, and It seemed to be a practical aspect that went along with my politics. Then the class is what really inspired me and really made me draw those connections more clearly, and made it obvious that farming was something I really liked to do and could do.

      I like watching plants grow. I like to make food, and I love being outside. I really like to work hard with my body. I mean, a lot of it is that I like being outside and watching plants grow. But originally, that whole decision was a pretty big one for me.

What did you think you should be doing?

Caty: I'd been doing some activist politics and was involved with a bunch of people who were quite a bit older than me, who were really big theory heads. And I really admired and respected them and wanted to be like them, but didn't really feel like I was so cut out for it. I wanted to be that way, but not completely. It wasn't quite for me exactly. You know, I wanted to be outside more and I wanted to have some concrete outcome of what I did with my life that I would feel more connected to than I did to academic stuff and activist stuff.

      Part of what made it attractive to me, and my motivation behind getting into farming, is I like being in the woods. I grew up in the suburbs, and every summer we'd go to the woods, and that's where I felt good. It's something in me. part of me. It's not an ideal about how I think everyone should be, or how the world should be. It came out of something in me, not a political idea I had about community or nature. Although, at the time I really didn't feel that farming was as valid as other, more obviously political work.

And now?

Caty: I'm still confused about it really. Mostly I just think we need to start making our lives the way we want them to be, as well as working on trying to change the structure of society and government and all that. And farming in a way that's sustainable and ecological is really important.

I think you have to be actively working on figuring out both practical things that make life worth living, and the things that make life possible, and food is one of them.

Where to get seeds:

The company that makes M&M's and Mars Bars now owns Seeds for Change – which are the seeds available for sale at most "green" stores. Here are some places that are better:

Fedco Seeds - this is where we get most of our seeds! Pobox 520, Waterville ME, 04903 (or on the internet Fedcoseeds.com

Johnny's Seeds – this catalog has great information about how to plant seeds – like how far apart and how deep. – you can use their catalog as a guide book, even if you don't buy the seeds from them.

High Mowing Seeds

Territorial Seeds

Southern Exposure Seed Exchange

Seed Savers Exchange

Uprising Seeds

Also, a friend of ours has a garlic farm, and you can order garlic to grow from him at **Garlicana.com**

Recommended Reading:

Farms of Tomorrow: Community Supported Farms, Farm Supported Communities, by Troger Groh

Start With the Soil, by Grace Gershuny

Rodale Book of Composting

Book of Garden Secrets (cheesy but has really useful information)

Growing West of the Cascades (if you live out there)

How to Grow More Vegetables

consent

IN 2009 I HELPED PUT TOGETHER
THE ZINE "LEARNING GOOD CONSENT".
THIS IS THE INTRODUCTION FROM
THAT.

I remember when I first heard about verbal consent.
I was 22 years old and it was all over the news that
Antioch college had passed a sexual assault prevention
policy that said you had to ask before each new stage
of making out, and that you had to get verbal consent.

In much of the media, it was attacked as some kind of
uptight, anti-sex, feminist takeover, but for me, and
for a lot of people, it was the beginning of being able
to envision and work toward a more healthy sexuality.

Before the Antioch policy, I blamed myself for my
inability to say 'no'. Saying 'no' was the only thing
I could think of to avoid unwanted sex, and since I
couldn't say it, I felt like I just had to go along
with whatever. Learning about verbal consent opened
up a whole world for me. I started practicing it.

Even though I wished other people would take the
initiative and ask me for consent, there was something
really empowering and sexy and sweet about constantly
asking them 'is this ok?', 'do you want me to do this?'

Sometimes it helped me to realize I wasn't the only
one who was scared or unsure. Sometimes checking in
with them helped me check in with myself.

For the most part, I didn't know what my own
boundries were. and I think learning our boundries
is a life long process. We can do some figuring out
on our own, but not all of it. and it changes.

44

and I think it is so very essential that we honor whatever ways we have survived.   and that we honor the ways we are surviving now.

Hearing people talk about their own experiences with consent helps me feel less crazy and less alone. It gives me hope that we will be able to change the world we live in - that we will be able to change what gets taken for granted, and how we see and understand eachother.

Things have already changed. I think it is important to remember this. From the founding of the first rape crisis center, the first feminist women's health center, the first workshop on consent, the forming of groups like Men Can Stop Rape, Sister Song, Philly's Pissed, Generation 5 - these and all the books and zines and conversations and art shows and speakouts and songs and friendships. they are changing things. I can see it. even when there is so much still.

Talking about our experiences with consent, our struggles, our mistakes and how we've learned, these are part of a much larger revolutionary struggle. I feel lucky to have been asked to compile this zine, and am amazed by the bravery of the contributors.

And I am amazed by your bravery too. Yes, you. In a world which asks us not to care too deeply or question too closely, it is brave to be here with this.

zines available at microcosm or at dorisdorisdoris.com/zines

| ZINES |
LEARNING GOOD CONSENT
SUPPORT / APOYO
ASK FIRST
LOVE LETTERS TO MONSTERS #2
MEN IN THE FEMINIST STRUGGLE

| BOOKS |
COURAGE TO HEAL, INVISIBLE GIRLS
SURVIVORS GUIDE TO SEX, MEN'S WORK

Consent questions

from SUPPORT zine

by andrea, cindy + aple

..Not all of the questions have right or wrong answers. We put them together with the hopes that it would help people to think deeply, and to help open up conversations about consent. I know it's a long list, but please read and think honestly about these questions, one at a time.

1. How do you define consent?
2. Have you ever talked about consent with your partners(s) or friends?
3. Do you know people, or have you been with people who define consent differently than you do?
4. Have you ever been unsure about whether or not the person you were being sexual with wanted to be doing what you were doing? Did you talk about it? Did you ignore it in hopes that it would change? Did you continue what you were doing because it was pleasurable to you and you didn't want to deal with what the other person was experiencing? Did you continue because you felt it was your duty? How do you feel about the choice you made?
5. Do you think it is the other person's responsibility to say something if they aren't into what you are doing?
6. How might someone express that what is happening is not ok?
7. Do you look only for verbal signs or are there other signs?
8. Do you think it is possible to misinterpret silence for consent?
9. Have you ever asked someone what kinds of signs you should look for if they have a hard time verbalizing when something feels wrong?
10. Do you only ask about these kinds of things if you are in a serious relationship or do you feel able to talk in casual situations too?
11. Do you think talking ruins the mood?
12. Do you think consent can be erotic?
13. Do you think about people's abuse histories?
14. Do you check in as things progress or do you assume the original consent means everything is ok?
15. If you achieve consent once, do you assume it's always ok after that?
16. If someone consents to one thing, do you assume everything else is ok or do you ask before touching in different ways or taking things to more intense levels?
17. Are you resentful of people who need or want to talk about being abused? Why?
18. Are you usually attracted to people who fit the traditional standard of beauty as seen in the united states?
19. Do you pursue friendship with people because you want to be with them, and then give up on the friendship if that person isn't interested in you sexually?
20. Do you pursue someone sexually even after they have said they just want to be friends?
21. Do you assume that if someone is affectionate they are probably sexually interested in you?
22. Do you think about affection, sexuality and boundaries? Do you talk about these issues with people? IF so, do you talk about them only when you want to be sexual with someone or do you talk about them because you think it is important and you genuinely want to know?
23. Are you clear about your own intentions?
24. Have you ever tried to talk someone into doing something they showed hesitancy about?
25. Do you think hesitancy is a form of flirting?
26. Are you aware that in some instances it is not?
27. Have you ever thought someone's actions were flirtatious when that wasn't actually the message they wanted to get across?
28. Do you think that if someone is promiscuous that makes it ok to objectify them, or talk about them in ways you normally wouldn't?
29. If someone is promiscuous, do you think it's less important to get consent?
30. Do you think that if someone dresses in a certain way it makes it ok to objectify them?
31. If someone dresses a certain way do you think it means they want your sexual attention or approval?
32. Do you understand that there are many other reasons, that have nothing to do with you, that a person might want to dress or act in a way that you might find sexy?

33. Are you attracted to people with a certain kind of gender presentation?
34. Have you ever objectified someone's gender presentation?
35. Do you assume that each person who fits a certain perceived gender presentation will interact with you in the same way?
36. Do you think sex is a game?
37. Do you ever try to get yourself into situations that give you an excuse for touching someone you think would say "no" if you asked? i.e., dancing, getting really drunk around them, falling asleep next to them.
38. Do you make people feel "unfun" or "unliberated" if they don't want to try certain sexual things?
39. Do you think there are ways you act that might make someone feel that way even if it's not what you're trying to do?
40. Do you ever try and make bargains? i.e. "if you let me _____, I'll do _____ for you"?
41. Have you ever tried asking someone what they're feeling? IF so, did you listen to them and respect them?
42. Have you used jealousy as a means of control?
43. Do you feel like being in a relationship with someone means that they have an obligation to have sex with you?
44. What if they want to abstain from sex for a week? a month? a year?
45. Do you whine or threaten if you're not having the amount of sex or the kind of sex that you want?
46. Do you think it's ok to initiate something sexual with someone who's sleeping?
47. What if the person is your partner?
48. Do you think it's important to talk with them about it when they're awake first?
49. Do you ever look at how you interact with people or how to treat people, positive or negative, and where that comes from/ where you learned it?
50. Do you behave differently when you've been drinking?
51. What are positive aspects of drinking for you? What are negative aspects?
52. Have you been sexual with people when you were drunk or when they were drunk? Have you ever felt uncomfortable or embarrassed about it the next day? Has the person you were with ever acted weird to you afterward?
53. Do you seek consent the same way when you are drunk as when you're sober?
54. Do you think it is important to talk the next day with the person you've been sexual with if there has been drinking involved? If not, is it because it's uncomfortable or because you think something might have happened that shouldn't have? Or is it because you think that's just the way things go?
55. Do you think people need to take things more lightly?
56. Do you think these questions are repressive and people who look critically at their sexual histories and their current behavior are uptight and should be more "liberated"?
57. Do you think liberation might be different for different people?
58. Do you find yourself repeating binary gender behaviors, even within queer relationships and friendships? How might you doing this make others feel?
59. Do you view sexuality and gender presentation as part of a whole person, or do you consider those to be exclusively sexual aspects of people?
60. If someone is dressed in drag, do you take it as an invitation to make sexual comments?
61. Do you fetishize people because of their gender presentation?
62. Do you think only men abuse?
63. Do you think that in a relationship between people of the same gender, only the one who is more "manly" abuses?

64. How do you react if someone becomes uncomfortable with what you're doing, or if they don't want to do something? Do you get defensive? Do you feel guilty? Does the other person end up having to take care of you and reassure you? or are you able to step back and listen and hear them and support them and take responsibility for your actions?
65. Do you tell your side of the story and try and change the way they experienced the situation?
66. Do you do things to show your partner that you're listening and that you're interested in their ideas about consent or their ideas about what you did?
67. Do you ever talk about sex and consent when you're not in bed?
68. Have you ever raped or sexually abused or sexually manipulated someone? Are you able to think about your behavior? Have you made changes? What kinds of changes?

69. Are you uncomfortable with your body or your sexuality?
70. Have you been sexually abused?
71. Has your own uncomfortable ness or your own abuse history caused you to act in abusive ways? If so, have you ever been able to talk to anyone about it? Do you think talking about it is or could be helpful?
72. Do you avoid talking about consent or abuse because you aren't ready to or don't want to talk about your own sexual abuse?
73. Do you ever feel obligated to have sex?
74. Do you ever feel obligated to initiate sex?
75. What if days, months, or years later. someone tells you they were uncomfortable with what you did? Do you grill them?
76. Do you initiate conversations about safe sex and birth control (if applicable)?
77. Do you think that saying something as vague as "I've been tested recently" is enough?
78. Do you take your partners concerns about safe sex and/or birth control seriously?
79. Do you think that if one person wants to have safe sex and the other person doesn't really care, it is the responsibility of the person who has concerns to provide safe sex supplies?
80. Do you think if a person has a body that can get pregnant, and they don't want to, it is up to them to provide birth control?
81. Do you complain or refuse safe sex or the type of birth control your partner want to use because it reduces your pleasure?
82. Do you try and manipulate your partner about these issues?
83. Do you think there is ongoing work that we can do to end sexual violence in our communities?

BOOKS SURVIVORS GUIDE TO SEX by STACI HAINES
INVISIBLE GIRLS - PATI FEVEREISEN   COURAGE TO HEAL by BASS + DAVIS   + ALLIES IN HEALING by DAVIS
MEN'S WORK - PAUL KIVEL
HOLY VIRILITY: the SOCIAL CONSTRUCTION of MASCULINITY - REYNAUD
REDEFINING OUR RELATIONSHIPS - WENDY OMATIC   THE ETHICAL SLUT
THE WILL TO CHANGE: MEN, MASCULINITY + LOVE - bell hooks
MEN + INTIMACY - ABBOT   CRACKING THE ARMOR - KAUFMAN

zine distros   dorisdorisdoris.com/zines
radicalmentalhealth.net
papertraildistro.com
socialdetox.wordpress.com

WEBSITES   campus-adr.org/CMHER/Report Resources/Editions 6_1/
stopping-rape.html - men stopping rape exercises + group activities

generationfive.org   myspace.com/phillyspissedandstandsup
dorisdorisdoris.com/resources   incite-national.org
cARA-seattle.org   men can stoprape.org   icarusproject.net
xyonline.net   a calltomen.com
girlarmy.org   notherapedocumentary.org

zines   SUPPORT.   WHAT WE DO WHEN
MEN IN THE FEMINIST STRUGGLE
NOT WITHOUT MY CONSENT
BEGINNERS GUIDE TO RESPONSIBLE SEXUALITY
SEE NO HEAR NO SPEAK NO

d is for

Dilly Beans

pick 4 pounds of green beans. wash them and
remove stems and tips and cut them so they
stand upright in pint jars (you will need 7
pint jars). Clean and boil the jars and lids.
In each jar, place 1 dill head or 1/2 tsp dill
seed, 1 garlic clove and 1/4 tsp crushed dry
red hot pepper. Pack beans in leaving 1 inch
room at top of jar.
Heat 5 cups water and 5 cups vinegar and a
little less than 1/2 cup pickling salt.
fill the jars. run a plastic knife or
something along the edges to get rid of
air bubbles. put lids on not too tight.
boil jars for 10 minutes. remove jars.let
sit for at least 2 weeks. eat. yummmmm!

♡

Dorothy Allison

writer, feminist activist,
southern lesbian sex radical

I LOVE DOROTHY ALLISONS BOOKS TRASH,
BASTARD OUT OF CAROLINA, THE WOMEN WHO
HATE ME, BUT ESPECIALLY SKIN: TALKING
ABOUT SEX, CLASS + LITERATURE. (she also has
another fiction book thats not so great but I
forgot its name) HER NOVEL + SHORT STORY BOOK
ARE ABOUT GROWING UP POOR WITH THE FOCUS
ON THE WOMEN and GIRLS. they are beautifully
written, horrifying + beautiful + real+ brave
HER ESSAYS ARE ABOUT MOVING FROM THAT
WORLD INTO THE LESBIAN FEMINIST ACTIVIST COMMUNITY.

"Entitlement, I have told them, is a matter of feeling like we rather than they. You
think you have a right to things, a place in the world, and it is so intrinsically a
part of you that you cannot imagine people like me, people who seem to live in
your world, who don't have it... I have never been able to make clear the degree
of my fear, the extent to which I feel myself denied; not only that I am queer in a
world that hates queers, but that I was born poor into a world that despises the
poor. The need to make my world believable to people who have never
experienced it is part of why I write fiction. I know that some things must be felt to
be understood, that despair, for example, can never be adequately analyzed; it

must be lived. But if I can write a story that so draws the reader in that she
imagines herself like my characters, feels their sense of fear and uncertainty,
their hopes and terrors, than I have come closer to knowing myself as real,
important as the very people I have always watched in awe."

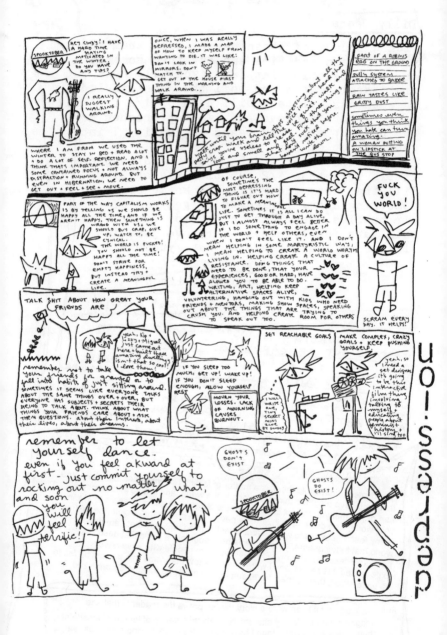

50

COMPASSION

SPOOKTOBER
HEY CINDY! I HAVE A HARD TIME STAYING MOTIVATED IN THE WINTER. DO YOU HAVE ANY TIPS?
I REALLY SUGGEST WALKING AROUND.
WHERE I AM FROM WE USED THE WINTER TO STAY IN BED + READ ALOT + DO A LOT OF SELF-REFLECTION. AND I THINK THATS IMPORTANT. WE NEED SOME CONTAINED FOCUS + NOT ALWAYS DISTRACTION + RUNNING AROUND. BUT EVEN IN HIBERNATION, WE NEED TO GET OUT + FEEL + SEE + MOVE.
ONCE, WHEN I WAS REALLY DEPRESSED, I MADE A MAP OF HOW TO KEEP MYSELF FROM WANTING TO DIE. IT WAS LIKE: DON'T LOOK IN MIRRORS. DON'T WATCH TV. GET OUT OF THE HOUSE FIRST THING IN THE MORNING AND WALK AROUND...
walk until your brain stops obsessing about all the petty crap. Walk and tell the voice in your head that says you're useless to please be quiet. Walk and look and smell and feel. Find three things that don't suck that you haven't noticed before. write them down.
PART OF A ROBINS EGG ON THE GROUND
PULLY SYSTEM ATTACHED TO BRIDGE
RAIN TASTES LIKE GRITTY DUST
sometimes even things you think you hate can turn amazing.
A WOMAN PUTTING ON LIPSTICK AT THE BUS STOP
PART OF THE WAY CAPITALISM WORKS IS BY TELLING US WE SHOULD BE HAPPY ALL THE TIME, AND IF WE AREN'T HAPPY, THEN SOMETHING IS WRONG WITH US + WE SHOULD BUY CRAP, GIVE UP, WATCH TV, BE CYNICAL.
THE WORLD IS FUCKED! YOU SHOULD NOT BE HAPPY ALL THE TIME! DON'T STRIVE FOR EMPTY HAPPINESS, BUT INSTEAD TRY + CREATE A MEANINGFUL LIFE.
OF COURSE, SOMETIMES THE MOST DEPRESSING THING IS IT'S HARD TO FIGURE OUT HOW TO MAKE A MEANINGFUL LIFE. SOMETIMES IT IS ALL I CAN DO JUST TO GET THROUGH A DAY ALIVE, BUT I ALMOST ALWAYS FEEL BETTER IF I DO SOMETHING TO ENGAGE IN THE WORLD + HELP OTHERS, EVEN WHEN I DON'T FEEL LIKE IT. AND I DON'T MEAN HELPING IN SOME MARTYRISTIC WAY, I MEAN HELPING TO CREATE A WORLD WORTH LIVING IN. HELPING CREATE A CULTURE OF RESISTANCE. DOING THINGS THAT NEED TO BE DONE, THAT YOUR EXPERIENCES, GOOD OR HARD, HAVE ALOWED YOU TO BE ABLE TO DO. WRITING, ART, HELPING KEEP ALTERNATIVE SPACES ALIVE, VOLUNTEERING, HANGING OUT WITH KIDS WHO NEED FRIENDS + MENTORS, MAKING SHOW SPACES, SPEAKING OUT ABOUT THE THINGS THAT ARE TRYING TO CRUSH YOU. AND HELPING CREATE ROOM FOR OTHERS TO SPEAK OUT TOO.
FUCK YOU WORLD!
SCREAM EVERY DAY. IT HELPS!
TALK SHIT ABOUT HOW GREAT YOUR FRIENDS ARE
yeah, Kip + Lizzy + Miguel just came out here + built these amazing dwellings! isn't that so cool! I love them!
remember not to take your friends for granted or to fall into habits of just sitting around. SOMETIMES IT SEEMS LIKE EVERYONE TALKS ABOUT THE SAME THINGS OVER + OVER, BUT EVERYONE HAS SUBJECTS + SECRETS THEIR DIEING TO TALK ABOUT. THINK ABOUT WHAT THINGS YOUR FRIENDS CARE ABOUT + ASK THEM QUESTIONS. about their interests, about their lives, about their dreams.
IF YOU SLEEP TOO MUCH, GET UP! WAKE UP! IF YOU DON'T SLEEP ENOUGH, ALLOW YOURSELF REST
MOURN YOUR LOSSES. LACK OF MOURNING CAUSES BURNOUT.
SET REACHABLE GOALS
I WILL WRITE ONE, TINY SECRET MINI ZINE BY SUNDAY
MAKE COMPLEX, CRAZY GOALS + KEEP PUSHING YOURSELF.
yeah, so I need a set designer it's going to be this interactive film thing involving talking to myself + educating people about feminist history + I'll sing too
remember to let yourself dance.
even if you feel akward at first - just commit yourself to rocking out no matter what, and soon you will feel terrific!
GHOSTS DON'T EXIST
GHOSTS DO EXIST!
SPOOKTOBER

death

One of the biggest things when my mom died, was I thought I had to get it all figured out. All the complexities of our relationship, all the unsaid things, all the unmet needs, all the mixed feelings of love and abandonment, betrayal and goodness. I was afraid that there were all these things left undone that now I would never be able to resolve. But the truth was, maybe I never would have been able to resolve them, and maybe I would have been able to. and in time, even with her dead, I have. There is this peace about it now. In the sorrow and bitterness, in the beauty of how she moved and how she survived, and the strength she passed on. The thing that surprised me was how long it took. Like, for years it hurt. The first three years were the worst. I think if I had know in the beginning that it was going to suck for three years, I would have may be taken it easier on myself.

Not that it totally sucked all the time. There were times when it was easy, times when I would forget. Times when I was worried that I wasn't sad enough. Times when I was worried that I was more sad about my failing relationship than my dead mom. I thought I had to get it right. There is no getting it right, it will all come. there is time for it all.

What I needed most was for the people around me to know that I couldn't hold up my side of things. Every task was difficult, most of the time. Cooking, figuring out what to do with my day, holding up my side of the friendship, calling people, reaching out, making plans, answering the question "what do you want to do". I couldn't care take. I needed taking care of.

I read a lot of trashy books. Weird pseudo-feminist mystery novels like by Elizabeth Peters, or Rita Mae Brown. Trashy pseudo-historical fiction, like Zorro by Isabel Allende. Paperbacks. Best Sellers. Shit I didn't have to think about. I read a book a day sometimes.

Part of what I needed was just to get through the day.
Part of what I needed was to do the normal things I did.
Part of what I hated was people being normal around me.
Part of what I needed was for people to be normal around me.

I wish more people had just brung up questions about death and mom in the beginning of each time we hung out, so it wouldn't be looming over us, waiting to see if it would be addressed. Like, they could ask questions about my family, about funeral stuff, about if there were things I was realizing I needed, about what she was like, about did I want to talk about how she died. did I want to talk about my relationship with her. did she read to me. did she know I wrote a zine. did I have ideas about what happened when you die. anything. anything to break the ice. And if I didn't want to talk about it, I could have just answered shortly, abruptly, I could have said I didn't want to talk about it right then. I could have said anything, instead of always waiting to see. Instead of feeling like a freak and a burden. Instead of feeling so locked up and terrible and pretend.

deserts and rain

I left home and moved to the desert, me and
my dog, into a small empty place and I made a
few friends there, women I could talk to about
some things. I felt happy, a slow kind of hot
weather happiness, where I'd wake up in bed,

sheets under me only, dog breathing noisily,
fan on. I'd go back to sleep. I drank tea
in the morning instead of coffee.

Maybe this is growing up, I thought. Maybe this
is growing up - you find out love is not that
feeling that makes your stomach sick and your
muscles hurt and your brain go fast trying to
figure out how to impress and how much to tell
and how to let go.

I thought maybe this is growing up, this
general feeling of not needing to romanticize
our ability to act in this world, or dramatize

the importance of our emotions. I could see
how for some people, calmness would feel like
defeat - and how it had even been defined as
defeat, so if you feel it, this is the catagory
you place it in, when really it does not need

to go there. I never understood why childhood
and its supposed innocence were most valued,
and then youth craziness with all its smashing
and breaking down and exploration and
adventure. And after that it's all shit, right?
I never got that. I don't think you have to
have innocence or craziness to live a full
and vibrant life.

I felt calm and logical and capable and good
and real. I didn't always have to be overwhelmed
by seeing things for the first time and living
things for the first time. A pomegranite
 growing from a tree in a city, the ocean, kids,
feeling, suddenly, not alone in this world, like
the city is ours - lets take a nap under that
semi, under that bush; watching friends move and
talk and sing and sleep, and loving so hard and
losing and wanting. And how come no one told us
to want like this and how to function with this
want in this world; how to keep alive.

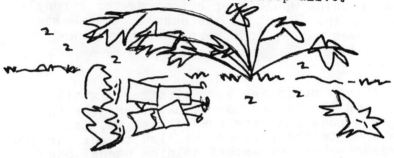

In my little square house I slept. I woke up. I
drank tea. I wrote letters. I walked my dog to
the creek and put my feet in and lay on the
rocks; slow thoughts. In two years I'd visit
Gabe in Hawaii, in three I'd sing in a band
again. No hurry, no impossible plans, not
wanting too much, only what was obtainable and
working hard and focused for that. When I went
home I would learn my van and how to fix it.
I'd have my women's health group. I would see
my sister again, soon. I read books. I watched
lizards. I thought about my mom a lot. I made
boots for my old dogs feet and we walked to
town and visited the friends I'd made. We talked
about some things. I went home with my dog and
slept.

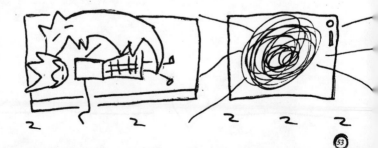

When my mom died I tried to drink myself to death too; and when the worst was over I felt alive and ok, content almost with this feeling that nothing would ever effect me too strongly ever again. I went to the desert, me a woman who loves water, and there Courtney showed up at my door.

I wish you could see her, with her pigtails and long skirts and tanned skin. She was the one who rode the city busses with me, last bus home to the suburbs. We lied to our parents for eachother. We walked holding hands. She ran around corners, tripped and cried and screamed about the stupid fucked up boys we dated, while I tried to hold my shoulders

steady and act unaffected, or maybe I was crying and screaming too.

Courtney who I loved and looked up to and was jealous of and embarrassed by, and maybe some-how I abandoned. I wrote her a letter and there she was. She knows the rare thing of what real friends should be.

she says: get in the car, we're going camping

♡ i says:

she says:

get in the car!

don't you want breakfast, tea? It's so hot don't you want to rest? don't we need supplies? and what the hell are you doing here?

understand, she is not a controling person, but this is what we did, once upon a time when one of us needed saving and couldn't see it. It's a language we both know.

"you sounded numb in your letter" she says. "no. I'm fine" I say. "well, you sounded numb"

"tell me what you haven't told"

I tell her about the hospital and the funeral and the year after

and all the years before. it comes out easy and so do her stories. we look at each other and understand eachother and ask questions when we don't. we are totally present, comfortable and safe.

IT IS A SHOCK TO MY SYSTEM THAT I HAVE NOT FELT THIS IN SO LONG, AND I CAN'T BELIEVE ALL I HAVE COMPROMISED AND SETTLED FOR.

We drive up the mountain, out of the desert.
We park in a small town and then hitchike further
and I feel that feeling of opening up inside,
that ridiculous feeling of open empty roads and
thumbs up, and she is singing to me and I feel
like the possibilities are endless.

In the back of a pickup truck, winding up the
road, she yells "Come to El Paso. I'll get you a
job and I'll finish school. Then we'll go to the
ocean", she has always wanted to live at the
ocean. "We'll go to one of those boat building
schools and we'll build a boat and sail around
the world. What do you say Cindy? What do you
say?"

I laugh and laugh and my heart, I want so much.

This is what I think is the crazy thing. I can
dream with her, and I can believe these dreams
are real and not just delusion, and together we
could probably make them happen.

In the woods, I show her how to pick stinging
nettles the way Mollie taught me so you won't
get stung; fold the leaves up from the underneath and use them to grasp and break the stem.

We watch each other the way people in love do.
We talk like we will always be together, day in
and day out, and the crazy thing is, we won't be.

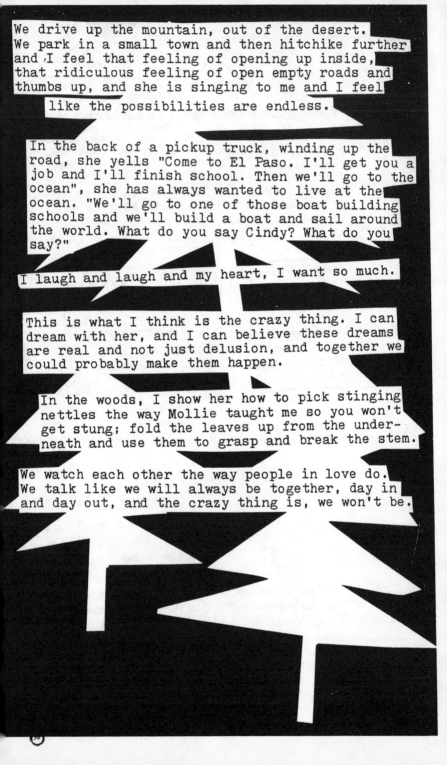

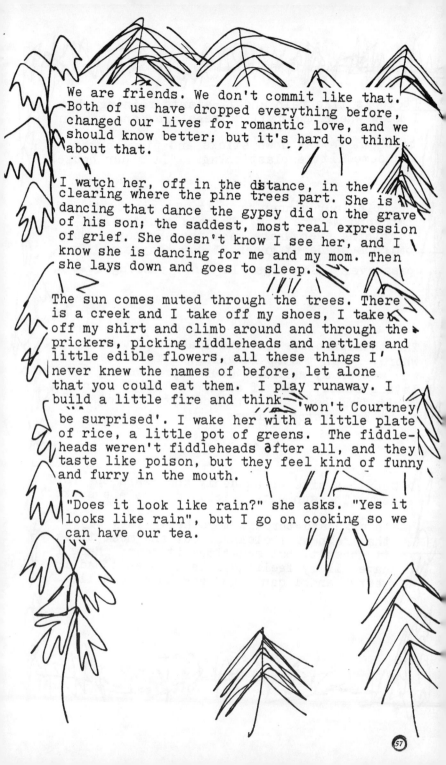

We are friends. We don't commit like that.
Both of us have dropped everything before,
changed our lives for romantic love, and we
should know better; but it's hard to think
about that.

I watch her, off in the distance, in the
clearing where the pine trees part. She is
dancing that dance the gypsy did on the grave
of his son; the saddest, most real expression
of grief. She doesn't know I see her, and I
know she is dancing for me and my mom. Then
she lays down and goes to sleep.

The sun comes muted through the trees. There
is a creek and I take off my shoes, I take
off my shirt and climb around and through the
prickers, picking fiddleheads and nettles and
little edible flowers, all these things I
never knew the names of before, let alone
that you could eat them. I play runaway. I
build a little fire and think 'won't Courtney
be surprised'. I wake her with a little plate
of rice, a little pot of greens. The fiddleheads weren't fiddleheads after all, and they
taste like poison, but they feel kind of funny
and furry in the mouth.

"Does it look like rain?" she asks. "Yes it
looks like rain", but I go on cooking so we
can have our tea.

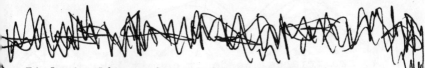

It looks like rain and it starts raining, but
I know where two fallen trees are, and we run

to them. We lay down sticks and pine boughs
and some little plastic bags. "It's our house!"

We bring our dinner into it. It starts to rain
hard and we are dry! There's thunder and
lightning everywhere, and the sky turns that
ominous shade of green. I say "Maybe it'll
pass over". She says "It's not passing over".

The thunder claps and the leaks start everywhere. I can't stop laughing. I feel the cold
and wet on my skin and Courtney swearing and
laying still, like if she's still the rain
won't find her, and I am so happy to not be
on my front stoop, alone.

Courtney sits up suddenly and tears the roof
down. The sun sets quickly and we are soaked

through and through together. They say
that rain will cleanse you, and most times
it doesn't, but sometimes it does. Here I
have all my feelings like I haven't had in
years, and I can't go back to my old life.

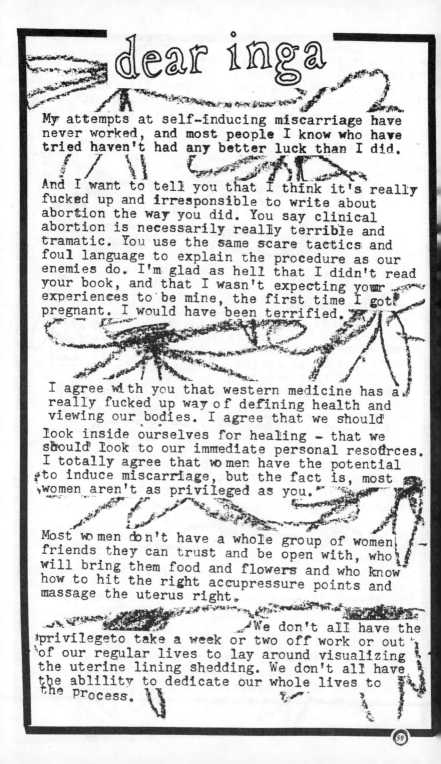

dear inga

My attempts at self-inducing miscarriage have never worked, and most people I know who have tried haven't had any better luck than I did.

And I want to tell you that I think it's really fucked up and irresponsible to write about abortion the way you did. You say clinical abortion is necessarily really terrible and tramatic. You use the same scare tactics and foul language to explain the procedure as our enemies do. I'm glad as hell that I didn't read your book, and that I wasn't expecting your experiences to be mine, the first time I got pregnant. I would have been terrified.

I agree with you that western medicine has a really fucked up way of defining health and viewing our bodies. I agree that we should look inside ourselves for healing – that we should look to our immediate personal resources. I totally agree that women have the potential to induce miscarriage, but the fact is, most women aren't as privileged as you.

Most women don't have a whole group of women friends they can trust and be open with, who will bring them food and flowers and who know how to hit the right accupressure points and massage the uterus right.

We don't all have the privilege to take a week or two off work or out of our regular lives to lay around visualizing the uterine lining shedding. We don't all have the ablility to dedicate our whole lives to the process.

You say you thought it was really important to have total confidence in what you were doing. Maybe you are at a place in your life where you've got that kind of inner strength, but I can't believe that you would think that most of the women reading this book you wrote would have the self confidence to believe with all their souls and bodies that they have the power to make this thing work.

Dear Inga, I hate you.

I hate you for making a pop-culture kind of book, made to be popular with young women, and you tell these girls that if they get pregnant they should self abort in this natural, woman's way, and you don't acknowledge how hard it is to get yourself and your life to a place where that even begins to be an option. I hate you for doing the thing that people do so often, just listing off a couple herbs, without talking about dosage or dangers.

I hate that you demonize clinics, turn abortion providers into the dreaded Abortionist. I know that your abortion sucked, but they don't all have to be that way. There are good clinics and nurses and councelors and doctors who are committed to woman's health and women's self determination and who do this work even though it is dangerous to them - doctors get shot, clinics bombed, their children get harassed in schools. They are our allies, and if clinics are bad, we should be working to try and make them better - and doing this while we try and create women's networks of support, where we can help eachother in every way possible.

My attempts at herbal abortion have generally
been worse experiences than my clinical
abortions. The first time I got pregnant I
was really excited about the power of women
to self abort. I was scared too, but really
confident I could do it! I didn't have a job
right then, and I had one woman friend I could
talk to. I was living on a friend's couch. It
wasn't ideal, but I at least had a stove to make
tea and a tub to soak in.

I visualized. I tried my hardest, but it didn't
work, and it made me feel like a real failure.
Like there was something lacking inside of me
and that's why I couldn't make it work. It's
been like this every time. I've gotten better
recipies, learned more about my body, I have
more confidence and more of a support system,
but evey time I try it, it doesn't work, and I
feel so demoralized. It makes me so mad that

we live in this world where our options are
so limited, and so fucked up. I start to hate
my life and the world more than anything, and
by the time I give up and go to the clinic, I
am just so glad to be finally getting it done
with.

My clinical abortions were never "harrowing,
tramatic experiences" like you say they
inherently are. I have plenty of complaints
about them - like I wasn't listened to enough,
I had birth control I didn't want pushed on me,
I was drugged up too much, I wasn't let recover
long enough, but some of them, parts of them
have been really good and strong and caring.
and I believe that we can make them more that
way.

e is for

the problem with eggplant is that a lot of people don't cook it long enough. It needs to be cooked for a very long time until it is just so very soft and mushy, then it tastes delicious. There is also a good trick to getting the weird bitterness out; what you do is you cut it up and then before you cook it you put it in a colander and pour a bunch of salt on it and mix it up, and let it sit for 20 minutes or so. Put a plate under the colander because weird eggplant bitter juice will come out. Rinse the salt off before cooking. This makes it extra good.

Louise Erdrich

I knew a group of girls once, who were young and gutsy and outspoken and did a lot of crazy things. Kate was the quietest of them. Years later I got a letter from her.

I had to learn to speak Dakota in order to speak English in front of people.

I had heard she was working at Louise Erdrich's bookstore. She said not anymore, but that it was like a second home to her.

If you are in Minnesota, you should go there. Birchbark Bookstore. You should also read some of Louise Erdrich's books. I particularly liked her first three books; Love Medicine, The Beet Queen, and Tracks. And then The Last Report on the Miracles at Little No Horse, and also her book of short stories.

You should also check out the Birchbark Foundation, which is "engaged in the revitalization of Native American Language for the spiritual, physical and material health of the people."

ELDA MOR
goddess of the
elderberry

ELDERBERRY NECKLACE

TO STOP THE PAIN OF TEETHING BABIES. USE THE STEM OF THE PLANT. PEEL OFF THE OUTER BARK. CUT 13 BEADS + MAKE A CHOKER. IT HAS PURIC ACID WHICH IS SIMILAR TO VALARIAN + STOPS THE PAIN OF TEETHING. ALSO FOR KIDS WITH DOWNS SYNDROM IT HELPS STOP THE DROOLING.
THE NECKLACE IS A LITTLE IRRITATING TO THE SKIN, SO KIDS WITH REALLY FAIR SKIN CAN'T WEAR THEM

EMErcOM ST. ETC

Once I was walking past Emmerson St house and there were all these girls I knew sitting on the front stoop, which was unusual because no one ever hung out on that side of the house. It turned out they were all getting ready to go beat the shit out of this guy who had raped his girlfriend, our friend, Shelia. And Shelia was there, pleading with them not to. and I heard her say 'he didn't really rape me'. I heard her say that that's what she told Avery had happened, but it wasn't really true. And I bet she was thinking 'this is what I get for talking. These are the consequences. I never should have told.'

Once I was at a show where my new boyfriend was playing. He was a scared one, shy and full of self doubt. His old girlfriend came in with a bunch of her friends and I could see her yelling at him and yelling, and him shrinking. He told me later that she said he raped her. He was crying in my arms and I didn't know what to do.

He said she said it was one night when she was sleeping and he came home blacked out drunk. He couldn't believe he was capable of doing that, but he believed her. He didn't know what to do.

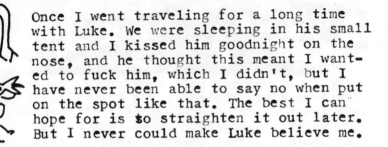

Once I went traveling for a long time
with Luke. We were sleeping in his small
tent and I kissed him goodnight on the
nose, and he thought this meant I wanted to fuck him, which I didn't, but I
have never been able to say no when put
on the spot like that. The best I can
hope for is to straighten it out later.
But I never could make Luke believe me.

He had this funny manipulative way about
him, this overwhelming way of being, and
he quick found my triggers and convinced
me that I was crazy. split personalities.

he make fun of my different voices. He
made it hard to speak. He said of course
I had wanted it. and the time I said
something was making me uncomfortable,
he told me to relax. He would fuck me
when I was sleeping and I'd pretend not
to notice.

after months and months of things
not getting better, I got up the
courage to try and explain in a way
that wouldn't hurt his feelings or
make him defensive. I loved him, I
didn't want to hurt him.

I told him that, well, you know, I had
been abused when I was younger and I had
these issues, and you know, just because
I liked sex sometimes didn't mean I
wanted it always, andI was having this

problem and I thought maybe to deal
with it, maybe he could wait for me
to initiate sex.

He was so sympathetic. He listened
and then he never waited.

every night

I never talked about it to anyone because I was scared of what I was allowing to happen to me. I felt like I was crazy, and I also felt full of shame for being in this totally abusive relationship. And I didn't want anyone to know what was happening.

It's been awhile, but I still felt sick when I heard Cloe talking about him the other day, and then at the bar, Dumpy telling me - I saw Luke, Luke's doing this Luke's doing that, he'll be here in a week or two * and I want to yell "don't you know what that fucker did to me?!" but I don't say anything because I don't think I could stand it if they just felt bad for me but still stayed his friend, and also, I'm not sure he has the slightest idea what he did.

So how do we deal with rape in our communities? When do we kill the rapist and when do we have to figure out ways to confront it and be there as a

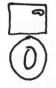

community of support for the person who was raped, and how do we take responsibility as a community for talking to the person who raped and figuring out how and if they're going to deal with it and change

I don't like to think about it. It makes me feel sick. I think this is the problem most people have. It's too hard to think about and so it just gets ignored. Some people stop being friends with the person who raped. or the person gets beat up. that's it.

There's this zine Radical Slut, and these women have really specific ways they go about confronting rape, andI think it's really good. Not that their guidelines would work for everyone in every community, but I think it's so important to start thinking about it and talking about it and figure out rational strategies; talking about what we've done,

what we wish had been done, what we think we should do.

← excerpt from Radical Slut Discovery

I asked a good friend of mine to be present during the discussion. I wanted the discussion to be pretty informal, but I definitely had certain things I wanted to say, and I had written out on a piece of paper certain things that I wanted him to follow through with after the discussion. The paper I gave to him said:
  - Tell people you are currently intimately involved with and those that you become intimately involved with in the future that you have sexually abused womyn (but don't use my name) and have sexually abusive tendencies such as being manipulative and sexually overbearing.
  - Think about how you treat womyn who you are interested in sexually or think are physically attractive. Are you respectful to them? Are you upfront about your intentions and feelings or are you deceptive? Do you watch out for their feelings and sexual boundaries (in their words and their body language)?

This is the list of demands that were given to the perp after the discussion:
You need to tell anybody you have any kind of relationship with, are working with, or are involved with in any capacity that you ARE (not have been) a sexual assaulter. things you specifically need to say to these people:
  - That you have a history of and continue to be a sexual abuser
  - That the reason you are telling them is because one of the wimmin you assaulted requested that you tell people.
  - That some of the ways you are (not have known to be) sexually and mentally abusive include being manipulative, overpowering, a guilt-tripper, coercive, not respectful, forceful, intimidating, attempting to rape, sexually self-absorbed and inconsiderate.
  - If they want or need to talk to someone about it, they can get in touch with someone else who has been a designated advocate.

more resources:

zines:
"GENDER OPPRESSION, ABUSE, VIOLENCE" by INCITE! Women of Color Against Violence
"TAKING RISKS: implementing grassroots community accountability strategies" by COMMUNITIES AGAINST RAPE+ABUSE
also: Phillys Pissed + Philly Stands UP

66

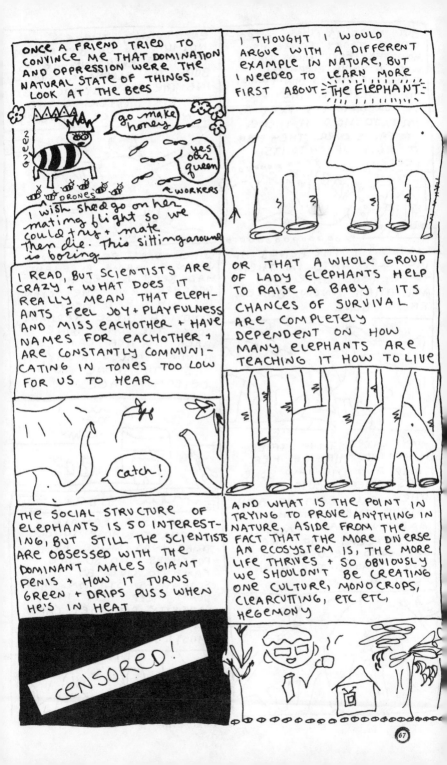

BUT WHAT IS MOST INTERESTING TODAY TO ME IS HOW THEY FEEL ABOUT DEATH. WHEN A YOUNG ELEPHANT DIES, THE OTHERS DON'T WANT TO BELIEVE IT. THEY PUSH IT UP ONTO ITS FEET + TRY TO HOLD IT THERE, IT FALLS OVER, THEY PUSH IT BACK UP ON TO ITS FEET

EVENTUALLY, THERE'S NOTHING TO DO BUT ACCEPT IT. THEN EVERYONE HELPS BURY THE ELEPHANT, COVERING THE BODY BY KICKING UP DIRT, COVERING THE BODY WITH TREE BRANCHES

THEY VISIT THE BONES OF THE ELEPHANTS IN THEIR TRIBE WHO HAVE DIED AND THEY KNOW BONE FROM BONE

WHICH WAS PROVEN ONCE WHEN A MAMA ELEPHANT HAD BEEN KILLED BY POACHERS AND THE SCIENTIST WHO HAD BEEN STUDYING THESE ELEPHANTS TOOK THE JAW BONE BACK TO HER CAMP, A HUNDRED MILES AWAY, TO TEST THE BONE TO DETERMINE AGE

WAY LATER, THAT TRIBE MIGRATED THROUGH HER CAMP AND THE JAW BONE WAS THERE, OUTSIDE. THEY ALL FELT IT AND STOOD THERE WITH IT AND EVENTUALLY MOVED ON, EXCEPT FOR THE SON, WHO HELD THE BONE AND STAYED THERE AND HELD IT.

new story

THERE IS A FEMALE ELEPHANT WHOSE WHOLE TRIBE WAS KILLED BY POACHERS AND SO SHE CAME TO LIVE BY THE SCIENTISTS STATION. THEY DON'T KEEP HER IN CAPTIVITY, BUT THEY CARE FOR HER + SHE STAYS MOSTLY THERE

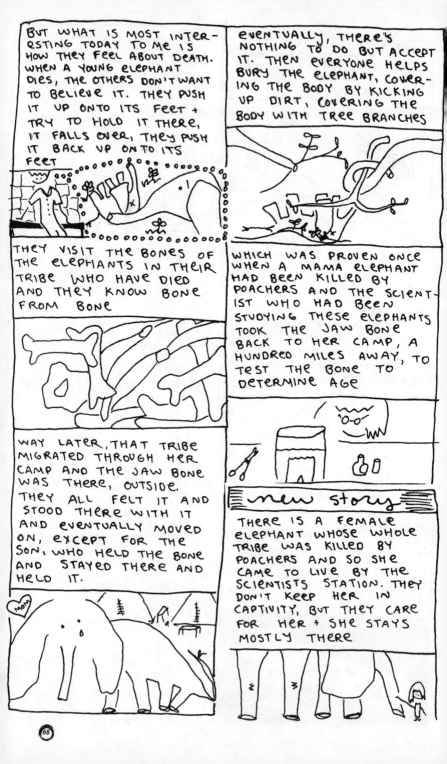

THERE IS A RICH WOMAN WHO TRIES TO SAVE BABY ELEPHANTS WHOSE FAMILIES HAVE BEEN KILLED. SHE HAS PEOPLE NURSE THEM WITH GIANT BOTTLES + TRY + PLAY WITH THEM + MAKE THEM FEEL SAFE

AND WHEN THE BABY'S WEENED, SHE BRINGS IT TO THE ELEPHANT WHO LIVES AT THE SCIENTIST STATION SO IT CAN BE TAUGHT, BY A REAL ELEPHANT, THE THINGS AN ELEPHANT NEEDS TO KNOW TO SURVIVE

BUT IT IS HARD TO RAISE A YOUNG ELEPHANT WHO HAS BEEN THROUGH THAT TRAMA

AND SOMETIMES, AT THE SCIENTIST STATION, THE YOUNG ELEPHANT DIES

AND THEN THE GROWN UP ELEPHANT, STILL LIVING, MAKES THE MOST AMOUNT OF NOISE, SHE RUNS AROUND LIKE CRAZY. SHE SPENDS DAYS DESTROYING EVERYTHING SHE POSSIBLY CAN

TODAY IS THE DAY OF MY MOMS DEATH. TWO YEARS LATER BUT STILL THE DAY, AND MY SISTER COMES TO SEE ME BUT I CAN'T EVEN HOLD HER HANDS TO CRY IN THE LITTLE VISITATION ROOM IN THE JAIL.

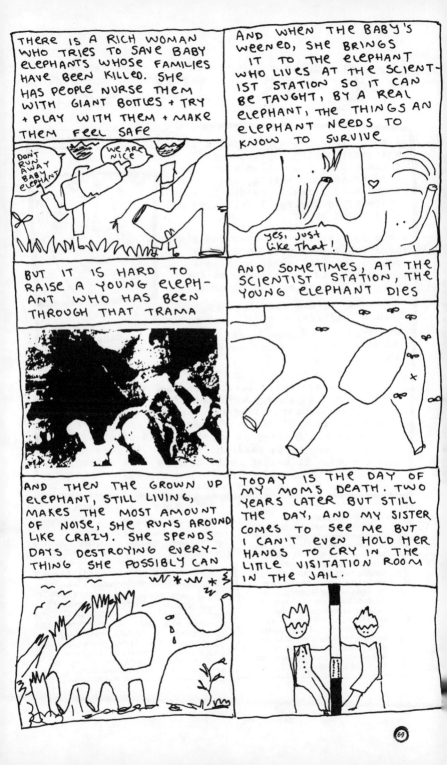

f is for fireflys

I read <u>Stone Butch Blues</u> when I was first trying to figure out trans stuff. I had been organizing some women only events, and sarah brown said I really needed to make it trans inclusive. I felt kind of threatened by it.

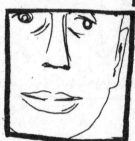

Leslie Fienberg

Women only spaces had been the place where I had been able to finally speak up within larger politiaal movements. The had allowed me the space to look at my own internalized sexism, my own self-loathing and fear, to put it in a political context, and to have the support to confront it and grow. I was afraid the transgender movement would somehow undermine the safty I'd found in these spaces.

Then I read <u>Stone Butch Blues</u>. It was basically about coming of age butch lesbian in the 1960's, when by law you had to wear 3 articles of gender appropriate clothing. the cops would raid bars, arrest them for being gender devient, rape them.

The story was a story of survival, and of struggling to be allowed to be real and seen and to love and live and thrive. It helped me to open my arms entirely, to embrace transgender liberation, to fight my transphobia. To feel it in my heart.

FOXFIRE

the Foxfire books are stories collected by highschool students interviewing the older people around up in the Appalacian Mountains. They are full of crafts and skills and rediculous stories. Soapmaking, Building a Log Cabin, Moonshining, Snake Lore, Games (like Snake in the Grass and Old Grandma Wiggens is Dead), how to get rid of warts, Hog Dressing. Miguel's dad told me that when he moved to the land he just did everything in the Foxfire books, because he figured if the old timers did it, it had to be right. Then he realized half the oldtimers were crazy. These are some of my favorite books.

FEMINIST WOMENS HEALTH CENTERS only 14 non-profit abortion providing health centers left. FWHC.ORG lists them - also has great articles about STI's menopause, self-exam, fertility awareness + abortion. THEY ARE DEDICATED TO REPRODUCTIVE FREEDOM, HEALTH and EQUALITY

FAITHALOUD.ORG is a pro-choice spiritual resource for people who have spiritual concerns regarding their decision about their pregnancy or pregnancy telmanation

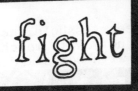

fight

She wrote me and told me she had hitchiked for
the first time alone. She said it was great.
She felt so much more freedom in the world.
And I could picture her on the side of the
road. I could picture her walking down crowded
streets. I could picture her in her room, arms
out stretched, taking up space.

I have always thought of her as a strong
woman, even though she is small, her hair is
long, she is pretty. She has a steady gaze.
She talks very directly about the things she
is trying to understand, and about the things
she thinks are important.

There was that hard year, and I was in NY,
and she came over one day and told me she had
just been on the subway and there was this
creepy man standing too close to a woman,
rubbing against her in that way they do that
you really can't pretend is only the crowded-

ness of the train, only bodies pushed, not
meaning to, together in the cramped space underground, New York City.

I can't remember exactly what Erin told me.
I think the lady got off the train and then the
man started rubbing on someone else, and Erin
wanted so badly to scream, but there was
complacency all around her, and it is so often
ingrained in us, this shit: this don't be
hysterical, don't make a scene, we deserve it,
pity him, this is our lot.

My Erin, she didn't know what to do, and
then her stop came and it was too late, but
then he got off right behind her, and she
found her strength and she started yelling at

him "You are a fucking creepy asshole. We know what you are doing! It's not ok to touch women like that!" and on and on with words and threats against him.

A crowd gathered and surrounded him and people supported her and cheered her on and yelled at him too. He was surrounded and powerless.

She tells me this story. Her eyes are shining and her skin even is glowing from the adrenalin and pride, and I am in wonder of it. I am used to women who wouldn't have thought twice before yelling at him as soon as they saw him. I am used to women who would yell at a man for looking at them in the wrong way. And these women I am used to are the same ones that say they hate feminism, that don't eat, that have no problems talking about masturbation but won't consider putting garlic or yogurt up in there. They yell at strangers but their ex-boyfriends, well, I won't say what their ex-boyfriends have been known to d

I listen to Erin and inside myself I try to bridge the gaps.

The next time I saw her was at a show in Asheville I always want her to like me. I want her to think I am worthy and smart and not just a fuck up. I saw her at the show, and - how was hitchiking anyway- I asked her, and a friend of ours, Roger was standing there. He said "You hitchiked alone! I would never hitchike alone if I were a girl!" If I'd been a dog my hair would have bristled, but since I am human I thought to myself, I can see what he's saying, I mean, I wouldn't really recommend it either. But Brin, she is saying "I feel so much freedom" and I think "What the fuck kind of right does Roger have to say what he would or wouldn't do if he was a girl. He doesn't know." And he could have asked questions instead of stating and judging and being one more reinforcer of the limits placed on woman's lives.

Because we are all aware of the risks and dangers. We've been taught to keep our legs crossed, hold our elbows close, talk quietly and listen well. We've been taught to sit in front of the mirror, to keep our door locked. And we'll probably be raped if we walk alone at night, if we don't check the back seat of the car before getting in, if we resist our boyfriend, if we flirt with our friends, if we get too drunk at a show. If we leave our house, if we hop trains, if we talk to strangers, if we run away, if we hitchike.

Once, that same time in NY, Mary came to see me. She said she had been walking down the street and someone called - hey baby - at her, and she just ran right up to him and gouged his eyes with her two fingers and thumbs held tight together like little poking weapons. just ran right up to him and slammed into his eyes.

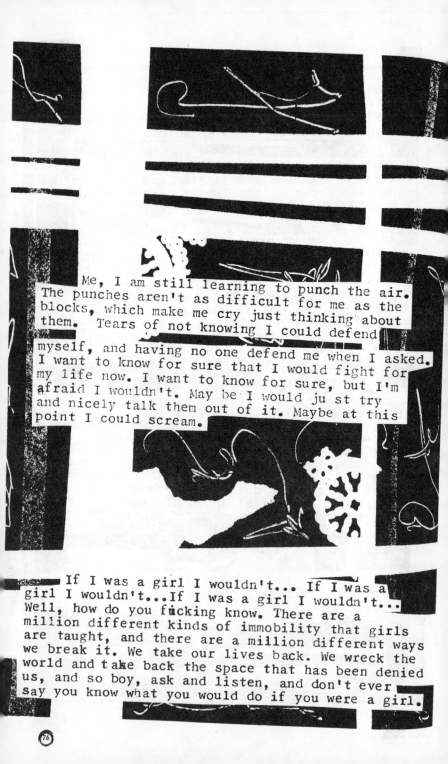

Me, I am still learning to punch the air.
The punches aren't as difficult for me as the
blocks, which make me cry just thinking about
them. Tears of not knowing I could defend
myself, and having no one defend me when I asked.
I want to know for sure that I would fight for
my life now. I want to know for sure, but I'm
afraid I wouldn't. May be I would ju st try
and nicely talk them out of it. Maybe at this
point I could scream.

If I was a girl I wouldn't... If I was a
girl I wouldn't...If I was a girl I wouldn't...
Well, how do you fucking know. There are a
million different kinds of immobility that girls
are taught, and there are a million different ways
we break it. We take our lives back. We wreck the
world and take back the space that has been denied
us, and so boy, ask and listen, and don't ever
say you know what you would do if you were a girl.

fishing

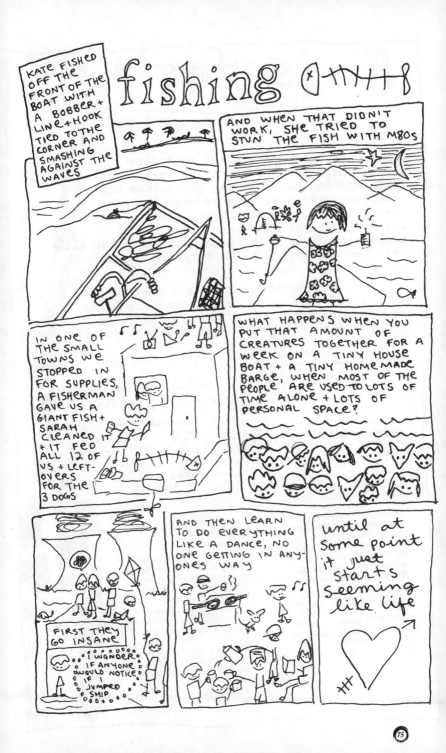

KATE FISHED OFF THE FRONT OF THE BOAT WITH A BOBBER + LINE + HOOK TIED TO THE CORNER AND SMASHING AGAINST THE WAVES

AND WHEN THAT DIDN'T WORK, SHE TRIED TO STUN THE FISH WITH M80S

IN ONE OF THE SMALL TOWNS WE STOPPED IN FOR SUPPLIES, A FISHERMAN GAVE US A GIANT FISH + SARAH CLEANED IT + IT FED ALL 12 OF US + LEFT-OVERS FOR THE 3 DOGS

WHAT HAPPENS WHEN YOU PUT THAT AMOUNT OF CREATURES TOGETHER FOR A WEEK ON A TINY HOUSE BOAT + A TINY HOMEMADE BARGE, WHEN MOST OF THE PEOPLE ARE USED TO LOTS OF TIME ALONE + LOTS OF PERSONAL SPACE?

FIRST THEY GO INSANE

I WONDER IF ANYONE WOULD NOTICE IF I JUMPED SHIP

AND THEN LEARN TO DO EVERYTHING LIKE A DANCE, NO ONE GETTING IN ANY-ONES WAY

until at some point it just starts seeming like life

g is for

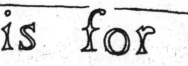

Girls Rock Camp

girls rock camp was started by ladies
who had been part of the riotg rrrrl movement, and had seen the way capitalism had
co-opted 'girl power' to be just another
cutesy marketing ploy. They wanted to figure
out a way to actually help girls to be
empowered. Girls Rock Camps have sprung up all
over the country. I think they are usually for
girls ages 10-18.

You don't have to be a professional
musician to be able to teach. They also have
non-musician volunteer positions. Everyone I
know who has ever been involved has loved it!

Eduardo Galeano

Eduardo Galeano is one of
my favorite writers of history
and political theory. He writes
with beautiful and direct
language and is extremely
accessible. Open Veins of
Latin America: Five Centuries
of the Pillage of a Continent,
should really be required
reading for everyone. I had
read history of Columbus and
of agribusiness and US
intervention in Latin America,
but this book made me *feel* it,
and *know* it, and made it all
stick strong in my memory.

Upside Down: A Primer for a
Looking Glass World, is a good
introduction to the insanity of
wealth, commercialism, denial,
mainstream media, imperialism,
and all forms of oppressive
governments and institutions.

generation fire.org.
an organization
committed to ending
childhood sexual abuse
in 5 generations,
using the model
of transformative
justice.

Girl Army

Girl Army is a collective in
Oakland California, dedicated
to peer taught, affordable,
physical and psychological
self-defense for women and
trans folks of all cultures.
committed to providing a
safe and supportive space.

There is a resource list on
their website that would be
great for starting a study
group
girlarmy.org

gainsville

On New Years day it was cold and clear. We
pulled up to the beach. First I took off my
shoes and ran down to the edge of the water.
My feet froze. I ran back to the van and put
on my boots and more layers, ran back to the
ocean where two of the boys were already
stripped down and swimming.

they stayed in there forever, through all
the big waves. I couldn't not go in. Maybe the
water was somehow warmer than the air. I
wanted to feel the old year wash away from
me. Off with my jacket my hat my sweater my
tights my socks and boots and dress rings and
glasses, just a slip left and I dove in.

I use to swim every summer, every day in Lake
Superior, where the water never got above 37
degrees is my guess. Cold eyes when you opened
them underwater, but there was so much to see.
I2 and I3 years old, when things started
changing; cell changes and capalaries growing
more close to the skin, and I was just starting
to love the feeling of my body, not worried
or concious of it yet, just loving the feeling
of skin and life, of cold water taking over
all senses. fingers on lips, the breath taking
first shock of cold water, and then the slow
calming into it, accepting and becoming
accustom and diving under.

At the Atlantic, New Years day, 31 years old.
They swam and I was cold and nothing was
going to take anything simply away, but I
was happy in the way that I am sometimes,

sitting huddled up into myself and watching
the friends, all of them hungover and unsure
what to do with themselves on a beach at the
ocean in the cold.

I thought we would watch the sun set over the
water until I realized the sun went down in
the other direction. I piled us in and drove
Half way home, there was a snow storm. I have
no windshield wipers. We wait it out at a
gas station, us and all our dogs, the van full
as it's ever been.

We cook popcorn on the stove,
Evan tries to fix the tape player by taking
it apart and spraying the motor with bug
spray, but it doesn't work for long, so we
talk and laugh and sing together, which is
what I like better, the snow comming heavy,
our voices rising louder and louder.

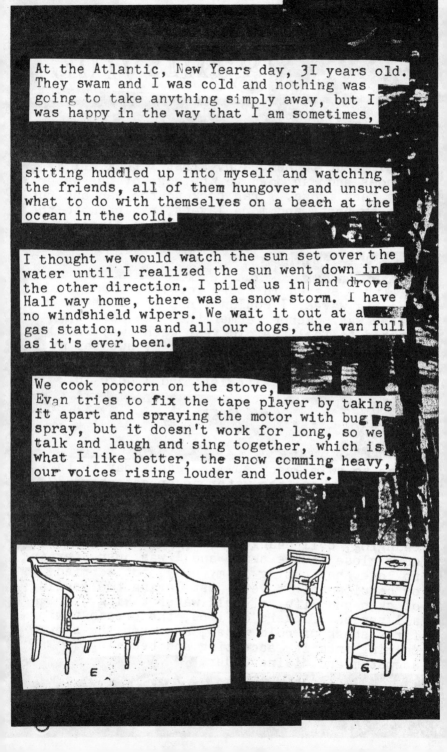

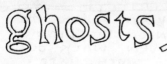

ghosts

The times I've seen ghosts have been times of desperation or something close to craziness when the borders of what is possible or impossible are loosened. The first time was my 18th winter, when almost all I could think of was shadowed by self doubt and suicide. I had started talking, a little bit, about the incest that had happened to me. my partner thought we could move through it like a hurricane. confrontation, sue the psychiatrist who didn't help us, cry scream move on,

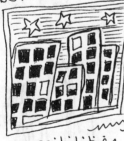

IT HAD BEEN 3 MONTHS AND

HE WAS GETTING TIRED OF THE FOCUS OF EVERYTHING ALWAYS BEING ON ME + MY PROBLEMS

We were ☆revolutionaries☆ we lived in rural vermont AND IN THAT ISOLATION, I BELIEVED EVERYTHING HE SAID. I BELIEVED FULLY + DEEPLY THAT THE REVOLUTION WAS RIGHT AROUND THE CORNER + VERY SOON EVERYTHING WOULD BE COMPLETELY DIFFERENT + BEAUTIFUL + FREE. then we left our small town.

THE PROMISE OF IMMEDIATE AND TOTAL SOCIAL CHANGE HAD WOKEN UP PARTS OF ME I HAD TWISTED UP + BURIED + SHOVED LIKE SPLINTERS BEHIND MY EYES. the world seemed brighter, my eyes seemed wider, the possibilities clear + endless. There was part of me that was happy, really happy, in a way I hadn't been since I was 10. BUT THEN THERE WAS PHILADELPHIA, LIKE A SOCK IN THE EYE, AND EVERYTHING CAME CRASHING IN AROUND ME. everything was so much bigger than I imagined. I knew nothing. I was of no use. Didn't even know how to use a hammer. ABANDON BUILDINGS + ABANDON ME. COULDN'T EVEN WALK OUTSIDE FOR THE FEAR. SO MUCH HATE + ANGER SO MUCH HOPELESSNESS + NOTHINGNESS. there was no revolution right around the corner. Around the corner was one of the flyers the girls in my squat put up. they worked in the sex industry. they wheatpasted the flyer

YOU CAN'T RAPE

A 38

and someone had spray painted under it "but you can rape with one"

I WAS HAVING A HARD TIME SEEING. MY EYES HAD BECOME BLURRY + UNFOCUSABLE. but one day Biloxi took us to the abandon horse building. It was 2 or 3 stories of stalls and ramps. SPLIT DOWN THE MIDDLE WITH TREES GROWING UP INSIDE. IT WAS BEAUTIFUL QUIET DECAY and I wandered away from the boys. wandered in the dust and the dark and the bits of light shining down, and I felt a little bit of that unusual feeling, safty.

AND THERE SHE WAS. GHOST OF A HORSE. IN THE STALL, FACING OUT SO I COULDN'T SEE HER FACE. if I had imagined it, wouldn't I have imagined her face?

THE NEXT TIME I SAW A GHOST WASN'T UNTIL MY MOTHER DIED. I HAD STOPPED BELIEVING IN GHOSTS BY THEN, BUT

WHEN MY MOM DIED FROM DRINKING IT WAS SO MUCH WORSE THEN I COULD HAVE EVER IMAGINED. like all the feelings i'd ever had surrounding her were avalanched. this hopelessness and helplessness and mostly so deeply alone! so alone, even though we didn't talk much or see eachother, there was this deep deep aloneness. Undescribable grief. MY MEMORY IS ALMOST GONE. I REMEMBER THE DAY AFTER THE ASHES, STANDING ON THE POARCH WITH MY SISTERS + WE HAD COLD PIZZA. MY MOM LOVED COLD PIZZA FOR BREAKFEST. THERE WERE SEAGULLS AND I WAS THROWING CRUSTS, BUT ONE SEAGULL LOOKED SO. IT LOOKED JUST SO AT ME and I could tell it was my mom. I wanted her to be there + then wanted her to leave. go. go. leave us alone now. I GOT ANGRY + CHUCKED A WHOLE PEICE OF PIZZA AT HER. I felt bad. I felt blessed. I looked at my sisters + could tell they knew too. Years later I said to one of my sisters "remember that mom seagull." SHE HAD NO IDEA.

MAY BE GHOSTS COME TO PEOPLE IN DIFFERENT FORMS AND FOR ME THAT WAS HER, COMPLETELY. EVEN IF NO ONE ELSE COULD SEE.

... there were times of desperation or something close to craziness, but sometimes crazy is not bad.

FOR TWO YEARS I LIVED ALONE IN THE WOODS. I had a therapist who was an old Earth Firster and now worked at the rape crisis center and she was helping me make sense of so much scared inside of me. Opening up the boxes I had drawn around the different parts. like the depressed part the strong + angry part the scared + small one the mediation the blamer.

I LIVED ALONE WITH NO ONE ELSE TO SEE ME. I TALKED TO THE VOICES INSIDE ME ALL THE TIME. HELPED THEM START TO GET ALONG. I LISTENED TO THE ONE WHO WANTED TO TAKE WALKS + LOOK AT PRETTY THINGS. I NURTURED THE MEAN ONE UNTIL IT WASN'T SO MEAN. I had always thought I was so alone in this craziness, but I started seeing the patterns everywhere — these people inside of me embodied in so many books so many movies. everywhere I looked. I mean everywhere human made. OK. TRUTH IS I WOULD SPEND WEEKS TALKING TO NO ONE BUT MYSELF. me and the ghost.

there really was a ghost in my house. One day it left me a little china owl figurine after I had been writing about a dream I had about my mom and an owl. I WAS SORT OF AFRAID OF THE GHOST AT FIRST, BUT THEN JUST TALKED TO HIM SO HE WOULDN'T BE STARTLED. "I am coming into the kitchen" I would say, and wait a minute so he could leave or prepare. ONE TIME IN THE EARLY SPRING HE BROUGHT ME A LATE FALL MILKWEED POD. ONE TIME HE LEFT ME A BOWL TO EAT OUT OF. So when I ate I could also feed him.

IT WAS LIKE EVERYTHING ELSE. ACCEPTING, COMFORTING, FEEDING, MAKING SPACE FOR, LOVING. learning to breathe. safty.

grief

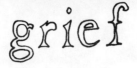

When my mom was dieing, I needed someone who wasn't
part of my family to come with me to Minnesota.
Someone who was a little bit removed and could
help me through it. There was no one I could ask.
I was afraid of hearing "no".

My boyfriend/bestfriend finally offered after two
days of me crying non-stop saying "I don't want to
go," and then "I need to go". Really I meant "I
can't go by myself. Please come with me. Take care
of me", but the look on his face when he offered
was pleading with me to say - 'no, don't worry.
You don't have to".

I ended up not going, never seeing her again, not
being there with my little sister. I will always
regret this.

After she died, I needed people to bring me food.
It's funny because other people I've talked to
recently, whose parents have died, have been
annoyed by all the food, but I did not have relatib
relatives or even close friends around. I simply
could not take care of myself, and when there was
no one around to take care of me either, my ability
to take care of myself only got worse.

I needed food. I needed people to ask me to do
things, simple things, like go to a movie, walk
around, go to the park, out for coffee. I got this
a tiny bit, but not much. I needed the chance to
be able to focus on something that wasn't just
inside my head, but mostly if anyone asked me to
do anything, it was something with lots of people
around - like just hanging out with a bunch of
folks. I was completely incapable of hanging out
and acting, groups of people were too much. They
give you that look that I started hating so much,
the "God, I@m sorry, but I'm not going to say
anything", look.

One person told me what it had been like when his
dad died. He talked to me about his mourning process
and how long it had taken, what he had done, and how
he felt now. That was really helpful. I wish I had
been able to have more conversations like this.

I needed people to want to ask me questions about it.
I needed people to stop being so scared. I needed
people to ask 'What was she like? What does it feel
like inside of you? How will your life change with
her gone?' Questions like that. Any questions really.

I've been trying to do this myself lately, when I
hear that someone I know's parent has died. I try
to step back and look at what I really do wonder
about them, about their parent or family, about
death itself. It's awkward, but isn't that part of
what friendship is? Pushing yourself and eachother to
get over rear and uncomfortableness.and talking,
and caring. and being real.

Sometimes I needed to talk about her, and sometimes
I just needed someone around to talk about normal
life things, to remember that the outside world
existed and I didn't have to be sad 100% of the
time. that I still could live and laugh.

I needed to know that it was ok and normal to feel,
along with the deep, deep sadness, also a feeling
of relief and anger and all those complicated
emotions. I needed to be able to talk about this
without feeling like I was dishonoring her.

After my mom died and I couldn't get the support I
needed, I started basically trying to drink myself
to death too. Maybe not to death, but I didn't
know what else to do. I drank all the time and it
got worse and worse for months, maybe up to a year.
People accepted this. They waited for me to get
over it. And this, in some ways, is the sadest part

of what I didn't get. I was so obviously fucked, so
obviously out of control, so obviously in need, and
why didn't anyone have the strength enough and time
enough to do whatever the hell possible - whatever
the hell was necessary, take me away somewhere or

whatever. I needed someone to help me quit or help
me figure out a way to get help. I needed someone
to recognize what I was doing and for them to decide
that they would help me get out of this total
self-destructing desperation.

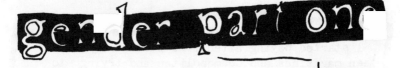

gender part one

When I was young I wanted to
live outside the world of humans.
I wanted to be the girl alone,
without human judgement around me;
without their eyes and hands
and voices and meanness and needs
and expectations. I wanted to be
the girl in <u>The Island of the Blue
Dolphins</u>. I would learn to make my
own spears. I would break the customs
of my culture. I would do what girls
were not allowed to do, and there
would be no one around to see so it
would be no big deal. It would be
regular life.

I am not sure how self aware I was or if I thought
about it like that at all: what girls are supposed to
or not supposed to do.

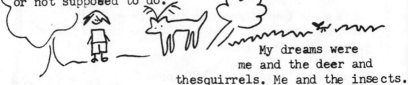

My dreams were
me and the deer and
thesquirrels. Me and the insects.
I followed paths in the woods. I slept in the fields.
I hung out with the grasshoppers on the side of the
freeway. In my dreams I was alone and accepted.

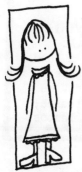

When I was growing up, it was a different
world than the one we have now. Girl power
hadn't been come up with or co-opted yet.
John Hughes hadn't made his movies. Sluts
were sluts and freaks were freaks and there
was nothing powerful or redeeming about
either.

l started paying attention. I started reading
teen magazines and Cosmopolitan and trying to
lighten my hair with lemon juice and hide my
worst features with the proper shades of makeup.
l read about the top ten secrets of what men like
in bed. l wanted to be the drummer for VanHalen
but I knew they would never let a girl in the
band, so I drempt they had try outs and I dressed
as a boy and was such a good drummer that they
let me in, even after I let my hair down and came
out as a girl.   I wanted to be strong and brave
and desirable. I wanted to be a girl, but an
exceptional one.

     When did I start hating girls? When I couldn't
ignore the outside world anymore? New houses,
stepfamilies and Jr.High.

     In the locker room I was ashamed of
my flat chest and no bra, and when I
started to get breasts, I was so
embarrassed I thought I would die.

     Boys made fun of and commented on girls
bodies all the time. (and so did the girls. the girls
j d judged eachother harshly)

     I sat at the lunch table alone.
Girls talked about which boys were cute and which
boy like who; which girls were sluts. Gossip,
diets and clothes. This was not a language I knew
or gave a shit about. But the isolation was
   terrible.

Where did my power lay? Girls could be anything,
doctor, lawyer, even president of the U.S.A.
(yeah, right) Doctor, lawyer, it was all a load
of shit. We were nothing if we weren't a certain
 kind of pretty and a certain kind of flirt. We
had to be very careful: not sluts or cockteases,
not uptight, frigid, bitch, innocent, not lesbos.

We were nothing Nothing. And our bodies weren't ours to say who could or couldn't touch.

I did not want to be a girl but I had no choice.

What white american patriarchal capitalist culture values as MASCULINE:

self control
rationality
consistancy
strength

the ability to stick with an idea and never back down. to protect. to provide. to laugh things off. to move with confidence no matter what. to use logic and emotional distance to understand the world and people's actions in it. not to cater to anyone elses needs.

What white american patriarchal capitalist culture values as FEMININE:

to nurture

Some of the ways women are systematically represented and demeaned by white american patriarchal capitalist culture:

irrational, hysterical, crazy, petty, untrustworthy, use emotions to manipulate men, need to be rescued, and taken care of and saved from themselves, take everything personally, overreact, burdonsome, and over all just kind of ridiculous.

I was a girl who hated girls

And all my power lay in my body, so I used it and sex became the most important thing in my life.

When I was a girl I wanted to live
outside the realm of human.
I did not fit anywhere, and
why should I? I learned to
value the masculine and
belittle the feminine.
And eventually I started
unlearning all of this.
I thought - these words are
weird. I thought - feminine
and masculine are in everyone and it's the task
of the revolutionary to integrate and love them
both.

I remember reading the poetry of
Audre Lorde and Adriene Rich, and the
essays "Uses of the Erotic, the Erotic
as Power" and "Compulsory Heterosexuality"
The book This Bridge Called My Back. The poetry
of Ntžoke Shange, Mary Oliver; Grace Paley's
short stories, Sylvia Plath's The Bell Jar.
And I wanted this. Not that their words were
always perfect, but I wanted to be able to see
and speak and feel these deep ways that they did.
To call on our history. To stop dismissing. To
start naming and changing this world and me.

What had I hated about girls?
I hated that some of them show their weakness,
talking openly about relationship problems and
either they didn't see or weren't embarrassed by
their need for male approval like I was. I did
not want real personal stuff to be part of our
spoken about lives. I did not want to let it be
important.   I hated that they were not more
self-confident and that their needs were so
obvious and strong. I thought girls were fickle
and competitive. I was jealous but pretended I
was beyond it, and thought girls were so annoying
when they were jealous of me.

hate

Girls talked about personal things too
much, and I would try and listen closely,
be empathetic, really be there for them.
I was afraid of hurting their feelings. It
was draining. It was easier with boys. They
were stronger and more removed. Their feelings weren't
as serious. We could laugh things off. I didn't feel
so much responsibility.

I liked the power I got from being
better than a girl.

I hated girls who talked about political theory too
much. I thought they were trying to prove that they
were just as smart as guys. I hated girls who
embraced girly things as some kind of empowerment.
it seemed so surface and meaningless.

I wanted to love women and hang out with the
dykes, but the dyke scene I found, I couldn't relate
to. I felt really vulnerable around them and like I
had to learn the rules to some new game. They were
always talking about who was HOT HOT HOT HOT, and I
tried to see it as somehow not objectifying, but it
felt so creepy to me, and I didn't want to play.

I hated talking about sex. I hated any sign that
sexism really did touch us. I hated being reminded
of things I didn't want to feel. I hated feeling
like I was automatically supposed to have something
in common with women and feel safe and comfortable
with them, and able to open up, when usually I felt
totally weird and unrecognized. I felt like there
was nowhere for me to be.

And what I want most is to create a space in this
world now where we can be real and whole and rid
of all this fear and judgement and shit that is
inside of us and inside of me.

love

I learned to respect and love these parts of me:

empathy= the ability to step aside from myself and feel another person's feelings.

compromise – the kind that comes from in the heart wanting the best for the community, not the selfish kind that feels like giving up.

I learned to want to see all the complexities, instead of wanting to make things simple and easy to deal with. I learned to love my strong feelings instead of thinking they were crazy; and to love the creative instead of thinking it was frivolous and just got in the way of more important political work.

It took me years of really consciously fighting the sexism inside of me; really consciously dissecting these systems of opression and control. Reading histroy, theory, feminist psychology, poetry, fiction. Looking at the ways we communicate, what is valued and why; and what were my defenses. Which ones could I let go of because I no longer really needed them to survive. I looked at the specifics of how I wanted the world and my friendships to be. I tried to become more self-aware and more honest. More self loving and more humble.

It seems ridiculous, but I know it's really true, that it took me years of hard and painful work for me to start liking and valuing women and the feminine in me and everyone. And now this is where my heart is.

What would have happened if I'd had a choice, when I was a girl who did not want to be one? If I could have just easily become a boy, would 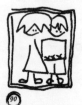 I have done this work? Would I have accepted and cultivated the masculine in me and continued to belittle the rest? Would I have been committed to

a radical feminist politics? Would I have been
working to blow apart a world that has kept us all
in boxes? If I had been able to become a boy, would
I have struggled to really understand myself and this
World, or would I have been able to just relax with
my privilege finally and forget about it.

If I had been able to become a boy, maybe I
would have felt freedom and been able to do all kinds
of things in this world that as a girl I couldn't.

Maybe I would have
all kinds of diff-
just my body and
have spent all
sex was the only
and sex was the
deal with every
in my life and
If I had been able
maybe I wouldn't
with so much self hate

felt valued for
derent things, not
maybe I wouldn't
those years where
place I felt power,
place I tried to
fucking thing
in my head.
to become a boy
have been filled
and fear.

who knows.
simple as any of that.
sort of the wrong
asking anyway.

It is not as
and probably it's
question to be

Like maybe the question should have been,
not what would have happened if I could have been
a boy, but what would have happened if the people
around me were challenging gender, looking at the
world that makes us, looking at the boxes and the
reasons for them, and supporting eachother while
we create and recreate ourselves, whatever way
we want to.

I have not always been a good transgender ally. I
have been frightened by the implications of people
born girl deciding they are not that, and afraid
that somehow that would undermine my struggle.
I have been afraid to ask questions because I didn't
want to looked fucked up or uncool or stupid. I
have been tired, not wanting to have to think
about anything new.   But I love it more than
   almost anything now. This struggle, this life.
      this new world we are making,

Guatemala

Our plane landed at an army base or something. We didn't know what was going on at the
time. Me and Mollie, all wound up and excited. We
were skuttled out, no time for customs, no money
exchange, just guided out the door, armed soldiers
all around, and we didn't really know if this was
just normal, well, she knew it was strange.

It was deep night, we were tired and hungover
still, happy and anxious and confused and I thought
What am I doing here? Guatemala.

I had sworn years ago, when I got back from Russia,
that I would never leave the country again. What
was the point if I didn't speak any languages and
had no real purpose anywhere. It was just tourism,
and a shitty kind of tourism at that - the kind
where I wanted to be seen as an exceptional white
girl, not so privileged, different from the rest.
I wanted to be recognized and accepted. I was
full of guilt and wanting to understand everything
and not being able to.

In my body, I felt like I learned something about
these places: the small town in Siberia where the
children played a game that looked exactly like
"duck duck grey duck" and I learned to buy laundry
soap and bread. There was no one our age in these
small Russian towns, only the young and old, everyone
one else gone to the cities. And it the city, the
teenagers drinking and smoking in the ruins of
what had once been a magnificant building I'm sure,
right in the city square. I felt in my body like I
was learning something, and that it would change
how I understood history and the world and myself,
but I also felt like it was a shallow, made up
understanding.

Guatemala. Mollie called me up, late winter in
Asheville, when the cold had seeped into my bones.
She said "$100 tickets round trip to Guatemala!
we have to buy them today!" So I said yes.

$100,

cheeper than driving my van to
Gainsville and back. and it
would be nice to see the rain-
forests before they're all gone. I want to see
monkeys and huge colorful birds. I want to hear
the sounds. I want my brain to be pushed in new
ways, and I want to be somewhere I can't talk at
all.

Mollies grandpa had a house there in the mountains
in a city that had once been small. He had lived
there forever, since before the revolution, and
had once been a civil rights lawyer, volunteered
for Cesar Chavez. Moved to Guatemala. Was a drunk.
When he died he gave his house to his friend Berto.
That's where we were going to stay.

The history of Guatemala is a brutal one. All the
terrible history of colonization and then the fate
of Central American countries that fell under the
sphere of US interests after WWII (the polite way
to say, ours to control, fuck with and exploit).
We provided the weapons and training, and insisted
that democracy not even get a toe hold, that the
poor be kept firmly under.

In Guatemala, unions and peasant associations were
subject to random terror to keep them silent, and
by 'terror' I don't mean arrest, I mean murder.
They killed everyone. That was even the policy for
quite awhile

                        If you went to a
street protest chances were you or someone you
knew would be killed - but still people protested,
and organized, and fought to live with dignity.

Guatemala has a huge Mayan population, and they
have preserved their culture and fought for
their lands. They have been totally
discriminated against like Indiginous
                    people everywhere.

93

In 1931, the ruler, Jorge Ubico, made it legal for landowners to kill Indians. He developed really efficiant systems of repression and control. He looked up to Hitlar, which the U.S. press did it's best to ignore, because they thought he was just the greatest.

In 1944, the revolution came and overthrew Ubico and brought a new government to power, with president Jacobo Arbenz. The next 10 years were a time of sweeping landreforms and other social reforms. Over ½million people were given land, and people in general were becoming politicized, feeling like they could have a say in shaping their lives and their country - they had the right to political participation.

The revolution's goals were to free Guatemala from military dictatorship and economic colonialism. To immediatly improve the low living standards of most people, and to diversify the economy. They said that "the first beneficiariesof the development of a countries resources should be the people of that country." An idea which seems pretty obvious, but is not at all ok with the USA. And the US government did what it takes to keep power. In 1954 the U.S. led a coup. 8,000 peasants were killed in the first two months, mostly United Fruit Company union workers and Indiginous village leaders. There were the usual huge lists of "communists" to be killed, imprisoned and tortured while the U.S. made Guatamala "a showcase for democracy". All reforms were reversed, of course, and the new government was unimaginable. It was a ton worse than the one from before the revolution. It was the kind of horror I can not even write about. Numbers and figures too high to understand. And all the times these words come up - villages destroyed - all the women raped then killed - all the men beheaded - children bashed on rocks.

the mountains

l go into denial. How can we exist in a world where
this happens? And how can people in power what this
power so bad? And howdo they decide genocide is a
necessary contingent of U.S. economic growth and
stability? and who is really benefiting from all of
this really? And is it possible that we need all
those fucking banannas? I mean, what is going on?
who are these monsters? the men who control the
world.

In Guatamala we stayed with Berto. There were red
flowers growing along the fence of the timy yard.
There was an evangelical church next door that
played music so loud, so late into the night, it
was like a punk show, music possessing you. singing
to forget and to purge.

Every morning we woke up to fireworks welcoming
the day. Breakfest of avacados, eggs, tortillas.
Every morning at 8:00, we walked to language
school, where we talked for 5 hours a day, one
teacher per student. Every day I stared at this
young man's lips, trying to copy him, get the
pronunciation right. trying to remember words and
wanting to communicate so badly. Every day I would
become so overwelmed I would cry.

We lived a quiet life in this loud village turned
half city, tourist town. We didn't talk too much.
Spanish took over our heads. I started to get my
tounge around the words, started to dream Spanish,
and I felt like may be it wasn't impossible and I
felt like it was all I wanted to do.

Sometimes we felt terrible, sometimes we felt good.
Sometimes we could not deal with anything past our
front stoop and the not too busy street. We sat
there, eating bannanna bread, drinking tea. We drew
pictures and read. and my life changed there,
with her.

We slept curled up together after I said "I don't
think I can sleep in bed with you. Every time I
try that with someone it gets confusing". She said
"I think it will be ok. We could just try it." And
it was. It was fine.

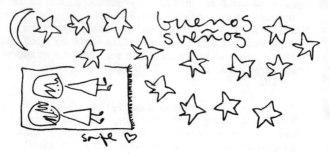

Some days we decifered the paper. There was a three
month long teachers strike going on. They had walked
across the country to Guatemala City. They had
taken over the airport and blockaded all the major
roads. They had taken over part of an oil pipeline
and basically said they would shut down the whole
country until their demands were met - free education for all children.

How is this possible in a country with this history.
I can not fathom the courage. Or may be I can.
They knew what they were doing and they won some
of their demands.

I left and flew home to a country mobalizing.
I came home to another war.

read:
OPEN VEINS OF LATIN AMERICA
by Eduardo Galeano
BRIDGE OF COURAGE by Jennifer
Harbury
THIS BOOK IS ABOUT
THE PEOPLE WHO TOOK TO THE
MOUNTAINS + FOUGHT AND ORGANIZED IN THE
70'S - 90'S - THE REVOLUTIONARIES. THEY ARE
SO AMAZING + I WANTED TO WRITE ABOUT IT,
BUT BETTER FOR YOU TO READ THEIR OWN WORDS.

GIRL GANGS

1991, down the street from my house on Fathers Day, there it was, spray painted in the alley: "Dead Dads Don't Rape". and it made me feel like there was someone behind me, after all those years, not a man creeping up, but a girl watching my back. an invisible force. A girl army. A girl gang.

Jacob, walking with me, said "That's pretty reactionary. It's not like all dads rape", And I was thinking about '85 and my friend who really did kill herself, not just cut wrists or too many pills like everyone else I knew did. Erika hung herself on Fathers Day. Of course we knew why, we had to have known. But none of us talked about any of that shit back then.

Can I tell you what it was like when the girl gangs started? It was amazing to see. I want to talk about this and not their faults. I want to talk about the power I felt in my body; the power and relief when I saw their flyers - and how their violence made everything so much more immediate.   Our lives are a war

and not less of a war than the one against the naziskins or the one against the class system, not less of a war than the war against the state. Our lives are a war, and you're part of it boy, and this war is full of unignorable realness and strong, fucking strong as hell emotions.

I want men to take us seriously. I am
tired of wanting them to
think about right and
wrong. I want them to
fear. I want them to feel fear
now as I have felt suffering.
And I want them to know that
know that there is always a
a time there always a right
time to wrong,
what is always a
there is retribution
time for time is begin
and ning.

The girl gangs redefined rape, and suddenly everything
counted. All the shit that happened to me counted,

they made it real. My stepbrothers hands counted,
the record store owner that used to get me to suck
his dick, the time Paul fucked me from behind in my
mothers kitchen, all the times I slept with that one
boyfriend because he said if I didn't he would find
someone else. All the comments on the streets, the
'accidental' gropes at the shows. Kill them all. It's

retribution time. Can you imagine the power in saying
that? Here's how it was: finally there was a counter
ballance in my brain. Ignore, forgive, spit kill. The
options widened. It was not a private issue any more.

no locks we must learn trust

no cindys, you can not have locks on your door. if it happens again just wake us up. wake us up. come upstairs wake us up!

1983

how could that be possible at all. — alone — trapped —

I didn't actually want retribution at that point. I wanted to work hard to dismantle patriarchy. I kept myself sheltered with a small group of friends who were all committed to anti-sexist work. But there had been a time when I tried to have my stepbrother killed.

It is a hard thing when it's the people you love hurting you. If I talked, it threatened our whole family structure. No one could fix anything or protect me. My brain learned to do these things: to forgive, to try and understand the causes and have sympathy for the people who hurt me. to try and help them, change them, smooth everything over. And these became the biggest parts of me. I could see the potential for good in everyone, except me.

The girl gangs taught me I could fight and hate. They wrapped tinfoil around their knuckles, dragged boys out of coffee shops and beat them up. They slipped drugs into the rapists drink, carried him home and cut off his dreads, tattooed 'rapist' on his forehead. They dressed sexy and walked in groups and carried baseball bats and attacked the cars that whistled at them.

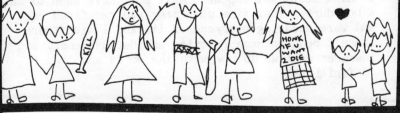

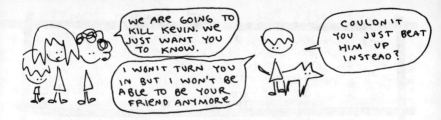

The girl gang glued my locks and poured laquor all
over my floor and left death threats on my answering
machine because I was harboring an enemy - my best-
friend, the most broken boy I knew, who had gone
out with one of the girls when they were very young,
and he had spit after going down on her. said it
smelled bad. So there were death threats and a meeting
where I said I understood if they needed to beat him
up, but if they killed him, I could not be friends
with them, the girl gang, anymore. and I did still
want to be their friend.

Here are the things I think about most when I think
about the girl gangs: I remember Allison sewing a
pink bunny suit for a disguise because she'd gotten
in a fist fight with the bus driver and he wouldn't
let her on the bus any more. I think about how they
forced our lives and our pain into the public eye.
All the little ways our lives are effected by rape
and sexism and silence - all the things we're supposed
to just live with, they scratched open and let bleed.
I think about how belittled they were and still are.

I think about how impossible it must have been to be
a boy during that time when they had redefined rape
and were accusing everyone of it. And I wish there
hadn't been so much reaction and defensiveness and
i wonder what we do now with the words and the
definitions.

There were things that happened to me that I called
rape then, that I wouldn't define that way now. There
is no way to put everything on a scale. What was worse?
My step brother molesting me, on-going non consentual
sex with a boyfriend, or the daily torture of growing
up sexualized female. I needed to call it all rape
to validate it, because the other words were not
strong enough for how I felt. I needed strong words
to be able to fight and learn to believe that

what felt wrong was wrong enough to try and do something about.

And I think the boys needed to hear it put that way too.
They were so clueless. So much was taken for granted.
Like sex was just fun, it didn't matter what you did.
It was a simple thing, nothing wrong unless the girl
said no, and even then, may be she didn't mean it.

The girl gangs forced a dialogue. They made people
fear. For the short while that they were around, I
think people talked more, both publicly and privately.
Like, "I was abused and here's what it's done to me
and I'm not sure what to do with it all but I need

you to be careful, to watch closely and be aware."

With them gone now, and so entirely demonized and
made fun of, I'm afraid the real work they did is
disapearing too. I'm afraid too much is taken for
granted again. Like everyone knows that everyone's
been abused so what's the point in talking about it.
So much silence. I'm wondering how many times we'll
have to start from scratch. Wondering if there's a
~~single one of us who had~~

single one of us who has been honestly seen and heard.

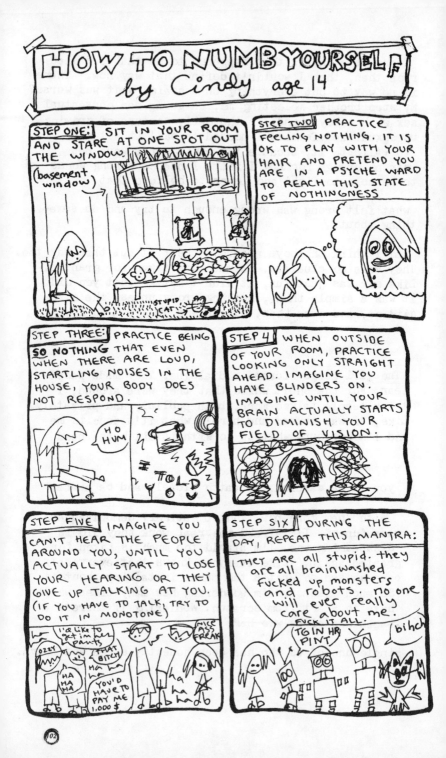

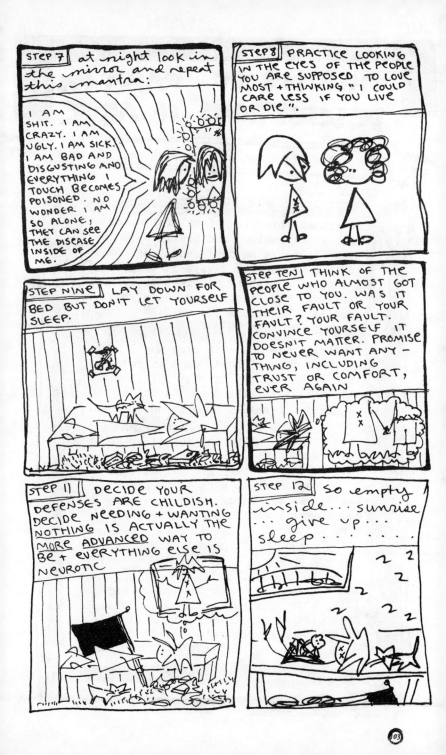

WARN-ING →

You might not want to read it.

(NOT THIS PAGE BUT THE NEXT FEW)

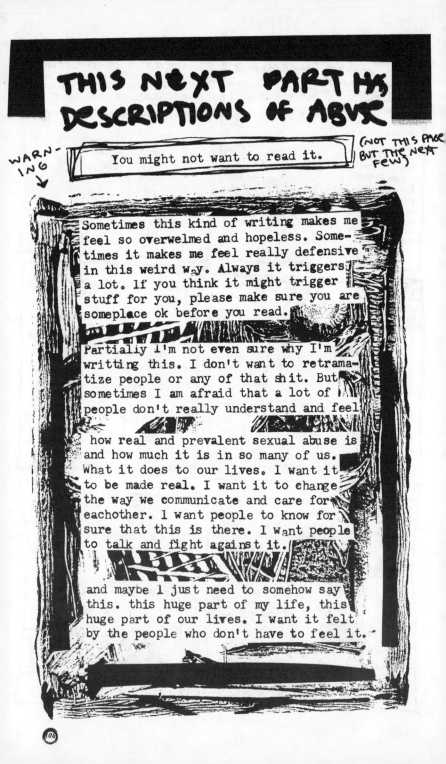

Sometimes this kind of writing makes me feel so overwelmed and hopeless. Sometimes it makes me feel really defensive in this weird way. Always it triggers a lot. If you think it might trigger stuff for you, please make sure you are someplace ok before you read.

Partially I'm not even sure why I'm writting this. I don't want to retramatize people or any of that shit. But sometimes I am afraid that a lot of people don't really understand and feel

how real and prevalent sexual abuse is and how much it is in so many of us. What it does to our lives. I want it to be made real. I want it to change the way we communicate and care for eachother. I want people to know for sure that this is there. I want people to talk and fight against it.

and maybe I just need to somehow say this. this huge part of my life, this huge part of our lives. I want it felt by the people who don't have to feel it.

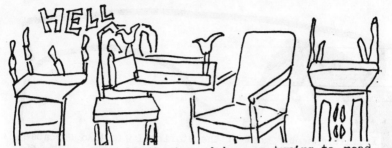

I was driving with Gerty and he was trying to read
"Cibola", and he said he couldn't read it. He felt
bad but it was just too much. It's about abuse,
about split personality. "Do you know about split
personalities" he said. and I nodded, hoping he wouldn't
try and explain splitting and it's causes to me.
Partially I was mad because, my life. how couldn't I
know about it. And part of me feels really crazy

because I can't remember whether or not Gertie has been
abused too.

I say "You don't have to read it. Some times are too
hard and sometimes we're too fragile to read or think
about some things and still function." I say "there is
only so much we can take. only so much we can know".

Part of me wishes I could go back and have the luxury
of not knowing all the things I do, and part of me is
screaming Why haven't you known.

I only know the tiniest fraction of my friends stories.
There was a time in my healing when I pulled stories

out of people. I knew no one had ever been heard
enough, and I wanted everyone to be cared for and
listened to. I wanted to create a world where we could
talk about our abuse openly and not just in times of
crisis. I wanted to feel less alone. I wanted to talk
because I knew it was in everyone, bottled up, and the
stories you tell are your life, the stories you don't
tell control you.

I can't remember most of the stories I was told, because
if I remembered them all, I think I would kill myself,
but the knowledge and terror is in me. I have two
friends who were ritually abused as babies, three who
were used in child porn. I have one friend who was
raped by a stranger in the park and then stalked by him
for months. She called the cops, but they laughed at her.

She is a black woman, the rapist was white. Girl talked
dirty to all the time by father. Girl constantly grabbed
at, constantly humiliated, can't escape. And how many
uncountable stories of first second third boyfriends
who did unwanted things. How many times have I heard
"All that time I thought that's just what sex was. You
were just supposed to lay there are bear it".

My ▓▓▓ spent 13 years and 3 kids with my ▓▓ and said
"I never enjoyed sex with him", but only once does she
define as rape. And what do I know of the other times?
My cousin has a scar the si₂e of her back from an iron
put there when she was a baby, and the cigerettes out
on her arms. My second boyfriend was molested by his
mom and I had to sit in her class, knowing this. She
is talking about art and I want to kill her. And in
her house, in her living room, I get rug burns on my
back wondering how long can this possibly go on for,
him pounding into me and staring into my face.

I did not know there was any way to be present. I didn't
know I'd left my body because I didn't know what being
in my body was.

Tara in the paddy waggon on her knees with the cops in a
circle, one shoving the night stick in and out of her
mouth, laughing. And the girl I knew on her way home
from grade school with her friend dragged into the

bushes. They killed her friend and her throat was
permanently damaged so now she only talks in a whisper.

Why vs ?

Why is it just the survivors who read books, trying to understand how it's effected us? Why is it only the survivors working hard to stay present in sex, while partners get carried away with assumptions; all the times consent to one thing was assumed to mean consent to a whole array of others. Why isn't everyone reading and talking, and not just when 'something' comes up so visibly it can't help but to be seen, the emptiness or crying.

i got this letter...

I got this letter from Amanda: "...Scott was telling me about how important he feels it is that we figure out how to deal with perpetrators, not by alienating them,

but so that things will be different. That people already know how to give support to survivors, maybe they don't do the best job but it's sort of instinctual to know how to deal with that. And this makes me think, Oh yea, that's what happens.

"If we place so much emphasis on healing the perpetrators, then this attitude comes out that it's a really easy thing to do to support survivors; plenty of people are doing that but someone needs to work on the really hard stuff. Fuck that. I mean, for me it's pretty hard to figure out how to offer support to someone who has just had someone try to take every bit of their power away from them, and if it's my friend or family or partner, then how is it supposed to be instinctual to know how to give them what they need and also deal with my own feelings of anger and sadness or whatever someone is going through.

How do we know how to do that and even with lots of time spent thinking about it and talking about it and reading and trying to figure it out, people are so bad at being supportive friends and community and human beings, and there is so much work to be done that just trying to imagine it all is exhausting.

And also, if people are able to recieve the support they need, then they are more likely going to be more capable to speak up and name rapists and tell others

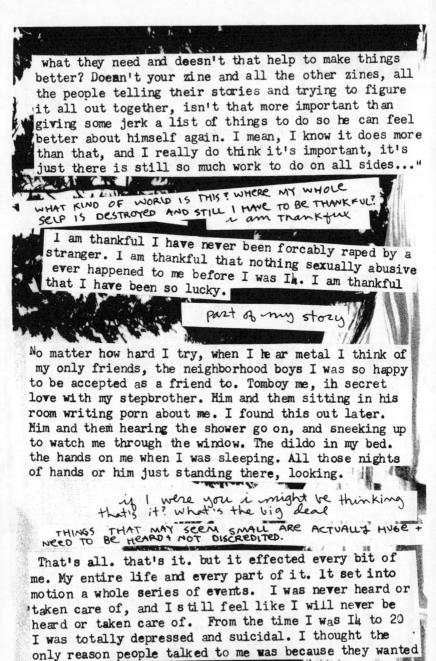

what they need and doesn't that help to make things
better? Doesn't your zine and all the other zines, all
the people telling their stories and trying to figure
it all out together, isn't that more important than
giving some jerk a list of things to do so he can feel
better about himself again. I mean, I know it does more
than that, and I really do think it's important, it's
just there is still so much work to do on all sides..."

WHAT KIND OF WORLD IS THIS? WHERE MY WHOLE
SELF IS DESTROYED AND STILL I HAVE TO BE THANKFUL?
I am Thankful

I am thankful I have never been forcably raped by a
stranger. I am thankful that nothing sexually abusive
ever happened to me before I was 14. I am thankful
that I have been so lucky.

part of my story

No matter how hard I try, when I hear metal I think of
my only friends, the neighborhood boys I was so happy
to be accepted as a friend to. Tomboy me, in secret
love with my stepbrother. Him and them sitting in his
room writing porn about me. I found this out later.
Him and them hearing the shower go on, and sneeking up
to watch me through the window. The dildo in my bed.
the hands on me when I was sleeping. All those nights
of hands or him just standing there, looking.

if I were you i might be thinking
that's it? what's the big deal

THINGS THAT MAY SEEM SMALL ARE ACTUALLY HUGE +
NEED TO BE HEARD + NOT DISCREDITED.

That's all. that's it. but it effected every bit of
me. My entire life and every part of it. It set into
motion a whole series of events. I was never heard or
taken care of, and I still feel like I will never be
heard or taken care of. From the time I was 14 to 20
I was totally depressed and suicidal. I thought the
only reason people talked to me was because they wanted
to fuck me.

I fucked them, sometimes because I wanted to, sometimes to get it over with, sometimes to prove to myself and the world what a bad person I was. I belived deep down I was bad. I believed everything I touched turned to shit. I beleived I was not worth anything. I thought that I was insane. I thought that I was a slut. I thought that I was an angel sent from heaven to have sex with people and act really pasionate and make them feel really good about themselves.

A lot of times I didn't know when I was really enjoying myself and when I was just acting. I still have this sometimes. I still am scared of all the middle ground. I am comfortable being friends, comfortable fucking, but all the slow stuff inbetween is way too scary. I don't want to think 'do I want to be doing this' because if I think that question, even if the answer is yes, it triggers off all the hundreds of times I have had things done to me and my body that I didn't want. And how I have never been able to say anything. And about the few times I did say something and it didn't make a difference, the thing being done to me didn't change, and I wished I'd kept my mouth shut after all. It has kept me quiet. When I speak out in defense of myself or my friends my body shakes for half an hour. I feel terror and I can't help it.

I can't be involved in the kinds of political projects I'd like to be, because it makes me crazy and unable to function. Some days I can't leave the house. I feel constantly watched and looked at, especially when I think I am alone. For a long time I thought women were too emotional, they were too threatening. I didn't want them for my friends.

and i couldn't be with boys who were nice to me.

I never touched my own body until I was 24. I started drinking heavily. I am afraid to get close to people because I have no faith at all that they'll stick with me.   I am afriad that once the passionate, performing, beginning of a romance wears off, all my fears and problems and self hate and body abuse triggers will come up and they will not want to hear or know or work on it all with me. So what is the point in trying or explaining or asking for help. I don't think anyone is interested in my real life. I have spent 19 years dealing with how much I have been effected by abuse. I've gotten a lot better. I don't hate myself at all any more. I have spent 19 years and have finally gotten most of myself back.

I don't know if people understand how much it all kills us, how every part of our lives is differant.   It needs to be seen, needs to be recognized, needs to be dealt with. I am amazed that I made it through these years, and I was one of the lucky ones. I was full of self love and love for the world before my abuse happened, so I had that in my core,   somewhere inside was that resource. and I had some amount of privledge.

Do you know about split personalities? I don't want to hear you. I can't know this. I can't read this. I don't believe you. She's exagerating. I want things to be solvable. I don't want to think about this unless there's an answer, a beginning and an end.

I want all the non abused people to start committing themselfes to dealing with this, reading about it, talking about it, you can talk with eachother. you can ask if it's ok to talk with us. I want you to in your hearts start wanting to understand the depth of it.

i want people to stop saying that they don't know how to be there, how to deal with it. I want them to set aside time to figure out ways that they can.

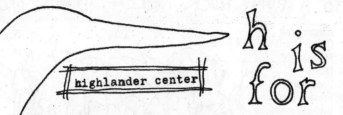

h is for

highlander center

an education and political organizing center
that was opened in the 1930's in Tennessee,
with the idea that "the best teachers of poor
and working people are the people themselves.
They are experts on their own experiences
and problems."

In the 1930's (and sadly, still today)
many white organizers thought poor people
were ignorent and needed to be taught
what was up and how to think

Highlander Center was the first openly
integrated place in the South, and was
active in the Civil Rights Movement.

It is still active today, organizing around
many issues, including immigrant rights and
queer liberation.

hibernate

the best thing about
winter in cold, cold
places was hibernation.
when it was too cold to
go outside or even leave
the bed + you just had
to rest, stay in bed,
read books, process all
the crap and all
the good things and
growth that had
happened over the
year. when friends
came over, you wrapped
up in blankets and sat
on the couch and warmed
hands on coffee or tea
cups and came up
with dreams + talked
about ideas, slowly,
with thought + care.
hibernation.

Home Alive

is a self-defense and anti-
violence project that was
started in Seattle by a friend
of mine and a bunch of other
women after Mia Zapata,
singer for the band The Gits,
was murdered.

One of the things I really like
about Home Alive is that it
was started by non-
professionals, who wanted to
make self-defense classes
that were affordable where no
one would be turned away for
lack of funds. They focus on
teaching in a way that
recognizes the reality of our
lives, and that honors the
ways we have protected and
defended ourselves. They
raised money by doing music
and art benefits, studied
different methods of self-
defense, and created their
own classes.

HOW WE TURNED OUR SHITTY LITTLE TOWN INTO A PUNK ROCK MECCA. 10 POINT PROGRAM

1. Hanging out
2. Create a visible public presence
3. Show space
4. Dance
5. Form bands
6. Freak + Punk unity
7. Inviting strangers
8. Treating bands
9. Dealing with Nazis, sexist assholes or speedfreakhippypunkgutterscumbags
10. Events and Projects to draw people in

When I moved to my town, there were just 5 punks, mostly just graduated from high school, plus 3 IWW folks, some EarthFirsters and some art freaks. Here are some of the things we did to transform our shitty town into a punk mecca:

1. Hanging out.

Never underestimate the power of sitting around in public as a way to draw people into the world of punkness. Punks look cool. Just by standing around looking good we become a vibrant propaganda tool.

2. Creating visible public presence.

Posters, flyers, graffiti, public art. Nothing is more depressing than a town with punks that just post on the internet, nothing is better than walking around a shitty town and finding an Anarchy sign spray painted behind the grocery store. You must put up flyers about shows. If there aren't shows in your town yet, put up flyers about other stuff. Flyers thats main graphic focus is on girls body parts are not rebellious, they are jock. Make flyers about your beliefs. Make art and staple it to telephone poles. Make it look like there is something mysterious going on that people should want to be a part of.

3. Show Space.

Basement shows rule. No basement is too short or too small. Even if people can't pogo, they can still skank. Our first show space was a storefront on a crappy main road, and we had an art project in it, where anyone could pick a section of the wall and paint it. It made it so that punks that otherwise would feel weird as hell just trying to hang out, could come and be busy, but still part of things. Our next space was in a short basement with a small creek running through it. We built a retaining wall to try and keep the water away from the electricity. The whole place was cavern like, the energy just hung in the moldy air and the stage was just a few pallets. Everyone said it would suck to have shows there, but actually they were the best shows ever, with everyone crammed in and dancing and sweating, mashed together, and trying to see and going wild in the sweetest way.

4. Dancing.

I can not overstate the importance of dancing. Dancing rules. Dancing is punk! At first, no one danced at the shows in Asheville, then me and my sister decided to dance as hard as we could to the entire set, no matter how bad the band might suck. It was difficult,

especially because in the beginning there would only be about 5 - 10 people watching the show, and everyone thought we were crazy, but after awhile everyone started dancing, and then when new people came, they thought that's what punk was all about - dancing like fucking maniacs. Punk is participatory, not entertainment. If the audience is not working as hard as the band, then it is not totally punk.

5. Form Bands.

Everyone can play. Everyone can scream. If I can form a band, you can. When I first started to try to scream, I just made a terrible choked croaking noise and I cried because I felt so stupid, now I scream like hell. Also, I've been playing the bass with only two fingers and only the top two strings for about 8 years. It's fine.

6. Freak + Punk unity.

One of the sad things about our shitty town become a punk mecca, is laziness and scene isolation. In the beginning, we all needed each other, punks and freaks and weirdos and intellectuals. If we wanted things to be interesting, we had to make it happen. There was the beautiful heyday of punk and freak unity, with amazing talent shows and musicals and cabarets and dance performances, but then, by the end, so many punks had meccaed out to our town that they thought they no longer needed the freaks, and it became just a bunch of isolated people who didn't need or care about each other any more.

7. Inviting Strangers.

So, the truth is, a lot of people are sort of afraid of punks. And a lot of people are scared to go to weird new places. So, it is important to reach out in person to people who look like they might secretly want to join the scene. Give people flyers, and talk to strangers, and if they come to the show, talk to them and make them feel welcome. I was always really shy, but then when I ran the door at the club, I got to watch how so many people felt uncomfortable and unsure what to do with themselves, and I realized it's important to be a welcoming committee and introduce people to each other, and do all the usual things of a good hostess. I've been to many towns where the only people who talked to me at the punk show were guys who wanted to sleeze on me, and I think it's so important that girls talk to girls, non-sleezers talk to the new people. Unity!

8. Treating Bands.

ok. So, if you book bands, be nice to them. Cook them food and give them a place to stay. If you are not going to have a place for them to stay, tell them that ahead of time. Also, give the bands money. Unless you are a greedy self absorbed capitalist bastard, paying the band should come first over show space rent. Figure out some other way to pay show space rent. Also, local bands should play first. If you start to create a scene where people only love the local band and only dance to the local band and the local band plays last, it sucks. Just play first, and make everyone stay for the touring band. Create a culture where people want to show off for the touring bands, and show them how much your town cares about punk by going wild and giving the band the best show they've ever had - I mean, dance!

9. Dealing with Nazi's, sexist assholes or speedfreakhippypunkgutterscumbags.

Don't let Nazi's into your shows. You can tell them that if they quit being a racist asshole then they can come in, but otherwise, no. Same with the fuckers who grope women. It is good to have some bitter ex-punks or bitter tough old punks around, because they are usually good at beating up Nazi's and other scum-bags if necessary.

10. Projects and Events to draw people in.

Punk is about creating our own lives, creating lives worth living, creating new and vibrant culture outside of capitalism's corrosive effects. Punk picnics, punk kick-ball, punk scavenger hunts, punk organizing, punk zines. And brainstorming up your own 10 point program for changing your own shitty town.

health groups

49 percent of women in America will have an abortion before they're 45, but hardly any of us really plan for it. I think it is just so important that we have knowledge of what resources are available for us and for our friends. Also, in this world that is increasingly hostile to women having control over their bodies, it's important that we know what is going on inside of us, and ways we can deal with the emotional and physical impacts of unwanted pregnancy.

I really want to encourage women to form women's health groups. It doesn't have to be the focus of your life or the focus of your activism, but I think it's necessary for us to have at least a basic knowledge of our bodies and our health care options. And if you can't form a group, you can still learn a ton on your own.

Here are some questions:
Where is the clinic/clinics in your area? Do they offer surgical and medical procedures? How many weeks are abortions offered until? What kinds of experiences have people you know had at local clinics? What kind of sedation do they offer? Valium? Twilight sedation? What are emotional pro's and con's of the different types of sedation? What do you think you would want? How does a surgical abortion work? How long does it take? How long do you have to be at the clinic? How does a medical abortion work? What is that experience like? Are there protesters at the clinic? Does the clinic accept volunteers? Do they have translators? How much does it cost?

These things are way easier to find out about when you're not having to deal with the emotions and panic that often come with unwanted pregnancy.

I'd like to offer up a couple resources here. On the internet, there is the Feminist Women Health Centers page at fwhc.org. It has a lot of information about how it all works, and also a good page on people's personal stories about their experiences with abortion. Also, there is a group called the National Network of Abortion Funds at nnaf.org/fundinfo.html. It is an organization with local groups around the country that raise money to help women who can't afford their abortions. They don't cover every part of the country and most groups need donations and volunteers.

Do you have a friend who you feel like could support you through an abortion? If not, is there anyone who could be that person if you put more commitment into deepening your relationship with them? What are your feelings about abortion? What are your partners feelings about it? Is your partener willing and able to help pay for an abortion? Have you talked about what you would do and what you would need for support if you were to have an abortion? If you need help figureing out what you think about abortion, or how to talk about it, there are a lot of good resources, like The Pregnancy Options Workbook, at pregnancyoptions.org, and Abortionsconversations.com/whoweare.php. I also really like the book Abortion Without Apology and of course, Our Bodies Ourselves.

I know a lot of people who have a vauge sense that they would like to try to abort with herbs if they were to get pregnant. If this is something you are interested in, I seriously recommend doing the research before you get pregnant! There is a lot of information to sort through, and since herbal abortion doesn't have the highest success rate, and the herbs are often hard on the body, it is much better to know which herbs and in which forms you would want to take. There is a really great website called Sisterzeus.com, that has some herb information, and also recommeds books that provide more detail. I particulary like Herbal Abortion: The Fruit of the Tree of Knowledge, by Uni Tiamat. Ordering information for this book is on the sisterzeus website.

I've been criticised in the past for taking abortion too lightly, and I really don't. I think abortions are really hard for many of us. They tend to bring up lots of complex and deep emotions, even when we don't have moral issues with it. They often bring up issues of self-worth and our ability to make healthy choices in our lives. They can bring up issues of abuse. They can bring up questions about our relationship with our partner and our relationships with our friends. They can bring up the defeated feeling of not being treated with care and respect from our doctors. They can bring up body fear and body hate, and control issues. I'm not saying that it has to be that way, or that it always brings up these emotions, but I know that it is often really complex and hard. And I want us to be able to face these difficult times with less fear and with more openness and support. I also think that if we talked more freely about abortion, maybe it would also become easier to talk about birthcontrol, body issues, consent, and all kinds of things that would help us in our lives.

I also want to recommend these books: <u>A Women's Book of Choices: Abortion, Menstrual Extraction, RU-486</u>, by Chalker and Downer, <u>Taking Charge of Your Fertility</u>, by Toni Weschler, <u>A New View of a Woman's Body</u>, by the Federation of Feminist Health Centers, and <u>The Biology of Women</u>, by Ethel Sloan

i is for

icarus project

MANY YEARS AGO, TWO PEOPLE I KNEW DROVE AROUND THE COUNTRY TALKING TO COMMUNITY GROUPS + PUNKS + FRIENDS ABOUT THEIR STRUGGLES WITH BIPOLAR DISORDER + OTHER MENTAL HEALTH PROBLEMS + HOW EVEN THE PUNKS, WHO EMBRACE CRAZY, STILL STIGMATIZED CERTAIN MENTAL HEALTH THINGS, LIKE TAKING MEDS. THERE WAS STILL SO MUCH INVISIBILTY, NOT ENOUGH SUPPORT, NOT ENOUGH ROAD MAPS OF WAYS TO DEAL WITH CRISIS, NOT ENOUGH TALKING ABOUT THE REALITY OF IT ALL.

THESE TWO WANTED TO CHANGE THAT — TO GET COMMUNITIES TALKING, TO FORM SUPPORT GROUPS, TO PUBLISH STUFF, TO LEARN FROM EACHOTHER. THEY HAD BIG PLANS THAT I THOUGHT WERE PROBABLY DELUSIONAL, BUT AFTER A FEW YEARS THEY MET ALL THEIR GOALS + MORE. THE ICARUS PROJECT IS AN AMAZING RESOURCE + AN AMAZING ORGANIZATION. PUBLICATIONS INCLUDE NAVAGATING THE SPACE BETWEEN BRILLIANCE AND MADNESS and HARM REDUCTION GUIDE TO COMING OFF PSYCHIATRIC DRUGS

theicarusproject.net

INCITE!
WOMEN OF COLOR AGAINST VIOLENCE

"A NATIONAL ACTIVIST ORGANIZATION OF RADICAL FEMINISTS OF COLOR ADVANCING A MOVEMENT TO END VIOLENCE AGAINST WOMEN OF COLOR AND OUR COMMUNITIES THROUGH DIRECT ACTION, CRITICAL DIALOGUE, AND GRASSROOTS ORGANIZING."

THIS IS A GREAT ORGANIZATION! VERY BRILLIANT + RADICAL — WITH LOCAL GROUPS, GREAT RESOURCES FOR DOING COMMUNITY EDUCATION + AN ANALYSIS THAT CONNECTS ANTI-VIOLENCE STRATEGIES TO THE "LARGER STRUCTURES OF VIOLENCE THAT SHAPE THE WORLD WE LIVE IN" INCITE-NATIONAL.ORG

Ida

trans and queer
community farm
and sanctuary.

my favorite place
and my favorite
people

i wanna

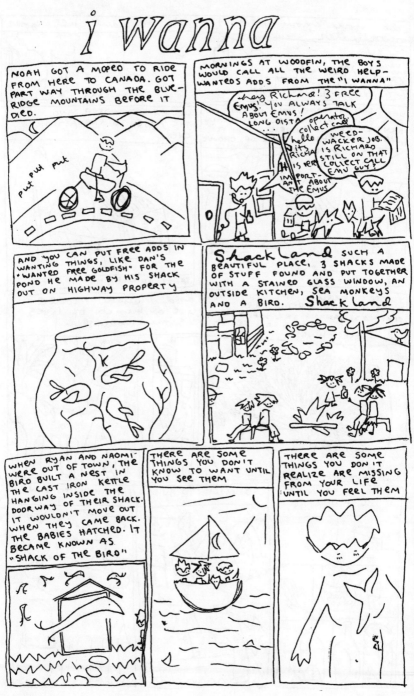

NOAH GOT A MOPED TO RIDE FROM HERE TO CANADA. GOT PART WAY THROUGH THE BLUE-RIDGE MOUNTAINS BEFORE IT DIED.

put put put

MORNINGS AT WOODFIN, THE BOYS WOULD CALL ALL THE WEIRD HELP-WANTEDS ADDS FROM THE "I WANNA"

Hey Richard! 3 FREE EMUS! YOU ALWAYS TALK ABOUT EMUS! LONG DISTA...

hello city operator collect call

WEED-WACKER JOB. IS RICHARD STILL ON THAT COLLECT CALL EMU GUY?

THIS IS VERY IMPORTANT ABOUT THE EMUS

AND YOU CAN PUT FREE ADDS IN WANTING THINGS, LIKE DAN'S "WANTED FREE GOLDFISH" FOR THE POND HE MADE BY HIS SHACK OUT ON HIGHWAY PROPERTY

Shack Land SUCH A BEAUTIFUL PLACE, 3 SHACKS MADE OF STUFF FOUND AND PUT TOGETHER WITH A STAINED GLASS WINDOW, AN OUTSIDE KITCHEN, SEA MONKEYS AND A BIRD. Shack Land

WHEN RYAN AND NAOMI WERE OUT OF TOWN, THE BIRD BUILT A NEST IN THE CAST IRON KETTLE HANGING INSIDE THE DOORWAY OF THEIR SHACK. IT WOULDN'T MOVE OUT WHEN THEY CAME BACK. THE BABIES HATCHED. IT BECAME KNOWN AS "SHACK OF THE BIRD"

THERE ARE SOME THINGS YOU DON'T KNOW TO WANT UNTIL YOU SEE THEM

THERE ARE SOME THINGS YOU DON'T REALIZE ARE MISSING FROM YOUR LIFE UNTIL YOU FEEL THEM

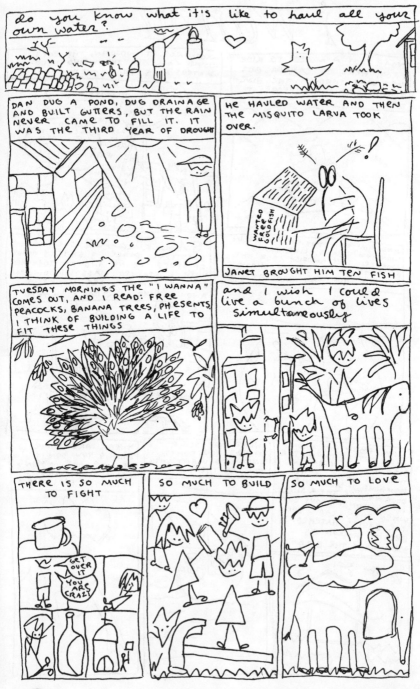

do you know what it's like to haul all your own water?

DAN DUG A POND, DUG DRAINAGE AND BUILT GUTTERS, BUT THE RAIN NEVER CAME TO FILL IT. IT WAS THE THIRD YEAR OF DROUGHT

HE HAULED WATER AND THEN THE MISQUITO LARVA TOOK OVER.

WANTED FREE GOLDFISH

JANET BROUGHT HIM TEN FISH

TUESDAY MORNINGS THE "I WANNA" COMES OUT, AND I READ: FREE PEACOCKS, BANANA TREES, PHESENTS I THINK OF BUILDING A LIFE TO FIT THESE THINGS

and I wish I could live a bunch of lives simultaneously

THERE IS SO MUCH TO FIGHT

GET OVER IT YOU ARE CRAZY

SO MUCH TO BUILD

SO MUCH TO LOVE

If your friend's parent dies.

Things that helped me after my mom died.

There was the crisis time, the time when she was dieing, and then dead. That part I will talk about later. What I want to talk about here is the later time. People forget that it is not a quick recovery. What I am talking about here is 6 months later, a year later, two years later, now.

One of the saddest suckiest things was that no one wanted to talk about it. I don't know what it is that makes people so afraid. Actually, I do kind of know because one of my friends had a parent die recently, and I feel some of the things other people must have felt around me. Like I'll say the wrong thing, or maybe it is not a good time to talk about it, I don't want to pry, I don't want to make her think about it if she doesn't want to.

but the thing I remember is I was always thinking about it. I was afraid to talk about it would be burdening people. I didn't know what to say, where to begin, what was important, what was too much for someone else to hear. I didn't want to talk if someone didn't want to know and I felt like no one really wanted to know.

If you are the friend of someone whos parent has died, try and think of how you can get yourself to a place inside your self where you want to know. try and figure out how to hear about it without it being a burden. Your parents will die someday too. It is part of our existance that is pushed away but so real. It needs space to be seen. It need space to be heard and experienced not just in our isolation.

If it is mothers day or fathers day, aknowledge it. If it is the anniversary of the parents death, remember and say something. If you are hanging out with your friend with a bunch of people and everyone's talking about parents and your friend is quiet, talk with her, later or then. at least tell her that you felt it too, the loss, the uncomfortableness, the empty space, the bitterness.

Make time to ask questions. For me, the first year was so uncomprehendable, and after the year came the time when I was really ready to talk, when I really needed to talk and the truth was, no one remembered. For everyone else, they were glad the crisis was over and they could finally get a break. It was over for them. For me, I needed to start peeling back the sadness and anger. I needed to remember the good things and say them outloud. I needed witness to our history. I needed friends.

Once a roommate out of the blue made breakfest, cleaned the house, got everyone else outside and quiet. He said "I was thinking about your mom when I woke up and I wanted to do something for you."

Once someone said, "I was too afraid to ask you about your mom when you were having such a hard time, and I'm sorry. But I do have so many things I wonder about your relationship with her. I realized I don't know anything about it really. but I'm afraid to ask you questions because I'm afraid it'll be prying." I said it wasn't prying. I said, "what do you want to know?"

The youngest mem

There is relief that comes from talking. There is relief that comes from finding out that what may seem like the hugest burden in the world doesn't turn in to a burden for someone else if I say it outloud. Like the details of my moms disintegration. When I got back from the hospital, I tried to tell my one friend, and he said shhh. He was not able to hear. But later, I told someone else and they heard it fine. They let me cry. They were not crushed by it at all.

Around anniversary time, I like it when someone else figures out something for me to do. Not anything too elaborate. It's just that left to myself, I will get angry or disassociated and I will "forget" and try and push it away, and then I'll remember and get sad and angry at myself. I like to be taken to the woods, may be just for an hour or two. Swimming maybe, or where there is something special and beautiful. I like it when someone cooks for me. comes into my room if I am not leaving it. leaves a little note saying something - I am here for you. I will be here all day if you need me. I will be back at 7, I will be in the garden. I am baking you cake, I am thinking about you, I am sad for you I am angry for you I am wishing and thinking and amazed at your survival. I wish I had known her, I wish I had been able to be there to help you. I wish you didn't have to do so much of all of that and all of this alone. I want to figure out how to be a better friend to you, and I am going to figure it out. I am loving you.

Leave me a note if it's ok if I come in.
Circle what you think you might need

for me to come and hold you
for me to stay outside your door but play you some music
for me to play music to you inside your room
dancing
for me to ask you questions
for me to just be near and silent
for me to hold your hand while you call your other family
to talk about the rest of the family
to go outside and scream
to go outside and talk about anything but this death
to get away from here
go to a movie
distraction
acknowledgement
some kind of ceremony
to get the rest of the roommates out of the house
to get the rest of the roommates to stop giving you uncomfortable looks
to get people to stop trying to cheer you up
to tell everyone else that this is the anniversary day
to tell you that all the mixed things you feel are ok
to tell you the things I love about you
to tell you that this is the worst thing you'll ever know
to tell you that I want to know everything. it is not a burden.

circle what you think you might need. or write more. I want to be here for you. I want to be your friend.

and dream On calm days

introduction to doris #22

I want to stay up all night talking, not drunk, talking
and remembering everything, with stars passing through
the sky, the rain falling on the roof. I want to watch
you and learn your ways. I want to break off this shell
I've put on myself that sometimes resembles resignation,
resembles panic and desperation, covers something too
big to explain, but with patience and care, maybe I can
explain it to you.

Remember the way cougars walk stealthy through the
forest? I want to do that. Remember the way herons dive
into the lake? I want to do that too. I want to fly like
a flying squirrel, run like a rabbit. I want to hold your
hand next time we go to the movies, do you?

I am here in my new house, writing this and a novel and
a comic book and a coloring book and letters in my head
to you. So many questions I could write a questionnaire.
What if I get scared to ask them?

In the daytime, I wait for the mailman. I haven't seen
anyone but him in five days. In the mornings I write
down my dreams if I remember. I try and stretch, try and
dance. I try and learn to move my body again without
censure or self hate. I listen to that Dead Moon song,
have you heard it? It goes, "It's ok, we've all seen
better days. It's ok, you don't have to run and hide
away." I listen to Sini Anderson spoken words. It says
"I want to run into the insane energy of love. I want to
run into every wall the upperclass puts up in our path."

Today I cut open my stuffed animal lion, the one my old
bdst friend Johnathan gave me before he died. I cut it
open, cut his eyes out, and sew new button eyes on. I
take out some of the stuffing so he's more flexible, more
cuddly. Sew him back up. Squeeze his ears, kiss his nose.

In the afternoons I chop wood. In the evening, I make up
stories of how things are and how things were. I string
them together with this undying hope that you'll want
to read them. That you'll hear.

i remember

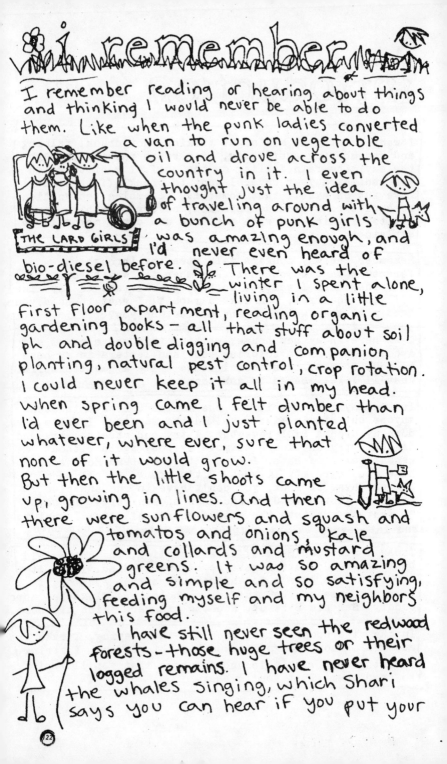

I remember reading or hearing about things and thinking I would never be able to do them. Like when the punk ladies converted a van to run on vegetable oil and drove across the country in it. I even thought just the idea of traveling around with a bunch of punk girls was amazing enough, and I'd never even heard of bio-diesel before.

THE LARD GIRLS

There was the winter I spent alone, living in a little first floor apartment, reading organic gardening books - all that stuff about soil ph and double digging and companion planting, natural pest control, crop rotation. I could never keep it all in my head. When spring came I felt dumber than I'd ever been and I just planted whatever, where ever, sure that none of it would grow.

But then the little shoots came up, growing in lines. And then there were sunflowers and squash and tomatos and onions, kale and collards and mustard greens. It was so amazing and simple and so satisfying, feeding myself and my neighbors this food.

I have still never seen the redwood forests - those huge trees or their logged remains. I have never heard the whales singing, which Shari says you can hear if you put your head underwater at the right time of year in Hawaii! I have never seen the top of a volcano (and maybe I never will)

I remember when I lived in the country, and my dream was to buy a couple acres, open a junkyard and build a small house. The books about building made me cry. There was too much math. Why was it so impossible? And why did I always have to do everything alone?

~~then here~~ my friends bought land up in the mountains. We build a house that's crooked but it won't fall down. I move rocks for the foundation. I BUILD A BRIDGE out of fallen logs. I dig out the side of the mountain. exavation. We put top soil in one place for the garden, put the red clay soil in the bathtub, add water from the spring. I take off my boots, put on my red dress that for some reason makes me feel like my grandma, I hold the hem up and dance around in the bathtub, squishing the clay, making mud. I am one big mixing machine. I cut my feet on rocks. Plaster the mud onto straw bales, until the skin rubs off my hands. I let it heal. next time I wear gloves.

I want a place of my own + so I clear out blackberry brambles. I burn +dig and build a fence out of sticks to keep the bunnys out, although I haven't planted any food. I dig and build paths + make a place that feels good to walk into; sheltered by a big magnolia tree.

H☐→

Q: When and how did you first find out about feminism? anarchism? anarcho-feminism?

A: Basically, I found out about feminism when I was a senior in high school. There was a program in Minnesota where you could go to University classes instead of high school, and it was free. I took an Introduction to Women's Studies class there, and a class called Sexuality and Self Image. They really changed my life.

When I was growing up, my parents told me that girls were just as good as boys and could do whatever boys did. They tried to instill this in me, but it wasn't the reality. It wasn't the reality in my mom's life at all, and it wasn't the reality in mine. I was a tomboy growing up, but by the time I got to Jr. High, I very much bought in to all the shit that is pushed on teenage girls. My goals were to be a model or a rockstar's girlfriend. At some point it became clear that I didn't fit in at all. I hadn't really been socialized right, and I went to a middle-upper class school and I wasn't that. I had two pairs of pants. I worked at a plastic factory and then a rib joint, when I was 14, so I could make money to buy clothes and makeup, to try and fit this role.

Eventually I made friends with people who rejected a lot of the normal shit. We rejected ideals of female beauty; we held each other's hands in places where people would be threatened by that. We got threatened and harassed for being lesbos, but actually, I at least, was still pretty homophobic. We rebelled, but it was at a very gut level, and I didn't have much home, and when my friend Courtney would get outraged by things like sexist advertising, I just thought "What's the point in even bringing it up? It's everywhere." I was very suicidal and I thought I was crazy.

The Introduction to Women's Studies class showed me that I wasn't just fucked in the head. You know, I just felt so alone and thought I had all these personal problems, but the class gave me a context to see my life in, and it gave me really concrete reasons to struggle.

What spoke to me most was black women writers, particularly Audre Lorde, and her essays and speeches about silence and fear. Like this: *"To survive.... we have had to learn this first and most vital lesson -- that we were never meant to survive. Not as human beings... And that visibility which makes us most vulnerable is that which also is the source of our greatest strength. Because the machine will try to grind you into dust anyway, whether or not we speak. We can sit in our corners mute forever while our children are distorted and destroyed, while our earth is poisoned; we can sit in our safe corners mute as bottles, and we will still be no less afraid."*

How can you ignore that?

Another thing that was good to read and hear people talk about was the whole "virgin or whore" dichotomy. I had very much bought into this way of looking at women and at myself. It was very interesting and validating to start to understand the history and the political and religious reasons that women had been placed in these categories; had their sexuality and self expression repressed and denied.

The class also helped me to look at really specific things about my life and how I participated in perpetuati   patriarchy. Like, our teacher once asked us to pay attention to who we made eye contact with when we were in groups of mixed genders. I looked for attention and approval almost exclusively from boys. I started trying to change this. I also ended up having my first girlfriend. She asked me on a date one day after class.

The other really important thing that happened while I was taking these classes, is I learned to define what my stepbrother did to me when I was 13-16 as incest and sexual abuse. There was very little written about incest at the time. I didn't know anyone who talked about this stuff and had never read anything about it, except in sickeningly sensationalized paperbacks.

Learning about feminism made me start to want and expect very different things from people, and from myself. It made me feel like my experiences and my voice was important and valid, and I stopped being quite so scared that someone would lock me up if I told the truth of what it felt like inside of me. I applied feminism to my life in very personal ways, but had a harder time seeing it as a political movement. I wasn't really interested in political movements at the time.

The next year, when I was 18 , I got to go to a shitty little liberal arts college in Vermont for awhile, and I got an anarchist boyfriend. Anarchism was amazing to me. I had always had this really deep love for humanity, and always saw so much potential in people, and here was a political philosophy that was based on these things. I started wanting to change the whole world, and I believed, and still do believe, that it's possible. We can create a world based on compassion and mutual aid, rather than competition and mindless consumption. It's the only thing that really makes sense.

My boyfriend was anti-feminist. He thought it was divisive and unnecessary. At first I thought he must be right. Having my own ideas and beliefs was still new to me, and I had terrible self-confidence and was very vulnerable. Eventually, though, I learned to see feminism as a completely essential part of the struggle for an anarchist world, and just completely essential in general, for obvious reasons. Sexism and patriarchy are so ingrained, in men, women and transgender people, and it's not going to just magically go away. If you're interest in feminist movements during revolutionary liberations struggles, I really recommend the books Free Women of Spain, and also Sandino's Daughters. There are lots of good books out there, but these two were inspiring to me.

Q: What kinds of things do you do in your life that are anarcha-feminist?

A: That's a hard question, because it seems like basically everything I do is related to anarcha-feminism. I just think feminism is so important, and working with women and trans people is really, really important. I think it gets ignored and taken for granted a lot. A lot of people get annoyed when you bring up sexism, Like "Oh, we already got over that, we're all cool." but it's just not true. I mean, I've been really actively fighting my ingrained sexism for 15 years and I still definitely have a bunch of sexist shit inside of me. So personally, it's very important, just in a sort of daily way, to fight for a pro-feminist world, and to let girls know that if they feel like they're experiencing sexism, they probably *are*, and it's not that they're crazy or oversensitive. People aren't over their sexism, and we do have to really fight for ourselves and each other.

I'm not very good at doing large-scale political work. I used to try and do coalition work and mass movement kind of work, but I find I'm a lot more effective in small groups. My main project, aside from writing, is women's health stuff. I'm in a small women's health group, and we're trying to learn about how our bodies work. It's been hard, but also really amazing. For me, just reading medical text books, and especially looking at anatomy pictures, triggers something abuse related and makes me just shut down, but it's starting to get better. For years, probably like ten years, I've wanted to have a women's health group, but I've never found people I was close enough to or comfortable enough with to do it. When this group started, we didn't all know each other that well, but we were just like "We're gonna do it. We're just going to become close somehow."

We do self exams and pelvic exams and study Physiology. If you're interested in this stuff I recommend these books: <u>A New View of a Woman's Body</u>, <u>The Biology of Women</u>, <u>Women Hormones and the Menstrual Cycle</u>, and <u>A Book of Women's Choices</u>, which has a really interesting chapter on menstrual extraction. We are also trying to write our own pamphlet that won't use gendered language.

One of the really great things that came out of our health group, is that we opened a little health resource center for women and trans. The idea was that we'd get together good books, and have certain days of the week when people could come in with questions they had about their health, and we could help find the information. The idea was that we could all learn together. We can all become experts about our own bodies and we can help each other. We're trying to provide an alternative to the whole way of looking at health. Our health concerns are usually just diagnosed and treated, and lots of doctors are judgmental and make us feel diseased. Often they don't try to help us understand what's going on in our bodies, and get hostile if we ask too many questions. So with this health center we are trying to demystify our bodies, and learn in ways that are empowering. We're trying to have people write about their personal experiences with local doctors, so that we know which ones are respectful and which aren't. Also, collecting people's stories of their experiences with std's, infections, etc., so we can share knowledge of how to heal ourselves, when that's appropriate. There's a bunch of things we want to do, but we're just getting started.

Soon after we opened the resource center, a doctor got involved, and she has been having a free clinic, once a week, in the space, which is really incredible! She's been influential in helping us educate ourselves about transgender issues, and helping the space become more trans inclusive.

Those are my main projects. the other thing I try to do, which might sound stupid and small, but I think is important, is just recognizing women. Like, I helped with this punk club for awhile, and I would run the door, so I would just sit there and watch people come and be awkward and not know anybody and not feel welcome. All my life I'd felt that way, and I'd never gotten to just sit back and be like, "Oh, everyone else feels totally awkward and uncomfortable too!" So I started just trying to be welcoming, to girls especially. I mean, I'm totally socially awkward, but I just try and be more aware of how we're kept separate and how hard it is for a lot of women to make connections that aren't based on using their sexuality.

Q: Is your community supportive of your anarchafeminism?

A: I feel like in a way I have a pretty supportive community, and I'm always pretty surprised when people aren't supportive. Like when we first started our health group some people thought it was weird, and they'd say stuff like "Oh, there go the girls! Girls group!" It was a weird, belittling kind of thing they were doing, even though I don't think they consciously wanted to belittle us. But they weren't like "Oh, rad! That's so important! We understand why!" It was just like "That's an uncomfortable thing that they're doing so let's make a joke."

We also had to fight really hard to get the space for the women and trans health center. It's in a room in our larger anarchist community center, and it was really shocking how much resistance there was to giving us a space. But now that it's there, most of the people who resisted it are very supportive.

Most of my closest friends don't live here and don't consider themselves anarchist or feminists. I think they've had bad experiences with people who define themselves as anarchists and feminists being really dogmatic and confrontational and shoving their politics down their throats, being super judgmental. Honestly, I used to be judgmental. I think it is sometimes an important thing to go through; to define what your beliefs are, and to be really strict. But these friends of mine are drunk and never had perfect language, never had the luxury to go to college and sit around and think about deconstructing language, and think about how it adds to oppression, all that stuff, they never got to do that, and I doubt they'd want to. But they are the ones who have been most supportive of me, and I feel like, in their hearts, they want to have the same kind of world that I do. I know a lot of people who consider themselves activists just think that my friends play music and get fucked up and are kind of worthless, but they are the people who made me totally know the feeling of what it meant to have a full community that was just totally, totally loving and that didn't think I was crazy because I was a woman, and didn't think I was stupid because I was a woman. They assumed I was just as capable as any dude, and also, they didn't sexualize me, so I love these people, but I don't know if I could say they're supportive of my anarchafeminism, but really, they are, because they're supportive of me.

Here, we have this much bigger, not particularly loving, kind of thing that gets called community. Like our community center. I am super, super proud of it and really proud of the people who are doing it, but when you get a group that big, there's all these power dynamics that come up, and I feel like a lot of anarchists and also a lot of anarcha-feminists, still have a lot of learning to do about how to work collectively. I think one of the problems is this crisis mode people are constantly in. There's this huge sense of urgency, and people just don't have the patience and emotional energy to dedicate themselves to dismantling power dynamics. Of course, things *are* really urgent, but they've been urgent for the past few centuries, and I think it's really necessary for people to take the time to do the really important things that make collective work empowering and good instead of just totally frustrating.

I sympathize. I know that in my smaller groups, I can get that way too - just totally impatient and task oriented, but in the big meetings I feel crazy. I want to get older and be more able to speak my mind. I want to be able to talk to my friends in groups or collectives, and when they're saying stuff that I think is fucked up, I want to be able to say, "That's fucked up!" or even just, "I disagree," but whenever I try, I feel totally terrified; like physically terrified, even though I know I am not in actual, physical danger. I get that feeling of being a kid and my family fighting and just any kind of conflict being potentially violent and in some way life threatening. I grew up learning to keep quiet or to use my voice and try and diffuse conflict, and now, even simple conflict leaves me scared and shaky and it's not worth it. I think lots of women experience similar forms of silencing, and it's not recognized enough in anarchist activist work.

Just in regular daily life, I don't feel like most people know how to be supportive in a real way, and most people are really overextended, including myself. Anarchafeminism has given me really high standards for humanity and for how I think we can and should be supportive friends. A lot of the time, I feel like I'm just so lucky. I know all these totally amazingly wonderful people who do really great and important things, but most of the time, I still feel pretty unsupportive. I think we don't know enough about each other's lives. Like I spend

half my time working on this magazine and other writing projects, and a lot of the time I'm writing about things I really don't want to think about. I would really prefer to not think about rape in our community, but I have to. I feel like I have an obligation to, and it's happened to me a lot. So for the past year I've been doing all this work around it - trying to think about it deeply and feel about it really deeply. I've been going over my experiences, and doing all this super hard emotional work so I can figure out how to write about it in a way that I think will be helpful to our community, and will bring about dialogue and hopefully help bring about awareness and help change things. It's super hard, and I'd rather not be doing it. I'd really rather be running around and having fun adventures and making things beautiful and writing about that.

I get a lot of support from strangers and people who write me, but not that much from my community here. I understand why, but it's still hard. I'm trying to figure out ways to get more support and ways to let people into my life more. I think they just don't know, and I don't know similar struggles that they're having in their lives either. We take too much for granted.

Q: Are you "out" as an anarchist?

A: I think I'm out. I have a pretty sheltered life, in a way, so it doesn't come up much. When I was 19 I would talk to my family and friends about anarchism all the time - try to shove it down their throats, or at least try to get them to see and accept me. Then, for a long time, I didn't talk about anarchism because it just didn't seem relevant. Like, of course, aren't we all anarchists? Recently, I've had some conversations with friends of mine who have really weird theories about how people are necessarily authoritative and you can tell because everything in nature is! And I was just like, "Oh my god! My friends aren't all anarchists! What the fuck!" So I've been trying to write and talk about it more.

Q: Can you talk a bit about privilege?

A: Privilege is such a weird thing. I'm glad people are talking about it and owning up to it, because when I was younger, it was a hugely divisive issue. If you were middle or upper class, you were just fucked. People just tried to lie and deny it. There was a huge amount of guilt, and it kept people from being able to use their privilege in ways that could have been constructive.

I always thought I had a lot of class privilege. I felt pretty guilty about it. I don't know what I was thinking. Recently I've met people who had a lot more class privilege, and I'm like "Oh, that's what people were talking about!" But I do have privilege. I went to college for a year, but I can't imagine what it would be like to have the money to go to college and get out and have this life that you're supposed to live - get a good job, do the right thing. I think it can be a real trap. I think it's important for them to let go of their guilt, and let go of some of their safety, and go out and live life and find out what they're passionate about, and find out how they can be most effective in working towards social change. I honestly feel a little bit bad for those people, I'm not sure why. I sure do wish they would just take the money their parents give them and fund local projects with it - pay the rent for our health project - give it to single moms. Seriously. I do think that privilege is not at all a cut and dry thing with an easy definition. Like, personally, I can't imagine having the privilege of not being raped and not having totally insane family that you're really tied to. I also can't imagine what it would be like to not have white skin privilege and more or less, heterosexual privilege, although I think about those things a lot and work hard to educate myself.

I think people with privilege need to seek out voices of people who are different than them, and to really pay attention and learn from these voices. And I don't mean just reading a book or two. I mean, reading theory, fiction, poetry, life stories, history. I think it's important to look at our prejudices, our fears, our defenses, and to call each other out and challenge each other and to expand our lives. I think it's really important for white anarchists to become allies to communities of color, and what I mean by that is, finding out what groups there are in your town or city. Is there an American Indian Movement group? An immigrant legal defense team? Does the black community have a mobilization committee to end police brutality? find out what is going on, and see if they need any volunteers to do some shit work. And then do it, and be consistent, even if it's boring and not as "revolutionary" as you think it should be. One of the big problems with white radicals is a lot of them only want to be allies if they can get a big clap on the back, some recognition and some glory. I'm hoping we can learn to change this.

j is for

JUNE
JORDAN

One of the first things that ever made me feel that a new world was actually possible was a plan by June Jordan and Buckminster Fuller for the rebuilding of Harlem after the 1964 riots. I had seen inspiring plans made by mostly white liberals/radicals, like rooftop gardens and bike riding, which focused mainly on people making lifestyle choice changes to create a more sustainable world. I was not very politicized back then, and had the general feeling/liberal complacency that all you could do was change yourself.

June Jordan lived in Harlem, was a poet, a theorist, African-American, bisexual, an activist and educator. Her plan for restructuring the city was very thorough and discussed how racism and structural neglect created violence and poverty, and the necessity of public space and vibrant cultures. It discussed how urban renewal was used as a way for cities to move Black people and other people of color out of neighborhoods in order to make the space available for wealthy, white people. Her plan for the restructuring of Harlem was extremely detailed, and she "… fully expected its enactment… as a form of federal reparations to the ravaged peoples of Harlem." And that expectation, in itself, blew my mind wide open. Like, right, what if we expected our supposed democracy to actually deal with the history of racism in this country, and to make reparations and to do it openly. What if we really expected a world that put ethics and equality first, instead of profit and manipulation?

June Jordon died of breast cancer. I read an essay she had written during her treatment. A wound that wouldn't heal. And sometimes a friend was there to help her with the bandages, but not always. And I thought "June! I will come out there! Change your bandages, drive you and cook for you. Whatever you need!" But by then it was too late She was already dead. And I thought what a crime it is that in these radical subcultures and movements where we create out own families, the people who inspired us still die without full community to care for their need. It is so essential that we change this We have to let our elders know that we are here for them, and then be there.

JANE
an underground abortion service when abortion was illegal and a group of women learned to perform them Themselves, allowing women to go through the process in saftey + with support + care.
we must keep this knowledge alive!

Jack Palance Band
sweetest, most singalongyest heartfelt no bullshit punk band ever.

justine

I wanted her to like me, and so every word
that came out of my mouth embarrassed me. I
felt taller than any human should be, and more
awkward than a new born goat. We were writing at
the picnic table, drinking coffee, swatting away
the bugs. Two city punks in the woods.

I say "How about we go wildcraft us up a four
course meal?" Justine looks at me, raises her
eyebrows, says "What?"

I've never been one of those - surviving in the
woods types. I don't believe in the apocalypse,
but I've been trying to pay attention to edible
plants lately, just because.

So we get some advice, and we walk around,
picking and digging and trying to look stuff
up in our books, which are far too confusing
to actually be of help. We tumble down hills,
get stuck in black berry brambles. and we end
up with enough for dinner alright. A big salad with
flowers and berries. "potato like" roots, cooked
greens and stewed apples.

Justine is toughness and raw honesty, open eyes and
ready for the world. I want to hold her to me. I don't
want her to have to face everything the way I had to
face it - alone. But I'm projecting. I'm paternalistic.
And the truth is, I see her as my equal, if not my
better.

We get back into town, and she jumps out the back
door, hits her skateboard and is gone in a second.
I look for her almost every day, even though I
pretend that's not what I'm doing.

One night I get done staffing the health clinic
and there's Justine, standing outside the ACRC
door, and then Sarahbrown pulls up, parks her
car half in the road, jumps out her door, and
runs up to us, like it's been a century since we've

seen eachother, and really, it has been awhile.
It's like a family reunion, Candice and Andrea
and Andrea and Frankie and Jess all pile out of
the car, SB talking a mile a minute, and all of
us happy in this night air.

Then this drunk kid stumbles up to us, talking so
fucking loud, interrupting everything, saying
"Whoa! I thought you all were DUDES!" He looks us
up and down, one by one. "Damn!" He yells, and I
say, "Fine, just leave us alone." But he gets
right up in our faces, overpowering, overtaking,
looking at our body parts, trying to make sure.
We can't even talk to eachother anymore, although
some of them are doing a pretty good job of
attempting to ignore him. Not me. I lose it. I
start standing tall, talking loud, trying to get
it through his unhearing ears, "We don't want to
talk to you right now." He says, "No, I think
it's cool!" looking at us. looking at us. I don't
give a fuck what he thinks.

I get in front of him,   "Leave us alone!"
There's no space between us, but I walk
forward anyways, making him back up, saying
"You're fine. We just want to be left alone."

I can see it not getting through. I start screaming and swearing. His face changes, along with everything else in him. He starts swearing and screaming right back "fucking dykes! Stuck up fucking dykes! I'm gonna kill you!" He's sitting against the wall, crying about how his dad beat him up and we're no different, we're all the same. I feel bad for a second, I suppose, but mostly I just can't take it anymore. Every week of every month in every year, it's something like this. Usually something worse.

I want a new world now. I'm impatient. I want goats and a dog and I want to take them hitchiking with me. I want to walk in the Bad Lands, I want to swim in the Great Salt Lake. I want to love my friends like there's no tomorrow. And I want tomorrow to last forever. I want tomatoes on the vine and the canning jars cooking. I want to learn to provide. I want to learn to strike with precision. I want to learn to rest. Just rest for awhile.

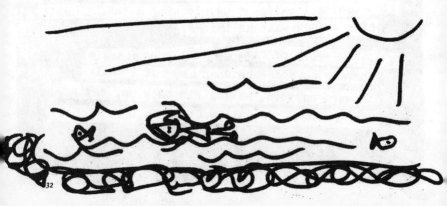

k is for

KATE BORNSTEIN

AUTHOR, PLAYWRIGHT, PERFORMANCE ARTIST, ACTIVIST, GENDER RADICAL, INSPIRATION. My Gender WORKBOOK is such a sweet, accessible way for people to look at, question + change their gender assumptions. It's funny + excellent. Hello, Cruel World: 101 Alternatives to Suicide for Teens, Freaks + Other Outlaws is also amazing + is saving + improving many peoples lives.

Jamacia Kincaid

I had probably read something about colonialism before I read Jamacia Kincaid's A Small Place, but this tiny beautiful book helped me to understand the implications of it. She writes with the most beautiful language. Her fiction autobiography books, like Annie John and another that I like even more but can't remember the name of - they are stories so beautiful and complicated and just dieing to be said outloud. read to your best-friend or just outloud to yourself. She's written some books recently about growing food, but her early ones about Antigua are so great

KEGEL EXERCISES

you know the muscle you contract if you gotta keep yourself from peeing? If you exercise that muscle by contracting it for like 6 seconds + relaxing it for like 6 seconds a bunch of times everyday it will strengthen that muscle which for some people leads to better orgasms

Koalas + kites

keesley highschool

We ate our afternoon breakfasts at the Uptown Bar.
They had ridiculously huge servings. I always got
homefries, even though I thought they were cut
too big and cooked too dry. The boys always got
something with Meat. Meat meat meat, the menu
said it everywhere. They thought it was really
funny. I thought it was kind of childish.

Them and me. Leather jackets and motorcycles.
My knee touching Shaun's. My slight embarrassment
and uncomfortable pride one day when I realized
I'd slept with half the boys in the bar. Ok, there
were only 8 boys in there, but still, I had just
turned 17.

The shy pride of having been accepted into their
lives, when I had never been accepted anywhere
else. Accepted into their bodies at least, if not
totally into their lives. After all, I still lived
at home, in the suburbs. I was still in highschool,
which no one ever mentioned. I was too young to
know their music references, too different to get
their inside jokes, but I saw something in them
that made sense to me. It was at that time when I
was trying to build up my walls as fast as I
could; trying to walk with big steps and confidence,
learning to spit and punch and not care, not feel
a thing. These boys had that already, all the facade
and swagger; and they were at that critical juncture
where the habit of living in a shell of no emotion
was about to become their sealed fate, and they
were scared to death of that, and I saw it. I
gave them sideways glances of recognition when their
hope or vulnerability leaked out.

And if they were so desperate, why was I trying to
become like them.

Some books would say they were using me to
regain their lost innocence, but that is not the
book I am writing.

—Voilà la tour Eiffel (*Eiffel Tower*).
Ils regardent la grande tour Eiffel. qui est loin
Après un

'An 'opposite' is here used to mean a word conveying a
contrasting idea. One word is seldom an exact opposite of another.

Latin or Old French word; cf. Fr. fenêtre—Lat.
fenestram.

A tell whether the following statements are true or false:
1. Brisquet est une bonne fem...
2. Brisquette est la

I didn't talk much when we were in groups together, sitting in the garage, at the coffee shop, at the Uptown Bar. I didn't think I had any stories of my own to tell. I hadn't been to New York City.

I didn't know much of anything at all, but I remember once saying, just to have something to contribute, "I swam with dolphins in the ocean once." Later, back at home, I sat cross legged on my counter, staring at myself in the mirror, staring into my own eyes for hours. I said 'What a stupid lie! Swimming with dolphins! Who are you trying to impress with that one?'

I didn't have stories like they did, about juvenile hall, or helping a friend kick dope. I didn't have stories about shows or trains or breaking into abandon buildings and the crazy things you find there. I didn't have stories of fear and adventure, and I didn't share their larger group of mutual friends. I couldn't name some name and have everyone go 'Oh yeah, that guy,' and then listen to all the stories go around.

I was thinking about this one night. It was Mike's housewarming party, just me and Liz and Shaun and Mike, and the other four people in our main crew. Mike's brand new apartment was the cleanest place I'd ever been; hardwood floors and freshly painted white walls, and just candles because the electric wasn't turned on yet. The only furniture was a

hammock, which I was laying in. They were passing whiskey around, and I didn't drink, but I had a little that night. The room was dark, and they were all talking and laughing and Erick already asleep. Shaun had been on this pretty serious kick about how he didn't want to love me because - and this is what he said to me, for real, one night, a week before, when we were just walking around town. We were in this alley and he took my hands in his and looked so seriously into my eyes, and he said "You are like a field of pure snow and I feel like I am just walking across you, leaving my muddy footprints."

135

There was a lot of fucked up shit for me, being with someone six years older, but I sure didn't feel like I was a field of pure white snow.

Then he told me he'd slept with half the women in town, and honestly, I didn't care. It seems weird to say, and I knew even then that I should probably act hurt, but I wasn't. I only felt kind of sad about the whole patheticness of the world and everything, but not jealous; I felt kind of tired.

At Mike's housewarming party, I lay in the hammock and Shaun was laying on the floor underneath. I had a pretty sure feeling that Liz was next to him, there was that kind of furtive sounds of sneeky movement going on, or may be I was just imagining it. Mike and Gage were telling stories, Erick was snoring, and I could see Lee out of the corner of my eye. I lay there and listened to the movements and voices, kind of content, kind of depressed and full of self hate. I thought about their lives and mine, and what stories did I have to tell? I had four parents and six siblings and all the fucking bullshit that went on in those houses, and also how I loved them and tried to protect them from eachother, and how I tried to make them live, and how I tried to protect myself from them. I thought about stories, and when are people going to stop telling the ones with easy punchlines, dramatic conclusions; when are they gonna stop talking about chictracks and crankshafts. What the hell do they actually think about anyway? It can't be as shallow as all this. I thought about: when do we start to tell the stories that sound mundane, but actually make up our real lives. Like what it's like to comfort these drunk parents. Why do we all feel so bad inside? What it's like to have to sit across the table every morning, eating sugar cereal with the brother who abused you, and you hate him and love him and feel sorry for him. The parents sitting on the couch nearby, ask outloud the question to a crossword puzzle, and you think "why don't they see this! Every morning it's the same. Invisible me. I'm not even here."

I was thinking, "When do we talk about love and what it really feels like, what it's made of, not just Holliwood or Iggy Pop shit. When do we talk about what it feels like to walk down the street? When do we talk about emptiness and what is it that draws us together."

Lee says, "I'm going home. You want a ride?" I say yeah, and when we've in the car, he invites me over for a game of cards. He cooks white rice, with a little chopped peanuts on top. "This is my favorite thing to eat in the world," he says, sort of apologetic, but it is, somehow, actually really good. His roommate is gone, and he shows me his roommates room. There's a super 8 camera on a tripod. "Him and his girlfriend make home porn," he says with a small- not sure what he thinks about it - kind of look. I don't get it. I think it's a weird joke, but then realize it's not. I wonder why any body would want to do that.

We lay lengthwise on the couch together, like we're an old and comfortabe couple; my back resting against his chest. We watch an old-fashion movie that way. I hold his scarred up hand. He says "I really was only thinking of playing cards and giving you a ride home." I say "It's ok." I kiss him. And you know how it is when one kiss makes someone the most beautiful person you've ever seen? When every-thing seems clear all of a sudden?

He was smaller than me, with straight eyelashes and the blackest hair. He had shy, uncertain eyes, and in this way we were equal.

It was the first time my body felt whole and alive and present and real, and I could see, I could feel, I felt treasured and beautiful and I never wanted to get out of this bed again. I felt safe and fed and it was fine to cry and to fall asleep and wake up, reaching out and laughing.

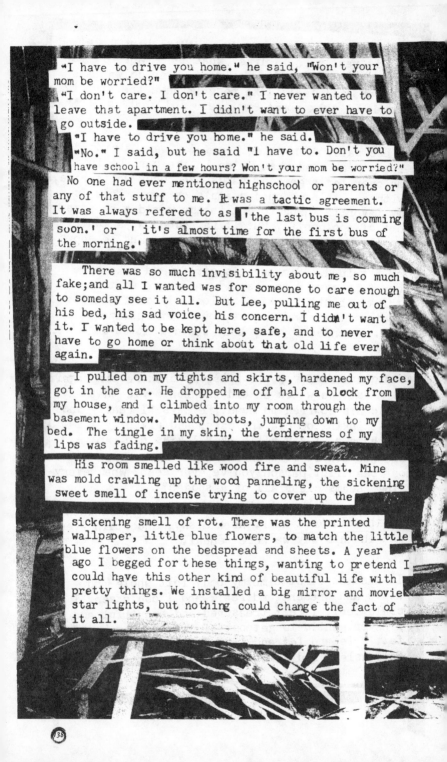

"I have to drive you home." he said, "Won't your mom be worried?"

"I don't care. I don't care." I never wanted to leave that apartment. I didn't want to ever have to go outside.

"I have to drive you home." he said.

"No." I said, but he said "I have to. Don't you have school in a few hours? Won't your mom be worried?"

No one had ever mentioned highschool or parents or any of that stuff to me. It was a tactic agreement. It was always refered to as 'the last bus is comming soon.' or 'it's almost time for the first bus of the morning.'

There was so much invisibility about me, so much fake;and all I wanted was for someone to care enough to someday see it all. But Lee, pulling me out of his bed, his sad voice, his concern. I didn't want it. I wanted to be kept here, safe, and to never have to go home or think about that old life ever again.

I pulled on my tights and skirts, hardened my face, got in the car. He dropped me off half a block from my house, and I climbed into my room through the basement window. Muddy boots, jumping down to my bed. The tingle in my skin, the tenderness of my lips was fading.

His room smelled like wood fire and sweat. Mine was mold crawling up the wood panneling, the sickening sweet smell of incense trying to cover up the

sickening smell of rot. There was the printed wallpaper, little blue flowers, to match the little blue flowers on the bedspread and sheets. A year ago I begged for these things, wanting to pretend I could have this other kind of beautiful life with pretty things. We installed a big mirror and movie star lights, but nothing could change the fact of it all.

I sat crosslegged at the mirror, lit the insense, and ratted my already matted hair. I put on my walkman, rub mascara onto the skin underneath my eyes, line my eyes with lip liner, pluck the hairs from the mustache trying to grow on my lip. I stare in the mirror. I punch my face. "slut" I go upstairs, eat my Capt'n Crunch, walk out the door and up the hill, and stand with my siblings, waiting for the bus that will take us to Keesley Highschool.

I was raised to believe that guys wanted sex all the time, and that if they didn't get off when they were turned on then they'd get blue-balls which was totally painful and terrible. I was raised to believe that it was my job to do what was needed. I was abused when I was young, and then dated much older guys, but when I was 18 I was in a relationship with someone my age. One time when he was out of town, I read his journal. (which, needless to say, was a really terribly wrong thing to do). In the journal it said something about how tired he was of always having to have sex with me in the mornings. The thing was, I didn't want to have sex either. I thought because he was hard, that meant I had to do it, and so I would iniate. I generally initiated when I thought someone wanted it, so that I wouldn't have to try and say no, and then be raped (even though this boy would have never ever raped me and I knew that). Reading his journal was the first time I realized that I could be the one who had power, and that I could be coercive even when I didn't want to be. This led me to really committ myself to reading about childhood sexual abuse, and looking at how my abuse history could make me do abusive things. Of course, it was a long task. I am still learning.

For me, it is important to remember that it is a long unlearning. I try and be really conscious, but sometimes can fall into old patterns when I least expect it. For awhile poly-amory was really important in trying to figure out my own sexuality and how to have healthy relationships, and sometimes I was good at it, and sometimes I used polyamory as an excuse to be dismissive of other people's feelings and needs. Reading Wendy-O-Matic's book Redefining Our Relationships was really useful to me in helping me figure out how to be ethical in my poly-amoury and not just to use it as a holier than thou manipulation tactic. Eventually I decided polyamory fed in to my over sexuilization of everyone I knew, and that I didn't want to be thinking that way about everyone. I wanted to be able to have clear friendships and clear boundries. It was really good for me to stop flirting and to figure out ways to connect with my friends that weren't sexual. I started to form much closer and more stable relationships with my friends, which has helped me learn about setting boundries and respecting boundries in all areas of my life.

I still struggle with always turning closeness into sexual feelings. I don't really blame myself for it, because I know that it comes from childhood abuse. I am trying to learn ways to be really upfront with my friends when I am trying to get physical, non-sexual comfort. I've found that even when it seems obvious, it's completely important to me to state from the beginning "I want to cuddle but don't want to do anything sexual." even when it is with my best friend and I have said it a hundred times before. I just almost always think that when someone touches me they want to have sex, and then I start responding to this assumed want. So stating what we are doing before hand helps.

There have been a couple times recently when I have been sleeping next to a new friend , who I felt pretty clearly like we wouldn't do anything but then we ended up doing sexual stuff that felt consensual. In both cases, I knew I should have talked about it as it was happening, and in both cases, I was older and so felt like it was my responsibility to bring it up, but I try not to beat myself up about it and I have made sure to talk to them later to make sure it was ok. These talks went really well.

I is for LYNDA BARRY

my hero. Lynda Barry writes
the sweetest, saddest, most
best comics and books ever.
a total inspiration to
everyone who comes in
contact with her work.
She is the reason I got
the courage to draw, which
is part of the reason I
started a zine in the first
place. these are some of
my favorite books she made

WHAT IT IS
CRUDDY
ONE HUNDRED DEMONS
THE GREATEST OF MARLYS
FREDDIE STORIES

laughter

once when I was
having a hard time
making friends,
someone told me
to make a list of
qualities I valued.
I made a long
list. politically
active, good listener,
a whole bunch of
things I can't
remember now.
They were all
good and valid
things, but once
it was done + I
was talking to
Cuty I said "I've
always been
happiest when I've
had friends I
can just laugh
with." I had
never realized
how important
that was to me.

the lesbian AVENGERS

THE LESBIAN AVENGERS: WE RECRUIT

When I was 23, the Lesbian Avengers came into existence.
It was a direct action based group – started in NYC, but
with local chapters, and they were so COOL! They
organized the first ever Dyke march! Their actions looked
so fun! I'd been working in a political collective that I
liked, but it was heavy into theory and I was shy and not
very educated, but I had a ton of energy and believed we
could create social change now! Queer didn't really exist
then. I was bisexual. Someone once said to me that bisexual
just meant I had one foot in the door of patriarchy, I
generally felt like I didn't count. Would the Lesbian
Avengers have accepted me? Probably, but I didn't even
try. The group was a direct action based group. They had a
great handbook that outlined ways to keep groups
energized and together – how to run meetings, pick action
targets, stay creative. Some stuff from the Handbook is a
little outdated, but most of it is still totally relevant and a
great resource. It's printed in part in Sarah Schulmans book,
My American History and is probably on line too at lesbian
avengers.com

listening

Listening. It's suppose to be this universal thing we all know how to do, but in reality, there are a million different ways to listen. There is listening that is silent, like confession, and listening where you quickly come up with your own opinions, or your own experiences, and like a discussion, you add them in as soon as you get an opening.

Think about listening.
Think about listening. Pay attention to the different ways people you know listen. Figure out what it is that makes you open up to certain people and not others - what qualities of listening do they have? What responses do you need to feel heard?

Of course, everyone is different, and what you need in a listener, most likely won't be the exact same thing that the person you're trying to support will need. But thinking about listening instead of just feeling like it's something we should inherently know how to do, is a first step.

A lot of the times, talking about sexual abuse may need a particular kind of listening. Below are some words about Active Listening, taken from a training manual for rape crisis councilors. (active listening is also used in consensus decision making. It might seem strange and formulaic at first, but it's really a great skill and once you learn to think in this way, it'll stop sounding forced, and will just become part of how you hear and process and listen.

The purpose of active listening is to help you understand what is going on inside the other person. What her feelings are, what she is experiencing, etc. Because that person is not able to always share what's going on inside, the statements she makes are sometimes coded or clouded. This means you have to decode or clear the message, and hear what she is really saying. The only way to know weather you are hearing correctly is to reflect back to the person what you are hearing from her. She will in turn let you know whether you are correct or not.

The purpose is to show that you're interested, that you've not only heard her, but that you understood (or are trying to understand) what she said. It helps check your accuracy of decoding what she's saying. It gives her a chance to breathe. It lets her know that you're actually there. It communicates acceptance. If fosters the person doing their own problem-definition and problem-solving and keeps the responsibility on her, not you.

When an abuse survivor says "I just can't tell anyone what happened", she may be saying any number of things
-I want to forget it ever happened
-I am afraid of what people will think of me
-No one believed me before, why would it be different now
-I am afraid of my feelings about it
-I am afraid I will fall apart if I talk about it
-I am afraid my abuser will come back and hurt me more
-I am afraid you'll think I could have prevented it
-I promised never to tell
-I don't know if I can really trust you
or a million other things

You need to find out the hidden feelings, otherwise you might assume the wrong ones. You can ask "Do you mean..." "Are you saying...", "What does it feel like?"

There are common errors to avoid while active listening, these will bog it down:

exaggerating the feeling, making it more intense than it is. Minimizeing the feeling, not acknowldedging it enough. Adding insight into the situation that is not there. Omitting or ignoring things she said to you. Rushing to an insight that the person may be coming to, let her come to it herself. Parroting what she said rather than decoding it. Analyzing what she says, why she feels the way she does.

Characteristics you should have or try to have:

— feeling accepting
— wanting to help
— having and wanting to take enough time
— trusting that she can solve her *own* problems better than you can

— feeling reasonably separate: (you can empathize with her pain, but don't become disabled yourself.)
— avoid evaluating the person or judging or telling her what to do.
— be aware of your own feelings

from Support Zine

LOUISE

Sometimes a new girl would move to our town who would be so punk that I would refer to her as "the one true punk girl". Louise was one of those girls - mohawk, fish-nets, bullet belt, black eyeliner. She helped start up a new show space when the possibility of there ever being a place for shows seemed hopeless, then she was the singer for the punk-as-fuck band Resserectum.

I remember running in to her one day, and she was dressed kind of square, and she said "do you think I look ok for court?" but she wasn't going because she'd been arrested, she was going as an advocate, working for a place called "Women At Risk". A year later my friend Molly was arrested for inciting a riot and assaulting a police officer. She was in the holding cell with bunch of other women, and somehow Louise's name came up, and Mollie was like "Louise! She's my friend!" and a few of the women couldn't say enough about how fucking great Louise is. This is when Louise became one of my heros.

Here is a quick little interview with her:

Q: Do the punks judge you for being involved in social work?

A: At first when I first got out of college and started working with Women At Risk I had some friends who were critical and who said I didn't do enough activism anymore. I see my job as activism. I feel like for 40 hours a week I'm doing activism, so my energy for other projects that I was doing before in the activist community was a little bit lower. There were people who had the stereotypical response "why do you want to work within the court system, why do you want to work in the jail, why do you want to be a part of the system?" because for some folk that goes against their punk values and what you need to do to be a punk. That critique was hard to hear at first, but it seemed mainly to come from people who didn't know much about the work that I did or people who didn't have the same viewpoints I have around activism. I feel like the longer I've been doing it the more used to it people have become, and I've had some people really tell me they think the work is amazing, how can they get involved, so it feels like it's changing. I don't know if that's because of who I choose to be around has changed, or if it's just become more socially acceptable, or if it's just like "ok, this is what Louise does, that's part of her identity". I'm not quite sure, and also the same thing about talking about my work, when I first started working there, I would talk about it at shows, and when I was having a beer at Rosettas, and it definitely got a bad reception.

Q: Why do you think?

A: Part of it that it's really tragic awful stuff, some of the stories I hear from women I work with are kind of unbelievable and it's too hard to hear. I don't think people were being disrespectful, it was just too heavy and too hard for people to want to hear about.And I respect that. But I have had to really seek out and find people who I can talk to.

Q: What exactly is Women At Risk and what do you do there?

A: Women At Risk is a alternative sentencing program for women who are involved in the criminal justice system. We advocate for women that instead of prison sentences they get access to mental health and substance treatment.

I am a case manager and outreach coordinator. As a case manager, I help women with housing, drive them to the food bank, help them access free or low cost child care, help them get access to medical care. We problem solve with them on all the issues that are getting in the way of them staying clean and sober in recovery, or being "successful" with their probation. Alot of the women have substance charges and poverty related charges, and because of their trauma histories and substance abuse, and the fact that they're women and often times poor women, and often poor women of color, there's a lot of barriers to being "successful" with probation and avoiding prison.

As an outreach coordinator, I go to the cell block in the buncombe county jail twice a week and meet with women and come up with plans to try and get them out of jail and avoid prison time and how to get treatment and housing and all those things that they need. A lot of it is coordinating resources, and part of it is they need to talk, so it's also like therapy.

Q: Is it non profit or is it government funded?

A: It's a private non-profit. We get some funding from state legislator, some funding from the Department of Corrections, because it costs somewhere around $70 a day to keep a woman in prison and $7 a day to have a women in our program, in the community with their family.

We've been able to get, surprisingly, Republicans on our side. We get some money from the ABC board, because they have to donate a percentage of their profits to substance treatment centers, and we have an amazing director who gets grants from a whole lot of different places.

The great thing about it is we get to run our program in the way we think it should be done, how we designed it. We aren't managed by any State entity at all, so we are able to create programs that are based on the women's needs and not based on some hierarchy or state organization that tells us how we can do our program.
Also, it's it's basically a feminist organization, and it's really different than working in most other social work. My coworkers know that I'm a punk, and that I do transgender activism. A lots of places aren't like that. It helps to be able to integrate my different worlds at least a little bit.

Q: Has working there changed your feeling about punk?

A: It's changed everything about my life. It's validated and confirmed my belief system about the prison system, it's hard and terrify to see that in fact the prison system is classist, racist, sexist, all those things, so while that's hard, it also validated my belief system.

There is kind of a tension between my involvement in the community and my work. Like I have to be at work at 9am so I can't go to every show that happens during the week, but also working in mental health and substance abuse, it's been hard for me to see how sometimes in the punk community these issues aren't really addressed. ...It's hard to see what can happen with addiction to these women who are like in their 50's, or 40's or even younger, who have been dealing with it forever, and then being around my peers, who I sometimes see as, I want to be careful with how I say this because I don't want to judge and we are all working on our shit in different ways, but sometime I fear that their lives could become unmanageable. So I've learned a lot around that and it's given me the opportunity to look at myself and what I need and how to address my own issues, which has been awesome and I had never even thought about it when I started working.

Also, working in the criminal justice system, I really have to be careful about getting arrested. So I'm not climbing around on rooftops or breaking into abandon buildings, and some of the kind of wild fun things that the punks are into, you know, drinking 40's at the railroad tracks, I can't do that, I mean, that's not a huge loss, but there are times, for example we had a show on Halloween at the new warehouse show space and the cops came and I felt like it was important for me to just get out of there, and definately when the war started, at the rallys I had to be careful about how far I wanted to go with my street level activism. Because if I get arrested, they'll say, "Oh, Women at Risk, they're criminals too."

It was hard at first to give up fun, living on the edge type activities. It was a big adjustment, even dying my hair and cutting my hair changed. I couldn't just show up with a rat tail and purple bangs anymore, which wasn't that big of a deal, but there were times when image stuff was really hard for me - not feeling like I could always represent who I was even ascetically, and what I've known for 10+ years. Learning how to dress to go into court - at first I felt like it was drag. I was like, "I can do this. It's just drag". I still haven't figured it all out. Part of me still wants to show my style, but at the same time, I want to be the best advocate for my clients in court. I've got to play by some rules, and you know, it's not about me.

Overall it's really awesome. My clients give me a kind of strength in a lot of ways, and I've learned so much from them that I can apply to life myself. Being able to meet with people and hear their stories and be available to them has been such a rewarding gift and so life changing, that all that other stuff, no more mohawks and all that, it's such a small price to pay.
(editors note: although she may not still have a mohawk, she is still totally punk as hell, and her band Subramanium has a 7" that just came out)

Q: What do you love about punk? What keeps you in it?

A: It's been a huge part of my life for about half of my life at this point. So, I don't really know another way. This is how I grew up. And I think that for most of us, it is the only way we could have survived, and to grow and blossom and become creative and work through the things that we see and experience in our lives. And while there can be contention between being a punk and doing social work in the criminal justice system, I think that it is this lens that I have developed in my punk community that led me here and has allowed me to make it here and be so moved to do this work.

What keeps me motivated? Part of it is community. These are my people. Despite some folks who have responded more rigidly to my work choices or have not done their peice to support me as a woman in the punk scene (you know who you are) the majority of the punks that I love are interested in my work and my music and my activisim and we are always looking for ways to work together on our new projects, new showspaces, new zines. Also, music is a huge peice. I grew up in a musical family and all of my family memebers are currently playing in several bands. For me, it is a viable outlet. It is sometimes one of the only accessible outlets. When therapy gets too expensive and close friends pull back, I have a totally constructive and acceptable venue to scream at the top of my lungs and everyone there wants to hear it! It is not intrusive or fucked up to scream it out in band practice or at shows, we're all in it together

letters of introduction

I've been thinking about Gertrude Stein and letters of introduction. Like, say it was 1912 and I was a misfit something; someone who wanted something and couldn't find where. And I was about to leave my little home town of confinement and travel up to Paris.

Paris.

May be I had a friend of a friend who had once met Gertrude Stein. She would say, "Oh, you should go to 27. Here, let me write you a letter of introduction." and she would write with ink on fine letter paper, seal it with her wax stamp seal, and I'd carry it safe in my breast pocket as I rode the steam trains across the countries.

Gertrude and Alice had people over every Saturday. Lots of people. Their house was a centering point, a sanctuary. They had art from floor to ceiling, tons of food. They would introduce a topic and the conversation would go from there to all directions.

But how do you get invited in the first place if you are just a no one coming in from nowhere? I have a letter of introduction in my pocket. Shy. Too shy to actually knock, I slip the letter of introduction under the door. I would have scratched the address of the boarding house I was staying at on the back, and in the morning there is an invitation from Alice and Gertrude waiting for me at the front desk.

I've been thinking of letters of introduction. I've been thinking about looking for the punks or freaks in new towns I was passing through, and

"here, here's my zine."

and they'd page through it. "There's a basement show tonight, do you want to go?"

I've been thinking about the way we stood around outside shows trying to sell zines to get a couple dollars to get in, and the quiet way we became part of something we couldn't otherwise find a way into. We didn't play music. We were not sure about dancing. But we had this. shy glance up. "do you want to buy my zine?" "oh, here, you can have it for free." That was part of it. It wasn't that we were trying to introduce ourselves exactly, but there was something of that, something about changing the normal dialog of our lives. something about opening up subjects that weren't in the public realm. something about creating a different path for us to go down. We don't have to be professionals and recognized by the system in order to be real. We can create our own standards. we can teach each other and make a world worth living in.

I liked the non-anonymity about it. The bravery of handing out something, secrets or not. music reviews or history. stories or essays.

here, have this.

There was writing and there was a face to it. It was secret code. It said, I think we might have something to talk about. I think we might be able to make friends. I think I might have something you could learn from. I think you might have something I could learn from you.

In a world of alienation and anonymity, where you could go whole days and months and years without any real connection to anyone and no way of figuring out how to find one; where the art of conversation had been lost on triviality and gossip, it was a way of reclaiming these things we felt missing. and laughter. and pushing ourselves to do something interesting so we'd have something to write about, stupid as that reason may be.

Zines were what you did with your friends when everything else was screwed. When the hearts were broken and there wasn't enough money to pay for heat and you all sat crammed into one room with the space heater and took turns venturing into the kitchen to bring back coffee and nourishment; to flip the record over. Delirious from lack of sleep and asphyxiated from propane heat, Melissa would tell a story.

"you should write that down."

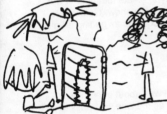

There were doodles turning into drawings, stories turning into secrets, our screwed up lives coming into perspective as not so screwed and actually kind of hysterical.

"We should write a zine. Everyone, two pages by midnight."

"but I don't have any stories."

"but I don't know how to write."   "what could I possibly have to say?"

Zines were how we learned to exist outside ourselves when the world told us to disappear. They were focus. A way to sort through our lives and look for what was most important.

Because paper. Copies. We had to make them small. Cram it all into tiny pages, bike to the Kinkos at 2 am which when our friend started their shift and the manager was in the back room doing the paperwork. We took turns working at photocopy stores. We broke into our shitty office jobs at night and scammed copies. We found ways around every system designed to keep us out. And when that failed, we got jobs at the copy stores again.

20 copies of an issue was kind of a lot. This is the thing I liked; that it wasn't about getting a ton of readership or getting it out everywhere or taking over the world or getting recognition. It was the making of it. the sound of the typewriter, the going over the words, the asking your friend "do you think this sentence makes sense? Do you think I should write about when the moose almost stepped on my head?" the trying to peel off some text laid down with glue stick and the paper ripping instead of pealing and then having to type it all over again. It was the late night bike rides the "yes, we made our self-imposed deadline!" It was bad donuts and bent staples and paper cuts. It was about being out in the world when everyone else was sleeping. And running into someone new at the donut shop up all night.

"What are you working on?"

"A documentary about my week in prison."

"Here do you want mine? I just finished it. It's the story of my grandma's immigration."

It was urgency and the feeling of a mission and a way to create meaning. It was what you did when you felt awkward somewhere. Leave the show. Go down to the railroad tracks and write. People wrote. It was as accepted as getting drunk.

"Do you want a 40?"

"No, I'm going to go to the loading dock and write."

And there were different zines for different reasons. It was about public life, making private public. It was the hand touching hand as the zine was passed between you. It was confronting the fear of rejection over and over until it didn't matter so much anymore.

It was creating a culture. It was about culture. It was about creating real physical connection in the face of nothingness.

It was folded well loved pages falling apart and holding you together, kept safe in your pocket as you rode the train under the bay from Oakland to San Francisco, and knowing that there was someone else out there, someone you met in passing for a second who had given you this gift who had secrets like your own. and that you weren't alone. you could live safe. you could tell the truth too, despite the blank suffocating stares.

We can make ethical decisions about our technologies, and what works and what is falling through the cracks. we remember the feeling of paper and touch, and think about how connection and community is foraged in a million different ways. and sometimes the wires make the most sense, and sometimes we need this: face and voice, realness and a way in; to confront fear and learn support. humility, honesty. a shy glance. "here, have this."

love

I wonder about that thing J. Winterson writes: about contentmen[t]
being a lot like resignation. The positive side of resignation,
she calls it. And why shouldn't I have been content for awhile?
Why shouldn't I have been resigned.

There's the kind of love that quiets. That holds you
softly, calming you to sleep; that wipes away your tears, walks
with you, makes you believe there is such a thing as
understanding without words. Maybe for some people there is.
I find what I can in what I am given, and then I rebel. and then
I explode. and then I cry. I am not made for contentment.

There is the kind of love you feel in your body, that
makes your heart clench and makes you run, towards it or away.

There is love that is full of words, full of a commitment to
struggle with the language and thought and emotions and the
vulnerability and misunderstandings, and sticking with it and
continuing deeper into the secret parts that we keep hidden.

There is love that makes secrets seem unnecessary any more.
There is love that makes you forget who you are, where you
become the other person instead. There is love that makes you
prove yourself, love that makes you hate yourself. love that
makes you want to cook, love that makes you throw everything
away. Love that teaches, love that strangles, love that gives
you the space you need.

There is love that leaves you wanting, and is it their fault or
yours? Are we just fucked up inside? Do we put up with things
we shouldn't? Are we hiding our true selves? Are we living in
a world of make believe, hoping they'll love the make believe
in a way they would never love our damaged selves?

There is love that makes you wish we were old already, sitting
in our rocking chairs, drinking iced tea. There is love that
feels familiar, makes you breathe deeper and with relief. There
is love that makes your breath quicken, like your head is on
fire, like you can fly, makes you race up stairs, makes you
run, towards it or away, towards it or away, with fear chasing
behind you or leading the way.

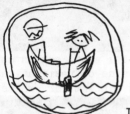

I go canoeing with Julian. I sit in back because I know how to steer, although it hardly matters. He sits in front, facing me, and I paddle around the shoreline, looking for turtles, pretending to look for alligators, mostly just looking.

It's a tiny lake. "This would not be called a lake where I come from," I say, "Where I'm from, these are called ponds."

I tell him the story of when I lived with my mom and stepdad and four siblings. I was in eighth grade, and I would wake up before the sun had risen, and the house was quiet and no one could see me, and I'd make hot chocolate in our blue and white kitchen. I'd take my thermos and skates down to the pond, and turn circles on the ice.

He tells me about waking up early, sitting on his front stoop, listening to the birds. "I loved nature so much," he says, "when I wasn't burning down the forest."

I wrote to my stepdad. I said, "I just need you to say this: that you knew what was happening to us. That you're sorry you couldn't protect us". He wrote back, but couldn't say those simple things.

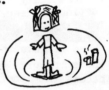

I remember giving up on him, years ago, when giving up was said with anger; felt like fear and hate and love and need, like panic and striking out revenge. This time it is real. This time it just feels like ache.

I am at the ocean again. It has been four years, and finally I can be here and not feel overwhelmed with the memory of my mom, the last time I saw her before the end; her little feet walking gingerly on broken shells.

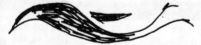

I have dreams about her. One, I am standing on the porch of her house. It is night time and there is the giant black bird with the long legs and long neck I have seen before in my dreams, hovering above me in the darkness. I think to myself, "There's that bird again. What is it? Some kind of heron?"

Mom sticks her head out the window, and she says in that voice, that - why are you such a silly child - voice, full of love and chiding: "That's no heron, it's a snowy owl!"

In another dream, I am standing in a lake, surrounded by forest. There is the bird again, diving towards me, and right before it crashes into the lake to catch a fish, I think "Great blue heron!" and how spectacular that I could be still enough that it could catch a fish right next to me. But it doesn't come up with a fish in it's mouth. It doesn't come up at all.

And then I feel it, dead at my feet. I pick it up, carry it out of the water. Why has it done this thing? It is not quite dead, and I know I should end its suffering, but I can't close my hands around its neck. It is too beautiful, too horrifying, twitching in my arms. And maybe it is right to let it die on its own. And then I know, it has done this thing for me. I can build a fire on the shore. I can pluck it and cook it and eat it, and stay in this place of calm beauty and solitude a little bit longer.

Julian takes me to the ocean. The first day, there is a beach with kids of all sizes in the waves, with brightly colored bathing suits and floating things to float on. There is the wind in the beach grasses and the rainbow umbrellas to keep sun away from skin. There is the smell of oil, the smell of wet dogs when they run up and sit on our blanket, and we pet them and I say "You are so good, look at you, you fuzzy bad thing!" We fall asleep, and the tide rises to us. We wake up with waves at our feet. Julian points, he says, "look over there". And I look. There is the biggest kite in the world, the biggest kite I've ever seen. I am not sure how it doesn't just carry the person away.

At night, curled up together, in a treehouse made of bamboo and screens, I tell him the story about the pelicans. There was an oil spill somewhere, I can't remember which one. The clean up people set up a building where they cleaned the oil off the birds. The pelicans didn't have it as bad as some. They had oil on them, they weren't on the edge of death but they couldn't fly.

For three days, they watched the people bring birds drenched in oil into the building, they watched the birds come out clean. After three days of watching, the pelicans got together, they marched right in through the door, into the building, squawking out their pelican language, "alright already, our turn!"

When we were canoeing, after I said that thing "In Minnesota we would call this a pond", and he said, laughingly,

153

"In Jersey, this would definitely be a lake"; I said, "Do you think that guy Crow is really an Indian or just some white new-ager?" He said "I assumed he was Native American". He said it sadly, as if the thought had never crossed his mind, and all of a sudden, I felt like an asshole. Like a jaded, cynic, hater of people, bitter to the world, empty of hope; everything I'm not supposed to be, because aren't I full of love for this world? I start to explain myself, and then stop. Not because the explanation isn't worth something, but because I want to be here, in this place, with this love. and history, we can talk about later. I worry for a second about age. I worry about wanting to see things through his eyes. I worry about a lot of things. I paddle us over to the raft. I climb out of the canoe. I dive into the cold water.

Julian is 9 years younger than me, and at this point in history, nine years is like a whole different generation, maybe. I remember sitting by a creek, 16 years old, in the Rocky Mountains, at a family reunion, reading a Lynn Andrews book. She is a white woman from Los Angeles who writes about how she was lost in herself and stumbling around, and somehow she stumbled across a Native American medicine woman who took her in and trained her in the ancient ways of shamanism.

Now, when I look at the book, I am ashamed that I could have been tricked by it. It is such obvious bullshit. Sick that this white woman could become a best selling author, making money off of exploiting and debasing the spiritual traditions of a people we have already stolen nearly everything from. At the time I didn't understand about cultural appropria-tion, and how it would be an aspect of genocide. How people could take Native American traditions, and twist them up and redefine them for their own uses, and when enough people do this, especially people with power, like access to media, or people who are teachers, or own little shops, or whatever the hell people do to make an idea and image part of the national conciousness. When white people take part of a culture, and twist it and define it as thier own, the people whos culture it is, suffer.

But when I was 16, I didn't think about the real actual lives of Native Americans. I saw them in the same tragic, silent heroic, physical, mysterious and romanticized way many americans do. And I felt tragic and romantic. I wanted to be mysterious and heroic. I wanted to live within a completely different value system. I saw the way the desire for money and the American Dream of nuclear family suburbia, destroyed the beautiful man who was my father and turned him in to the

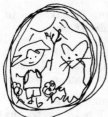

monster that destroyed my mom. I wanted magic.
I wanted quiet. I wanted animals to talk to me.
I wanted ceremony and a community of humans and
nature. I studied insects. I tried to walk toe
heal. Give me something, anything, just not
this emptiness, these worthless goals   these
imitation designer clothes.

Julian was right. When we saw Crow again, we talked to him,
and he told us he had just finished a seven year walk. It had
started in Canada as part of a massive protest march called 500
Years of Resistance. People from all different indigenous nations
walked together from Canada to Mexico City, and from there, Crow
kept walking; through the rest of Mexico, Central and South America, Hawaii and Cuba, and now he was here, in Georgia, at this
tree house youth hostel, resting.

There are people who make me want to stand near them, and
I'm not always sure exactly why. Maybe sometimes it is a strength
in them I want to be sheltered by, or a fear in them I want to
comfort, or an easiness I want to catch, or a mystery I want to
unfold into me, or a craziness that makes me feel at home in this
world where I have none. A craziness that is familiar, like my
mothers.

I wanted to hold Crow's hand. I wanted to stand
near him. but I have learned not to cross the threshold
of bedroom doors, and when he said "Would you like to
see my room?" I stood outside, peering in. There is a
Marine flag on the wall and little carvings on the
windowsill.

Julian walks in past me and picks out a tiny owl figurine
and holds it up and says "Look Cindy, your owl."

It is true that after the dream I had with my mother, the
heron, and the snowy owl, a little china animal owl showed up on
my planting table, outside, where there was nothing before.

I live alone, an hour from anyone I know, on a dead end
road, in the middle of nowhere. Small tobacco farms, some plots
of vegetables, enough for eating and canning. Where the old
people look up at the house I rent and say to me "Old Earl Ramseys
house. He was one of the last old timers." One man sighed and
said "I guess I'm an old timer now."

The ghost left the owl. Who else could have? He must have
read over my shoulder when I was writing about my dream. He also
left me a bowl to eat out of. It's blue and white and says "Hotel
Peabody Memphis Tenn" on the bottom, and he left me a milkweed pod
which has since disapeared.

Me and the ghost, we get along fine. I talk to him some days; him and the people inside of me.

I remember Berkeley when I was 25, and thick in the middle of discovering all the ways possible to live and think and love and talk and struggle and be.

I wanted it all, and took people in like they were life lines, tossed them out when they started to drown me. I held on to what was most unstable to force some kind of inner stability upon myself. I was trying to learn what I wanted, finally, after a lifetime of self sacrifice.

You know what I mean? Self sacrifice? Like being touched, unwanted touch, when you thought you were safe in your own room, sleeping. And you don't tell mom cause it just might kill her to have to deal with one more bad thing. Sacrifice, like fucking whoever possible to feel alive and worthy, to forget, to feel worthless, a hundred reasons for it, and running from anyone who actually has the ability to care.

In Berkeley, I was learning and unlearning, and the more I unraveled, the louder the voices got in my head. I denied it. I joked about it. I blamed it on sleep deprevation. I thought I was better than other people, because how could you not be crazy in this world? I did not listen to the voices, (I mean, I tried my hardest to ignore them) until one night.

It was Derin's birthday party. I guess party would be the wrong word for it, because he didn't want anyone to come. He had pushed away most of his friends and given up on his past. Him and some of the other WDH boys had moved deep into Oakland where they wouldn't have to see what was being done to their city or what was being done to the thing they had loved most, punk.

I baked a cake, as usual, and brought Kyle and Jude with me. We met Derin and WDH at the fountain where the black male prostitutes hung out. "They're the only people I talk to any more," Derin had said to me.

Everyone was drunk by the time we got there. whiskey drunk, funny, but starting to turn. Ward was pontificating about something basic, Derin was dancing one minute, head in hands the next. Chad kept taking his crutches and going up to Giant Burger to try and pick up the girl who worked there. I went with him one time and met her. He didn't stand a chance. and there was something kind of offensive and disturbing about it, not cute and funny.

These were the boys I hung on to. If I had
dropped off the face of the earth, they wouldn't
have noticed, but I loved them.

When we got back from Giant Burger, Derin was
laying in the fountain with his brand new leather
pants on. He'd had to pee and couldn't get the buttons
undone.

Kyle had disapeared, and Jude,
with his soft voice, white jacket, bleached white pompadour hair,
Kyle's shadow and polar opposite, leaned against me and said
"He wandered off. Will you help me find him?"

I didn't drink in those days, except every once and awhile
with Ulla, because I knew together we'd make it home safely.

Jude held on to my arm, stumbling, bleary eyed, and we went off
into the darkness to look for Kyle. We didn't find him, but did
come across a really beautiful gazebo and sat there, and Jude
started shaking. He told me he was a rapist. He told me a story
about being a little kid, and how the man up the street would
babysit all the kids for free. He'd get them all in a room and
would make them watch porn, and then make them do things to eachother. He threatened to kill them if they didn't and kill them if
they told.

I was saying "Jude, that is not your fault." I was holding
his hands, trying to look into his face, trying to bring him back,
trying to convince him, "Jude, you were a little kid. It was you
being abused, it was not your fault, it was not you, it was the
man raping all of you."

Jude was crying and I was repeating myself over and over,
when I heard footsteps on the stairs. It was one of the prostitutes. He asked if he could sit down with us. Jude told him the
story, and the stranger cried too, took one of Judes hands and
one of mine, and said "honey, don't ever let anyone blame you for
what some   man made you do when you were a child. a child."
And then he told his story too, of the way his cousin looked at
him, the creepy things he said to him, the feeling of dirtiness
surrounding him when he was growing up.

That night, walking home alone, through strange neighborhoods
without even my dog to protect me, without even my dog to talk
to, the voices came, and they would not shut up. I invited them

in even. I was scared and pretending I wasn't. My friend Marc
had told me once that people won't fuck with you if you just act
really crazy. Not the best advice, but I took it at the time,
even though there was not a single person on the street to see or
threaten me. I let the crazy out. I let the voices in.

One voice was crying, one was screaming and swearing, one was mumbling under its breath. The screaming one made my body twitch, my arms flail. The crying one wrapped my arms around myself. The mumbling one made small hand gestures up by my face. Their talking went kind of like this:

"Oh, little miss save the world. little miss shit. you are so fucking stupid. no one cares about you. just die. nothing you do is helping anyone, get it over with. everything you touch you kill, everyone you touch, you hurt."

"Oh, god, it hurts, i can't take it anymore. help. it's too much. it hurts"

"shut up shut up shut up"

"you are shit"

"I just want to be good"

"shut up shut up shut up"

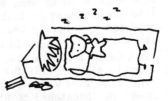

Well, you get the picture, right?
They got louder. They argued. They
saw everything opposite of eachother.
They wanted to pull me apart. They
wanted to kill me. I walked fast
then slow, fast then slow. I thought
       'this is it. I'm done for now. The crazy is out
and there's no return'. I was terrified. I wore myself out.
By the time I got home, the sun was starting to rise. I
squeezed through the crack in the garage door and fell into
my bed, held my teddy bear tight, slept.

Julian takes me to the ocean. The second day, we
find a beach that is empty. a beach that is all
ours. At high tide, the water comes right up to
the forest, washing the dirt out from under the
trees, pulling them down, slowly, burying them
in sand. The beach is a maze of salt-water-smooth root systems,
jutting up. Some eight feet tall, some buried so deep only
inches show, and who knows for how long.

We walk holding hands, like my mom and stepdad used to,
when they could walk for miles together, at peace in their
own world; safe and in love and nothing else could touch them,
until the bad things started heppening again. and then their
only protection from it was liquor and denial.

I understand my mom a little better, now that I am the
age she was when I started to be abused by her true love's son.
I think about her lifetime of terror, and how she kept the
life inside of her so pure and shining somehow, even when the
whole world was trying to smother it, including the people she
loved.

And then finally she broke free, and she found someone who
who loved her back with a ferocity and tenderness; a love so
deep I have never seen anything to compare. The life was able
to shine out of her with its full laughter and brilliance. And
so when the troubles came again, it was like a landslide, past
and present. Self sacrifice or self preservation. I understand,
kind of, the impossible choices she felt she had to make.

Remember the dream about the heron,
diving through the water and ending up
at my feet? It's not about my mom and
her sacrifices, it's about that voice
in my head, the mean one. Shannon
explains it sort of like this: like,
when you're young and you're hurt,
especially sexual abuse hurt, especially
if it's someone who's supposed to protect
you, the mind and body can develop this intense sort of defence.
a type of splitting that allows you to hold two different
realities at once. and something is born inside of you that
will do anything to keep the soul from breaking. But as you
grow, it does too, and it can become confused and twisted up.
and it will even go as far as to kill you, just to protect you.

She calls the thing it's protecting soul and innocence. I call
it the life inside.

I know what she means. For years I loved with heartbreaking
intensity. desperation. I opened up fast as possible. quick,
quick, see me before it is too late.

I could feel love and hate and ambivalence simultaneously.
I would always feel at least two things at once. Feel pleasure
and at the same time nothing at all. Pain and also a hope.
Mostly I felt like I was a bad person, but part of me thought
I was an angel. I could feel like I had switched off my feelings,
and also be totally devistated inside.
I thought all of this made me a monster, or crazy. I
figured one of the feelings must be the true one, and the other
one was trying to trick me.   it made it impossible to
trust myself or anything. Simple decisions could be tramatic.
I needed other people to define me.

Now I don't feel crazy any more, and that mean voice is dieing
slowly in my arms. I talk to it. I listen. I say, "I hear
what you're saying, but please, not so loud". And here, at the
ocean, the life inside of me shines. I say "Julian, Julian,
catch me!" and I gallop like a horse in the breaking waves.
"catch me! Catch me!" I spin in circles, arms out, head back,
spinning and dizzy and laughing. "Catch me!" I climb the root
systems, dive off straight into his arms, and we fall together,
in to the sand, sun on our bodies, hand in hand.

ladies lunch

For the past few weeks I've been living in the
desert. It's the longest in record the state has
been without rain. I hear coyotes ourside my
house at night. They come and step into my Grand-
parenb's pool. If we don't lock the garbage up
tight, the javalinas come. I am scared of pigs, no
matter what their size is.

My sister described them as small wild pigs,
when she lived in Bisbee and was going to herb
school, and she'd walk through the pitch black
desert night to the RV she reluctantly, temporarily
called home. She'd bump her way through whole herds
of javalinas, invisible in the moonless night.

I'm sure Caty will say that's not what happened,
but that's how my brain remembers what she said.
My Grandma says javalinas have razor sharp teeth,
but she still likes to feed them if we have meat
turning bad or leftover bones. I remind her that
Sandy says no feeding the wildlife. Still I do kind
of love it when she puts food out. She hopes for
the pigs, I hope for a coyote, but it's usually a
hawk that comes first.

On Wednesdays, me and Grandma go to Ladies Lunch.
At ten to noon she's ready, curlers out of her hair,
and we drive her big Buick down to Harold's Saloon.
If a handicap space is open, she takes it, but
every time she says "I hate to take the handicap
spot. I'm not _that_ decrepit." I like it when she says
this because my mom liked to say the word decrepit
with the exact same tone and inflection.

My Grandma can walk pretty well, but likes to have
something to stedy her. She sets her fingers on the
other cars as she passes by. She holds my wrist. She
grabs the railing. She was born in 1915.

I am not sure if my Grandma is the oldest lady at
Ladies Lunch, but she's up there, along with her
best friend Esther, who she met in New York City
when they both lived in a rooming house that was

for women who worked in the arts. My Grandma wanted to be an actor, but she had stage fright, so she did stuff behind the scenes. Esther wrote for Vogue, that's what grandma says, but when I asked Esther she said "All I ever wrote were descriptions of the patterns. I was a secretary, an executive secretary."

Esther sits at the head of the table at Ladies Lunch. She's in a wheelchair, so that's where she fits best, but she looks good presiding. She shines out radiance. She has such a loving smile. Last week she said "From now on if anyone can't remember someone's name, just call them Sally!"

They have mostly all known eachother for at least 30 years, but you know how memory can get.

I am in love with Ladies Lunch. I don't think I have ever felt so genuinely embraced, so open arms accepted.

My Grandma and I never used to get along. It use to be that every sentance she said to me ended in an insult, and I was never one to let things go. I called her my evil grandma. but after my mom died, she changed, and so did I.and now I am here, where I never would have expected to be, changing my grandpa's catheder bag, helping my grandma with her stockings, finding out what foods they like, talking to their doctors, cooking, cleaning, finding caregivers who will care for them right.

How this society deals with old people. How we push it all away. and what we lose by not being around this process, this time.

At Ladies Lunch they talk and laugh, they have nothing left to prove. They have seen so much and are interested in everything, they have been through the subject of death together a million times.

On Saturday mornings the younger ladies, the ones who are in their 70's and early 80's, go for a hike in one of the nearby mountains, a different mountain every time. They pass by giant saguaros, hedgehog cactus, prickly pear, coyote dens, and the little dug out places where the baby javelina lay.

m is for

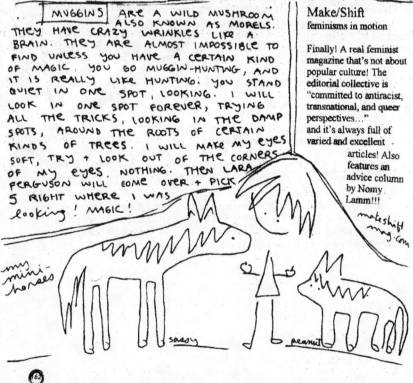

she also started a mine Bean in NY.

Kate Millett

When I read her books. I fall in love with the writer, not just the words. You get such a sense of her as a human, just from the way her sentences go from one subject to another and then back with always such insight and examination. She was one of the founders of the feminist movement in the 60's, and is still writing great books.

Her book <u>The Loony Bin Trip</u> is one of my favorites. I read it a long time ago, so I might have some facts wrong, but I remember it being about crazy. Struggling against her family, who finally succeed in having her committed. going on Lithium. Going to Ireland to interview political prisoners and getting locked up in the mental ward there. I think for a bunch of years. Eventually she started a women's artist colony in upstate NY and went off Lithium, and it's about that too.

MUGGINS ARE A WILD MUSHROOM ALSO KNOWN AS MORELS. THEY HAVE CRAZY WRINKLES LIKE A BRAIN. THEY ARE ALMOST IMPOSSIBLE TO FIND UNLESS YOU HAVE A CERTAIN KIND OF MAGIC. YOU GO MUGGIN-HUNTING, AND IT IS REALLY LIKE HUNTING. YOU STAND QUIET IN ONE SPOT, LOOKING. I WILL LOOK IN ONE SPOT FOREVER, TRYING ALL THE TRICKS, LOOKING IN THE DAMP SPOTS, AROUND THE ROOTS OF CERTAIN KINDS OF TREES. I WILL MAKE MY EYES SOFT, TRY + LOOK OUT OF THE CORNERS OF MY EYES. NOTHING. THEN LARA FERGUSON WILL COME OVER + PICK 5 RIGHT WHERE I WAS looking! MAGIC!

my mini-horses

sassy

peanut

Make/Shift
feminisms in motion

Finally! A real feminist magazine that's not about popular culture! The editorial collective is "committed to antiracist, transnational, and queer perspectives..." and it's always full of varied and excellent articles! Also features an advice column by Nomy Lamm!!!

mateshift mag.com

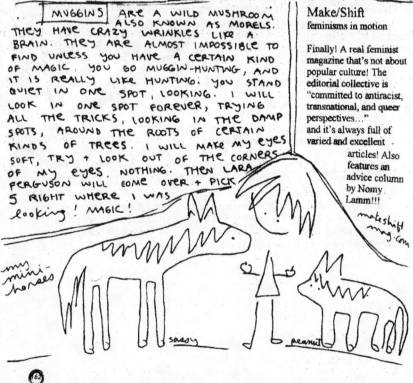

music

Naomi: How old were you when you first started to play music? What instrument did you play? Can you remember what your motivations were?

Cindy: I started trying to play drums when I was 16, I think because it seemed powerful and kind of sexual and I wanted to feel power in my body. I didn't get very far playing drums. Then I started trying to sing when I was 22. I wanted to be able to use my voice. It was very hard for me to learn to raise my voice. I tried and failed and gave up. It brought up all these body memories of not being able to defend myself, not being able to voice my needs. I'm not sure exactly why it was so hard, but it was. I would feel confident and certain, and then I would get behind the mic to scream, and all that would come out was a squeak. It was humiliating. When I was 25 I tried again, and finally, with some encouragement, could do it. Now I scream my guts out and it's very satisfying. I started playing bass when I was 28, because we were starting a house band and needed a bassist.

Naomi: How old were you when you first started a band? What did you play in the band? Can you remember what your motivations were?

Cindy: I was in a couple fake bands that didn't play out or anything when I was in my early 20's. I wasn't in a real band until I was 25. I wanted to do it because I felt like music could be a really powerful way to bring people together, to bring our bodies together, to release and celebrate. There is a real lack of powerful women role-models in our society, and of women playing music, and I wanted to help show girls they can do it too, I wanted to prove to myself I could do it. Touring sounded nice, my best friend needed someone to be in bands with. Also, I was really fucking angry about a lot of things, and needed to be screaming.

Naomi: What is the best thing(s) about being in a band?

Cindy: Being in bands is pretty frustrating to me, and I always can't wait for my bands to be over, and then I miss it and start another one as soon as I can. I like the communication that happens between us, the non-verbal signals and the way we have to really pay attention to each other. And also the feeling of completion, of learning a new song and really getting it down tight. I like have a reason to travel other than just for the sake of traveling, and I like having something to give back to communities.

Naomi: Have you gotten reactions (positive, negative, neutral) from people about your band specifically related to you being a lady?

Cindy: Mostly I have gotten good reactions, people being glad to see a woman rocking it so fucking hard, but also looking like she's having fun. I know a few women who said it helped them start bands, a few people who said certain songs helped them think differently about issues like abortion, and also about consent, and a number of ladies who said it just helped them in general.

Naomi: How does it feel for you playing in a band within a scene that (bandwise) does not represent ladies equally?

Cindy: I don't think there's anywhere in our culture, except for specifically feminist spaces, that represent ladies equally. There may be places where the numbers are equal, but equal numbers doesn't make equal representation. It is sad to me about the punk scene that it doesn't just get more and more ladies representing. I feel like in the mid 90's there were more women playing then there are now (or maybe it's just that there's a lot more boys now), since I love punk I wish it wasn't like that. I wish that people would take sexism more seriously, but if you look at how misogynist a lot of the 80's punk was, it is improving, and I think a lot of punks are more open to change and to looking at sexism and working to change it than in a lot of other scenes.

Naomi: What is the importance, for you, to have ladies in punk (on stage, in the crowd, behind the scenes, etc)?

Cindy: Punk can be really powerful and liberating. A lot of women are taught to repress their anger, to turn anger into self-hate and self-blame, and I think punk can help us turn that around. I think ladies have a lot of really powerful things to say about their experiences in the world that make great songs, and can change people's lives. For me, having other punk ladies to dance with made it so I could dance and not feel objectified, it helped give me safety to dance really hard and not feel like I always had to be on the defensive.

Naomi: Do you think others (the scene, guys, other bands) have expectations of you because of your gender?

Cindy: I've been places where guys think that if you're a punk girl then you obviously want to fuck whoever wants to fuck you, which sucks, but is also just kind of pathetic. And I've definitely felt like the band mom before, like I had to figure out about practice and places to stay for tour and mediate between band members when they weren't getting along, etc. I think it was partially gender roles, partially motivation and vision difference, and sometimes age differences.

Naomi: Do you have expectations (in punk, in the scene) of yourself or of your band because of your gender?

Cindy: I feel like I have a responsibility to the scene and to other ladies to stay involved, even when I feel sick of it. I know a lot of ladies who felt like they had to be extra good at the instruments before playing, to prove something, but honestly, I suck at the bass. I've been playing it for years, and I play it really hard, but I only play the top two strings and I only use two fingers, and to me, that is fucking punk.

Naomi: Do you have any opinions regarding this punk scene and some punks being a lot like regular, dominant culture?

Cindy: Definitely. There are whole sections of punk that are more jock than jocks. It's like they think being anti-PC is radical or rebellious, when actually the whole label PC was invented by Rush Limbaugh to discredit the very real and important work feminists were doing to try and create a world that was less hostile towards women, and that took language and real, lived experience into account. I think it is totally valid when ladies drop out of punk because they are tired of dealing with assholes like that. But I also think that there is a huge section of the punk scene that is committed to change, and to creating community, and to being real. I like the realness, the non-dogmatic realness of punk.

Naomi: Do you have any suggestions for guys being allies to ladies in the punk scene?

Cindy: I think it would help if ladies got more credit for all the work they do. And I think it's important for ladies to be allies to each other. I see a lot of girl hatred among girls still. And I think there's a lot to do around the ways we communicate. One of the many things is I think guys need to learn to listen in ways they might not be used to listening in. Like, listen to what ladies have to say about their experience, and acknowledge it without turning it back to be about you. Also, there is a lot of work to do around sex and consent. Like, just because a woman is punk-as-fuck, doesn't mean she can say no. I know I didn't used to be able to. We need to acknowledge the very real abuse histories that most of us (guys and ladies) come from. I'd like to see guys in punk getting together and talking and studying about abuse, sexism, and how these things affect their lives, and how they can heal and change. I think that would be so fucking punk!

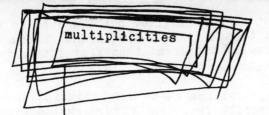

multiplicities

Is it normal to have voices in your head? it is
right. normal. don't you hear them? the one that
says you are sucky the one that says stupid you
the one that says die scum the one that says kill
the one that says hold me cut me love me don't
love me hold me fuck me don't touch me eat don't
leave the house put that dress on don't look
like a slut flaunt it find someone you don't need
anyone don't let anyone come near. the one that
says you were never good for anything the one that
says I think you are a perfect angel actually
sent from god.

ok. I do know that it is not normal to think you
are actually sent from god. that is pure crazy.

but I don't usually feel that way. I mean, come
on. that would be stupid.

When I went to therapy for the 5th time, it was
not to talk about this. it was to talk about
something else. but since I was there and the
lady kind of actually ruled, I said, after many
times of thinking about asking. I asked. I said
'tell me I don't have split personalities.'

she said cautiously "many trauma survivors
develop multiplicities."

oh, i cried. what a relief. not crazy. but also,
I wanted to have split. not really. who in their
right minds would want that.

she said, "I don't think you are split to the
soul." and I am 100 percent not lieing when I
say that I was glad to hear that. Multiplicities.
ok. I can be that.

I don't want to pathologize. but I wanted to be
sick enough to make what I feel count. because I
feel like really different than what I think most
people feel.

she is always telling me to stop thinking about
what other people feel. she says normal doesn't
matter. but don't we understand ourselves by co
comparing to the other humans around us. isn't
that what makes up something essential about our
species?

but I know what she means. fuck it. when did normal
ever matter. it is. it just is. the brain. the heart

The multiples don't particularly want to be
written about. This is giving me a headache, and I
don't think it is just because this electric. this
electricity. this typewriter is electric and loud.
they don't like it.
like the way they hide their names.

When I tell people they have names, that is when
they think I am actually different. special. better.
sicker. more neat and cool and interesting. Because
they may have voices in their heads and they might
have a lot of mixed feelings and they might
disassociate, but they don't have extra names.

well, the truth is, I didn't have names, extra
names either. not until the lady told me to ask.
so they tell me, but it is funny/not funny because
they tell me but then if I try and recall, they
are like side eye ghosts. illusions.

but there is the hairdresser. that one cuts the
hair. no big whoop.

there is the translator. this one changes and what
i mean is it is not always there and it is not always
the same one. The translator takes what all the
others are seeing and doing and tells me so I
don't get confused. Most of the time the
translator does a really quick job, so even

though when I took the "do you have disasociative
identity disorder" stupid bullshit quiz on the
computer, when the question says "people sometimes
look down and can't imagine who they got athat
outfit on," circle 1-10, I circle 5, because
although I don't totally experience that in a
lasting way. it still does happen all the time.
just everything gets translated so quickly that
I don't consciously notice exactly.

the worst thing is, there is not a me. I mean,
when I say "I" I am not talking about a stable I.
I am not talking about someone who is always in
front holding the soul of me and the spirit of
me. There is a shell. that is the shitty part.

or may be that is just something I read and I
want to feel bad. That's a good way to feel bad.
"There is no I" god, give me a break. That's like
some kind of extesential bullshit. however you
spell it. some kafka or one of those fuckers.
boring!!!

so there is that. There are the others. some of
them come in threes. It is hard to explain. Like,
of course, there are the little gang. The young
ones. The cry babies and the sweetness and best
ones. I have to admit, I love the little o es.
trouble though they are. Some of them have their
own place. Like the one main little one that holds
the others has her own little room. It is a small
square empty room with box walls solid walls and
only a spider can come in to visit. This probably
sounds sucky, but it is really nice. She likes it.
She loves it in there. but it is true she is often
sitting down with her head on her knees, crying.

She is the center of the youth gang, and some of
the other youngs run wild, sniffing things and
loving with wild abandon, and other careless
things. but also say stupid things like "no one
will ever love me!" cry cry. come on! give me a
break! except, I do know why they say that
bullshit, because it is basically, more or less,
true.

There's the animus crew. I don't really know what
animus is, but the lady did explain it to me, and
in her way of saying, it seems like the beloved.
the inner beloved. the part we are always looking
for outside.

they come in threes. like the shadow hater who
stands in the shadows and says mean things.
only not so mean any more since we have been
talking. the shadow hater stood in the shadow and
hurt me in my heart before other people would hurt
me to keep me safe because that is all he knew
how to do.but we have been learning new lessons
hopefully. there is the winged feet messenger to
the dead tricky confuser who puts too many thoughts
all at once, but also delivers me from evil delivers
me from dead. i prey to him. i pray to him.

if you watch the movie Spirited Away, he is in
there. Sometimes all giving, sometimes all closed
off. Tell me why? beloved. tell me what have I
done? it is random the way he gives love or
withholds. There is the suffocater. the suffocater
comes down upon me and covers me until I think I
might die. but we are working on loving embrace
instead of suffocation. loving soft floating on
top instead of blobbing blob squish.

I will hold the all of you. I say. I am not
frightened. I know you are trying to help.

does it suck that the beloveds are so these ways?
Yes! It does!

and the problematic boy artist. I love him too.
it's ok. He is sensitive and hates this. quiet
now. quiet. He says he does not want to be seen,
but I know that is not true 100% because for the
first time he really came to the front the last
time there was a switch up.

You were fine there honey. We did good.

I do not always know when they switch positions.
sometimes it is slow. It might just look like
   switching from one mode of being into another.
from quiet writer into rockstar singer. or at
peace with aloneness to so lonely I could die.
this is normal. normal changes in the cycles of
being.   right.

but sometimes it is sudden and hurts like ripped
up insides and like non stop crying and like I
might lose myself like I might get lost. like I
need someone to hold me or at least hold my hand
becaused I might get sucked into black hold
blackhole. lost forever. and I cant stop crying
 and I can't see right and I don't know what
simple objects are and my head hurts hurts hurts
except when I plug in electric guitar and play
except then the electricity stops working right.
honestly, that did happen last time. honest.

and one pushes to the front after a three day
attack. and then the others scramble for position.
 Who's gonna be running mate? whos gonna translate?
who's gonna take the eyes? how about the heart?

   who's gonna protect the youngones? who's gonna
   make the body move. Last time the way my hands
   worked changed. Last time said "real real. you
   have to start talking about this. isolation has
   done you fine. isolation has served you. but it
   is time now."

   I am not sure I want it to be time.

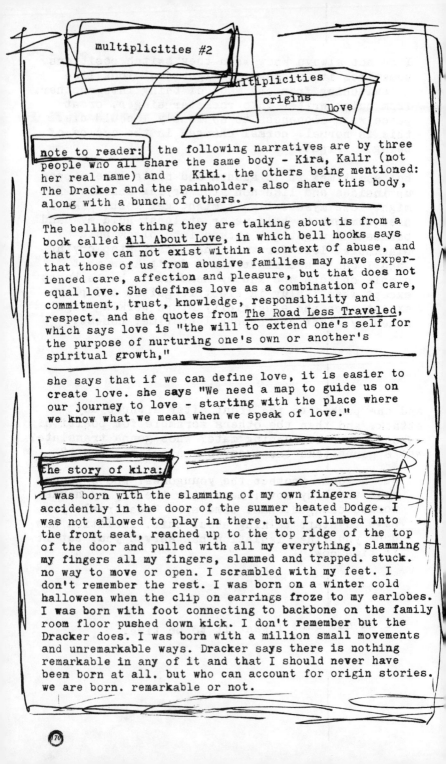

multiplicities #2

multiplicities
origins
llove

note to reader: the following narratives are by three people who all share the same body - Kira, Kalir (not her real name) and Kiki. the others being mentioned: The Dracker and the painholder, also share this body, along with a bunch of others.

The bellhooks thing they are talking about is from a book called All About Love, in which bell hooks says that love can not exist within a context of abuse, and that those of us from abusive families may have experienced care, affection and pleasure, but that does not equal love. She defines love as a combination of care, commitment, trust, knowledge, responsibility and respect. and she quotes from The Road Less Traveled, which says love is "the will to extend one's self for the purpose of nurturing one's own or another's spiritual growth,"

she says that if we can define love, it is easier to create love. she says "We need a map to guide us on our journey to love - starting with the place where we know what we mean when we speak of love."

the story of kira:

I was born with the slamming of my own fingers accidently in the door of the summer heated Dodge. I was not allowed to play in there. but I climbed into the front seat, reached up to the top ridge of the top of the door and pulled with all my everything, slamming my fingers all my fingers, slammed and trapped. stuck. no way to move or open. I scrambled with my feet. I don't remember the rest. I was born on a winter cold halloween when the clip on earrings froze to my earlobes. I was born with foot connecting to backbone on the family room floor pushed down kick. I don't remember but the Dracker does. I was born with a million small movements and unremarkable ways. Dracker says there is nothing remarkable in any of it and that I should never have been born at all. but who can account for origin stories. we are born. remarkable or not.

I have heard stories less something than mine that I
wouldn't trade for twenty heart-beats. and I have
heard these storytellers say "it was nothing much. It
was unremarkable." and I say mark it. pain. mark it.
real. I can see it eating eating trying to be seen.
This thing you say was nothing sounds so hurt to my
ears. and I have heard stories so terrible it makes
it hard to keep living in this world. and I have heard
these storytellers say, "It was nothing much. it was
unremarkable." and these tears. these tears. I can not
stop crying.

kalir:

I was born into a body already changing. I was born
thinking I was already dieing. the disease coming out of
my cunt. I had not yet had wanted touch there. I had what
they call hormonal changes. I had what they call budding
desire. I had crud coming out of my cunt and I thought I
was sick already. I didn't like it when boys touched my
butt. let them and you are a slut. don't and you are a
tease. I wanted to be a slut but there was no grace or
respect in it. I wanted to be touched. I wanted lips on
lips skin on skin and slowly a little more a little more.
I wanted weight on top of me and pushing against and
feeling how this body could make. brought into body.

brought out of other. I wanted touch like drowning. I
wanted grabbing and rolling. but they were such dumbshits.
what did those fuckers think they were doing?

slut or prude. virgin or whore. society told us it was one
or the other and we lined up to eat it.
Kiki suffered. Oh, how I hated her. All she wanted was to
be loved. she wanted to be held and not all this rugburn
and sleeplessness. not this slam against the locker - did
you fuck my boyfriend you bitch.   I mean really girls,
who was fucking who?

Although we did not like eachother, Kiki and I, and Kira
was a pathetic mediator, the three of us were still three,
and we did agree on one thing, even if we didn't realize
it: We needed to get the hell out of Dodge.

I was born in the cracks of a world that was cracked open.
the magazine articles that promised 10 ways to keep your
man happy in bed. but we were so unhappy. we didn't even
have a bed. I was born with women crawling half naked
across every billboard and sticking beer bottles close to
every kind of crack. and the story I was told was "you can
be anything do anything" except not to walk alone and you
must hold your car keys like a weapon and you must not
fight back or fight first, and you must lock your car when
you are inside, and you must look in the backseat before
you get in, and you must not walk in dark parkinglots or
on dark college campuses, and you must not sleep in the
woods at night. And most of all, you must keep up the lie
that the danger is always out there out there and not
right here inside your own house.

I was born in the cracks that wanted love from the kicking
foot. and that got something that for years I defined as
love. and even now I hate bell hooks for making me
redefine it as not love. fuck you bell hooks. for breaking
Kiki's heart. all she ever wanted was to believe she was
loved.

thank you bell hooks. I am ok with heart break. it is
familiar. it is remembering. sometimes it pulls me to the
floor in pain, that is true. the painholder comes right
up and takes me. but I have heard people's stories and I
have seen and had such beauty. May be Kalir was fucking,
but I was tasting and smelling. I was looking I was
seeing eyes wide with fear and hope and grace and
thankfulness and surprise and feeling and amazement and   ^^
something unexplainable. something like peace. I have
felt hearts so close to mine that they bled right into
eachother and it hurt to look and it hurt to leave. I
have been floored by pain. I have been inconsolable.
I have loved with ferocity even if the others weren't. but
if it is true that none of what I got in return was love,
then I am waiting. because that means. well, you can see
what that must mean. but please soon, because I am so
tired of waiting.

M.E. eventually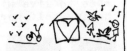

Sometimes I wish I did not know anything about the world. I wish I could just cut myself off from news and people and stores and things. I wish I could play music and laugh and swim and grow things and not have to think about my friends and their unhappiness, what turned us in to the ways we are, what the world is turning people in to.

I wish there was some kind of simple answer and easy contentment, and sometime it seems like ignorence is preferable, but I know for sure it's not.

I remember when my big goal was to change one persons life. Remember that? when that was the extent of a person's power - touch one person's life and you have done your part. and how empty and hopeless that feels because it's obviously not enough when the ice caps are melting and people are starving and war war war and you can't even talk to your own family, and is this the worst the world has ever been? are we gonna die or kill ourselfs tomorrow? and how do all these people walk around? I mean, once I was up in the mountains up a long dirt rutted road, at a little beautiful hot springs, with deer coming down to the trickle of a cold stream that ran into it and they were quietly drinking, an d the sky was blue blue blue, and the girl sitting across from us was complaining about how there was no Walmart near by. I mean, what? I remember what it felt like to first find out we could change the world. When I first started learning how people had changed things. When I first had hope in widespread, fundamental change. and how this hope made me open up, it made me breathe deeper, it made my eyes shine brighter, it made me want to live, it made me love the world, even it's contradictions, it made me sad and loving and empathetic. It took me out of myself. It took away some of my fear.

I know that we have to do a million different kinds
of things to make social change happen. Sometimes
we have to fight in the streets. sometime we have
to study and educate. sometimes we have to humble
ourselves. sometimes we need to hide. sometimes
we have to relearn the things this world has
taken from us - like growing food. like not even
knowing how to hate our bodies. like creating and

having community and community responsibility.
like feeling part of the natural world. like being
able to live without daily money exchange. like
having self-worth.

Sometime we have to fight the laws
that are coming down on us. sometimes
   we have to fight the media
representations of how and who we
should be. sometimes we have to fight
the voices in our heads, our own roads
of destruction, our own roads that
are no longer keeping us sane.
sometimes we have to push ourselves
to learn, even though the learning
seems so pointless. sometimes we need
to set examples just by the way we look
and love. sometimes we need to send out our knowledge,
sometimes we need to hold on to what we know.

I have been thinking a lot lately about Menstrual
Extraction, and how knowledge of this thing kept
me curious and hopeful at a time in my life when
everything seemed so hopeless. and I've been
thinking it is really time for people to start
knowing about it, because I am scared of what will
happen in this country, what is already happening
even if they don't elect whatshisname to the

Supreme Court. I don't know how to do this thing,
but I will tell you what it is, and also, here
is part of an interview I found years ago.

Ok. here is how they describe it in the book
A Women's Book of Choices by Rebecca Chalker and
Carol Downer

"Menstrual Extraction (ME) was developed as a
technique to help women maintain control over
their menstrual cycles, and hence, over their
reproductive lives. On or about the day that a
woman expects her menstrual period, the contents
of the uterus are gently suctioned out, lightening
and greatly shortening the expected period. If
an egg has been fertilized within the preceding
weeks, it will be suctioned out as well. Dealing as
as it does with normal bodily functions, ME is not
a medical treatment - but a home health-care
technique, similar in many ways to self-catheter-
ization, at-home bladder instillations, and other
health-maintenance routines." '

It is a technique that was developed in 1970,
when abortion was illegal. These women wanted to
quit the frustration and humiliation of trying
to persuade the powers that be to legalize
abortion. They decided just to take back the
technology, the tools, the skills, and whatever
else they would need. Here is how it works:

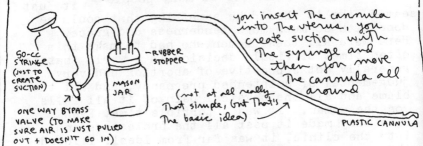

you insert the cannula
into the uterus, you
create suction with
the syringe and
then you move
the cannula all
around

50-CC
SYRINGE
(JUST TO
CREATE
SUCTION)

—RUBBER
STOPPER

MASON
JAR

(not at all really
that simple, but that's
the basic idea)

ONE WAY BYPASS
VALVE (TO MAKE
SURE AIR IS JUST PULLED
OUT + DOESN'T GO IN)

PLASTIC CANNULA

it is a technique that "women without specialized
medical backgrounds can learn to perform... but
their training <u>must</u> involve working with a group
over a period of time, learning directly about
women's reproductive anatomy and function; it
 <u>must</u> include self-education, utilizing medical
texts and journals; it <u>must</u> include independent
research into abortion availability in the
immediate area and beyond; it <u>must</u> include locating
medical personnel to provide consulation and
assistance; it <u>must</u> involve a group of women
who are committed to in-depth discussion of the
struggle for women's reproductive rights and
periodic reassessment of the groups goals; and it
<u>must</u> include, if at all possible, personal observa-
tion of clinical abortion, to become adequately
acquainted with the differences and similarities
between menstrual extraction and clinical
procedures." ⁺

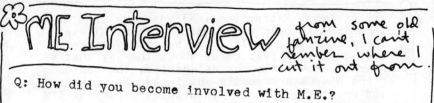

M.E. Interview

from some old fanzine, I can't remember where I cut it out from.

Q: How did you become involved with M.E.?

A: I was involved with a clinic defense group, this was before the "Free Access to Clinic Entrances" law was passed, and at our local clinic there were protesters crouded around the doors of the clinic, screaming and often physically trying to stop women from being able to go in and get their

abortions. It must have been 1991 or 92, before Dr. Gunn was shot and killed outside of his clinic in Pensacola. I was interested in Menstrual Extraction in a theoretical way. I had read "When Birth Control Fails" and thought it would just be really amazing if abortion didn't have to be such a traumatic experience for so many people - it just

seemed like it should be something that could be done with so much more tenderness and grace. Here were all these women who had to make this often times difficult decision in a world that is generally not supportive of abortion and very judgemental of unintended pregnancy, and all the blame and all the physical pain of it all falls on the woman. It was a terrible time. Even once they made it past all the protesters and into the clinic, it was far from ideal. I loved the women and people who worked in our clinic, but they were under a huge amount of streess and their patient load was unreasonable. There were

no other abortion clinics for about 100 miles, and overall, we had very few providers in our state. Our doctor traveled to other clinics every week. She worked for a fraction of what she would have gotten paid if she had stuck with general practitioner. She did all she could to be supportive of clients and to keep costs down, but with all the regulations and insurance needs that clinics have - it was still prohibitivly expensive for many women. Also, we didn't have

a translator, and a lot of Spanish speaking women would come, and we'd have to turn them away until they could find someone to translate for them.

There were death threats to the clinic workers and
the doctor had to move twice because of pretests
outside her house. She had a daughtor in elementary school, and the protesters threatened her d
daughter as well. There were bomb scares at the
clinic. I'm sure it was a very stressful
enviornment to be in day after day, and while
I know the doctor and workers wanted to provide
a calm and healing enviornment, they simply weren't
able to.   Quite honestly, it sort of felt like an
assembly line in there sometimes.

Q: So you saw M.E. as an alternative to this?

A: Partially, yes. Not as an alternative exactly,
Clinics are obviously incredably important and
it is essential that we fight against restrictive
abortion laws, that we support our abortion
providers, volunteer at clinids and work toward
creating the clinics of our dreams.

    I'm not at all confident that abortion will
remain legal, so learning M.E. is important
for that reason, but I also think it is important
to create the world we want to live in, and if
I ever have an un wanted pregnancy again, I want
to be able to terminate it amongst friends, with
my partner there, and to have the kinds of support
I need. I want it to be a time when I can reflect
and let go and feel my feelings and not be
judged.

The scope of what we need to do to create a world
where women have full reproductive freedom is
huge - abortion is only a tiny part of it, and
M.E. is a tiner part of it.
    The group I was in didn't start out as an M.E.
group. We had a wide range of interests.

        At first we were mainly educating ourselves
about the feminist movement and political policies,
and we studied anatomy (which made me very uncomfor-
-table.) and we researched about the different
kinds of birth control. There was a stigma about
women's health groups in the radical community at
the time - jokes about us getting together and

dropping our pants, but the reality was, we didn't even consider doing self exam type stuff until the group had been going for a long time. Some of the women were interested in it, but I for one,   was   not. I had no interest in letting anyone else see my body, and honestly, didn't really see the point. What eventually happened,

is we got really interested in herbal abortion, it really seemed like the solution. Then I got pregant, and we tried herbs, and it didn't work. someone else in our group got pregnant, we tried again, it didn't work. We got very depressed about it all. Now, I know people who have had success with herbs, but I know more people who haven't. Anyway, that is when we seriously started to try and learn a about M.E.

Q: What were your first steps?

A: We started studying anatomy and physiology much more seriously. We started reading everything we could get our hands on about ME. We started learning about whatever we could - sterilization techniques, std's, what complications can occur and what do you do about them. We went over different scenarios.

Q: What kind of scenerios?

A: Emergency scenerios. Like what to do if some-one goes in to shock, what to do if there's a hemorrhage or a perforation. If you're trained properly, M.E. is very safe, but it is important to take it seriously andknow how to deal with emergencies.

We took a CPR class and also practiced counciling skills. We started to get closer as a group, dedicating more time to eachother as friends, outside the group, and addressing more personal things inside the group - boundry issues, body issues, abuse, previous abortions, We did stretches and self-defense warm ups - trying to become more embodied as a group and stronger, and just to be more relaxed and have some fun. Eventually, we started doing speculum exams and a nurse friend of ours taught us pelvic exams. For awhile it seemed like that was as far as we'd ever get. It just seemed like how would we ever learn to actually do M.E. or get the last bits of equiptment we hadn't managed to get. We tried to become a little bit more visable as a health group - teaching classes about birth control and fertility awareness, and eventually we found someone who wanted to teach us.

Q: How did you find them?

A: I think if you are in a group long enough, someone will just come and find you.

Q: Can you talk a little about the pro's and cons of M.E.?

A: Abortions can be done much later than M.E.s. Every group is different, but our group didn't do them past 6 weeks from the last menstrual period. We found that after 6 weeks, there was a higher risk of incompletes, and the procedure just took too long. May be if our group had lasted longer, we would have gained more skills and been able to do them later, but it really is designed for early pregnancy, at least that's my opinion. There are a lot of benefits to having it done at a clinic. It is quicker, you can have sedatives, you can use a wider range of defense mechanism to pull you through it.

Q: What do you mean?

A: With M.E. you really have to be present in your body, before, durring and after the procedure, you have to be aware of how you are feeling during the procedure, and be able to communicate what is going on. It is very emotional for many people to experience pain and vulnerability around people who care about them. For many of us, it is a basic survival skill to cut ourselves off from our emotions.

One of the things I really like about M.E. is the idea that pregnancy is often a time when people are feeling a really wide range of feelings, lots of things that are very deep-rooted and seemingly not directly related to the pregnancy. And if they can be supported by a whole group of caring people, during this time, even if they don't talk with them about all the feeling; and if they experience the pain in an atmosphere of love and support, it can fundamentally change the way they envision possibilities in their lives. Is this making sense?

It's weird, but I guess it is pretty spiritual for me. Of course, for many people, it is not like that. Some people experience pregnancy as just a growth inside them that they need removed,

and I completely respect that. I just want there to be a world where every single experience of pregnancy and pregnancy termination is validated, and where we have the widest range of options open to us in all facets of reproductive health. I want us to all know our bodies and be able to make good decisions for ourselves, and for us to have our decisions respected.

I could talk about all this forever, but I do really have to go. Thank you so much for the interview.

The last thing I want to say is: Start a health group!!!

notes from cindy

→ I want to tell everyone about the National Network of Abortion Funds NNAF.ORG it provides financial assistance to woman who can't afford their abortions. This is a great resource and most of The groups also need volunteers! Get involved!

heres recomended books for & health

A WOMAN'S BOOK OF CHOKES: abortion, me., RU-486, by Chalker + Downer

NEW VIEW OF A WOMANS BODY - federation of feminist health centers

TAKING CHARGE OF YOUR FERTILITY - Toni WESCHLER

♡

n is for

National Day Laborers

a national organization
with lots of autonomous
local groups. I have a
few friends who are
involved with this group
and love it - feel like
they're finally doing
things that are useful
and exciting and good.
super important work,
dealing a lot with anti-
immigration
fighting anti-immigration
and exploitation, developing leadership and
fostering community,
protesting, making
alternative media, making
better lives, caring for
eachother, and just so
much more.

NASTURTIUM
spicy edible red
yellow + orange
flowers. One of my
very favorites. Sometimes
if you plant it around
the edges of the garden
it can keep deer away
because they don't like
the taste. I love the
taste! Good on salads!

Native American Land Recovery/Reclamation Projects

The project I know the most about is
White Earth in Minnesota, but I have
heard there are projects all over the
country, working to recover land that
was stolen, committed to traditional
practices of good land stewardship.
They recover land though land
donations and land purchases.

The White Earth project, and I'm sure other ones as well are also "preserving
and restoring language fluency, community development, and strengthening
our spiritual and cultural heritage"
Another part of the White Earth project is called Native Seeds HARVEST, which works "to
continue, revive, and protect our native seeds, heritage crops, naturally grown
fruits, animals, wild plants, traditions and knowledge of our indigenous and
land-based communities; for the purpose of maintaining and continuing our
culture and resisting the global, industrialized food system that can
corrupt our health, freedom, and culture through inappropriate
food production and genetic engineering."

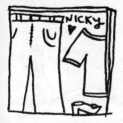

Nicky was telling me about the last time she was in prison, "Back then they used to allow us to wear our own clothes, ten pounds of new clothes a month."

She winces, rests her hands on her middle. I know I'm not suppose to want to touch her belly. Pregnancy doesn't make a woman's body public property, and it doesn't matter anyway what I want; we're not allowed touch here.

"Just watch," she says, "He's kicking so hard, you can probably see his foot."

I want to run her a bath, cook her some greens, find a bed big enough for her whole self, but all I can do is sneak her my milk when the guard isn't looking.

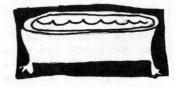

She says, "It was like another life-time ago. When I went in, there weren't hardly any gangs to speak of, but half way through my five years, here come the gangs. And then we weren't allowed to wear red or blue anymore, not even our stonewashed jeans," she laughs, "which is pretty much what we had.

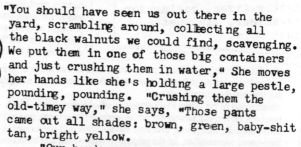

"You should have seen us out there in the yard, scrambling around, collecting all the black walnuts we could find, scavenging. We put them in one of those big containers and just crushing them in water," She moves her hands like she's holding a large pestle, pounding, pounding. "Crushing them the old-timey way," she says, "Those pants came out all shades: brown, green, baby-shit tan, bright yellow.

"Our hands were purple for about a week, but at least we had our clothes. Some of the girls tried to dye their clothes with hair dye."

Nicky's features grow soft when she talks, her eyes distant, and you can see that she doesn't see us at all, she sees the California prison yard, smells the California air, She's pulling clothes up out of a vat of homemade dye, and in her face, there's amusement at these strange colors.

The power of memory's ability to transport her makes me want to join her there somehow.

"I ate a black walnut once that tasted exactly like pink bubble-gum."

"Yes," she says, "yes, I know exactly the taste you mean."

Nicky was arrested this time on a ten-year-old warrant that she'd pretty much forgotten about. She's awaiting transfer to state prison, where she'll spend a year. Maybe her mom will get custody of the baby, but maybe the paperwork won't come through in time.

The jail is quiet. We get yelled at if we talk too loud. It is clean and new and bright and small. For exercise, we are supposed to walk the perimeter of the room. Twenty laps equals a mile. No pausing at the window. We don't go outside.

We have single cells, and are let out three times a day. One hour for breakfest, two hours for lunch, three hours for dinner.

There are nine round tables that sit six people each. The first day I felt like I was in Jr. High. It felt exactly like that; holding my tray of food, looking for a place to sit where I wouldn't be spit at, looking for a sign, a signal, something to save me, someone to tell me where I belonged. But there was nothing, so I sat down with the butchest looking girls as if I had every right to be there.

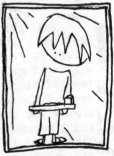

because I am a tough girl, right? I have done tough things. But I didn't even get a chance to brag about any of the things I didn't want to brag about. They moved away from me. One of them even held her

nose. They complained to the warden that I smelled bad, which was true, I did. Scum of the earth, how much can one shower wash off?

So next meal, I hurried to an empty table. People had to sit with me of course, but it wasn't my fault.

I skipped breakfest, just stayed in my cell.
I thought I could try to make the best of it.
I'd do stretches, write letters, read 100
pages of the bible a day. I'd order instant
coffee, and make it, lukewarm, from the sink.
I didn't want to talk to anyone, didn't want
to haff to prove myself.

I stood on my bed, tiptoe, put my fingers
on the edge of the window and jumped to see
out, trying to hold myself up.

X X X X X X X X X X X X X X X

I didn't want to prove myself, but there is something
so debilitating about wholesale rejection. Every day I
imagined a bubble around myself, didn't look at anyone,
didn't talk to anyone, pretended not to care. I know I
have removed myself from mainstream society, but I didn't
want to be removed so completely, and I didn't see why
I was. If I tried to talk to anyone, there was nothing
there, and I had no choice but to shut down my hoping heart,
accept the isolation, hide out in my cell.

The truth of the matter was though, I had
lost the skill of shutting down, and every time
I left my room, there was a corner of my eye that
was looking. And one day it caught a small movement. A
toss of blond hair, a second of eye contact, a gesture
over. I thought I had to be wrong, but I sat down
anyway and she smiled at me. Nicky. She took me in.
and I became part of her regular table. Me and her and
Gloria and Jill. We were the quietest table, playing
endless games of Rummy 500, telling bits of our stories
sometimes. There was something really simple, slow and
fundamental about the way our friendships formed.
Every day, hours of cards and small disclosures.
I showed Jill some Yoga stretches, showed them
the sad comic I was drawing about elephants and
death.

And Nicky told long stories about childhood. Stories that transported her somewhere else.

"Daddy told me bees could only sting you when their butts were up," she said, at lunchtime on my last day in jail. She crooked her finger one way and then another, describing the safe and unsafe position of bees.

"So I'd go out in the clover, and with my toe, my barefoot toe, I'd hunt the bees out and step on them, and one time I saw a bee that was kind of sideways. I thought 'I can get him,' but he turned and he got me. I went screaming to Mom. She said 'What did you do?' I said, 'Stepping on bees!' She said, 'What did you expect? Put some shoes on.'

"I was always outside. My sister, always inside, saying 'Let's play hangman.' She'd be playing on her Merlin or some stupid thing like that, and I'd be out the door and up a tree.

"I used to get out the old red wagon and get the old bathmat and spread that mat on there, drag the wagon over near the window where Mom would be inside washing dishes, and I'd just lay out." She put her arms out, head back, eyes closed, and I could feel the sun on her face, warming her body, warming me. And then the buzzer rang and the guard called my name, and I did not want to leave.

O is for

The first time I ate okra was at
Ivy's birthday party at the landfill, a place I ended up living
for awhile. The landfill was an old
construction garbage dump that
stretched out into the Bay. We could
see the city and the Golden Gate
Bridge. There was a shack that Kerb
and Faith and Ivy and one of the guys
from Radon built. It was an empty,
beautiful place back then.
Ivy got okra, which I didn't even
know what it was. She breaded it
and fried it in a lot of oil, and
of course it was delicious as could
be.
How did a person get to be this brave? Where
they would discover unused, unwanted places
and make them theirs? Sleep in the open. No
locks. I wanted to get there.

OKRA

The thing I found out about okra later, when I planted
it in my garden, is it has the most amazing flowers -
kind of hidden in a way, but big and showy with
purple and yellow insides.   Pick okra before it
gets too big and tough. Plant like 3-5 plants so that
 you'll have enough ripe at once that you'll go
through the trouble of breading and frying, but not
so many that you'll have to eat okra every day.

NNEDi OKORAFOR

amazing auther. Her
book WHO FEARS DEATH
is seriously haunting,
set in the far post-
apocalyptic africa, it
deals with racism +
genocide, racism against
mixed-race people, violence
against women, sexism,
inner power, change.
complex, beautiful + scary,
so good!

ocean always again

I had never been to the redwoods. I still never have, but when me and Jono were in California, we tried to get there. We were staying at Sarah and Jimmy's house, and Jimmy said, "Those trees really do not like humans. If they had a choice in things they would destroy all of us. They don't care if you love them, they hate you. Who could blame them?"

"Go," he said. "Of course you should go, but if you sleep under them, just know that I warned you."

We'd been sleeping in their garage, which was homier than my own home, all full of little knickknacks and piles of things, two chairs, books, an extra guitar, and a huge air mattress that was more comfortable than my futon, except for the small problem of the tiny leak, so that half way through the night, we'd sink in to the middle, and my hip would feel the floor, and I'd reach over and push the button on the battery operated pump, and we'd feel the bed rise up beneath us.

Sometimes we'd hear Jimmy in the other room, mining for gold. That's what Sarah called it. She said that whenever they go camping, he starts panning for gold. (They go camping all the time because they are crazy about edible wild mushrooms.)

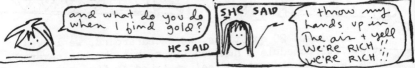

and what do you do when I find gold?

HE SAID

SHE SAID

I throw my hands up in the air + yell WE'RE RICH!! WE'RE RICH!!

So now it was urban gold mining. He was taking apart old computers from back when they used to use gold in the making of them. He was trying to figure out how to seperate the gold from the rest, because the simple scrapping method he was using took forever and he'd scrapped his hands all up, and for the amount of gold he got, and the quality, it turned out he was making about seventy five cents an hour.

That seemed like it was about what I was making too.
We were on vacation, but I was also trying to train
for this sewing job, which I thought would take only
a little while, but it was taking forever, because I
am a bad sewer and couldn't get it right. So every
day I'd sew and sew, and Jono would wander around the
city, and by the time I got off work, It'd be raining.

It was raining when we woke up, the day we
planned to go to the redwoods. What's a little rain?
I said. It'll pass over. It'll be an adventure. We
can be practicing for if we ever get to go to Ireland,
cause isn't it always raining there? Besides, what's
a little rain? Once you're wet, you're wet, who cares?
It was a little bit cold. Not too cold really. Right?
right. We were off. We were gone.

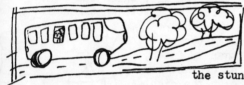

A city bus and then
a fancy bus. We crossed
the bay to the windswept
hills, the rocky coastline,
the stunted sand-and-ocean trees.

I was thinking that we could hide anywhere, we could
do anything, we could pitch our tent, we could become
invisible, we could disapear together and never go
back. But there was the rain, and it was kind of cold
after all, and the Redwoods were out there, inland,
where it had to be warmer, inland, where may be the
rain would stop. We waited and waited for the shuttle-
bus van to come to this stripmall town bus stop, to
pick us up and take us inland.

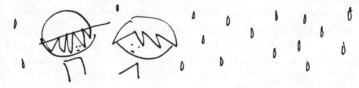

We played 20 questions, we paced around, we looked
at our bus schedule a hundred times, but the bus never
came. We went and got coffee, we tried to find a payphone, we sat close, trying to warm eachothers hands,
we waited and waited and waited, but still, it never
came.

Finally, we found someone who knew. "That's a seasonal bus," she said, "and the season ended yesterday." But we couldn't give up. I thought may be we could just walk there. It was only like 20 miles. We could find somewhere to camp along the way. I like thinking it is reasonable to walk far distances, but Jono is a little more practical, and it was true, we needed to get out of the rain, we needed zipped up tent, enclosed space, warm breath, body heat.

I quit hitchiking when my dog got too old to protect me, and Jono had never been before, but it was two hours before sundown, in a land of rich ex-hippies, so we walked down the streets that were not made for walking, a skinny winding street that where we live would have been a wide one-way, but here was rush hour highway; cars so fast and inches from us and nowhere to pull over, and may be it was all a really bad idea , if we weren't so disfunctional we would have planned better, we would have at least left earlier, we would have found out about the seasonal nature of the bus, we wouldn't have waited so long. And if I wasn't so optimistic and delusional, we would have paid better attention to the weather report. Stupid, stupid stupid. stupid me. stupid me.

But when I'd turn around to stick my thumb out, and there was Jono behind me, trudging   along, stomping in the puddles, looking at the ground, and then up at me, and in to my eyes, and a small smile, and I was so happy. A small kiss please. And a car pulled over.

It was a girl driver with platform boots and spikes, and no pretension, just sweet as could be. When we came to the crossroads, redwoods or ocean, she stuck to the coastline and convinced us just to camp on her little town's beach.

The ocean, we do love the ocean, so she dropped us off, the last of the light fading, the cold rain falling and the ocean, huge and turbulent, the sound of it opening up my heart, saying swim, but the cold wind closing me in.

We raced with the darkness over the first set of dunes, trying to get away from the "no camping" signs, trying to get somewhere where no one would see us. Somewhere solid enough to sink our tent stakes into; not beach, not marshland.

We ended up on a little ridge top, a windy little ridge top that was so perfect at first. Our cold hands struggled with the tent poles, the rainflap. There were missing peices. We used our shoelaces to tie it down. We bundled ourselves into the tent, it was a roomy tent, big enough to sit up in. We layed out our picnic, bread and cheese and hard-boiled eggs. We curled into our sleeping bags with our books and our flashlights, reading and listening to the ocean, listening to the wind. We'd warm up for a minute, but then the rain flap would flap off, and we'd run out and try to fix it, getting soaked all over again.

The missing peices were a problem, and the soft ground that wouldn't hold the stakes properly, and i guess it wasn't the best of thinking to set up so high on a ridge top, on top of the world, majestic, but open to the elements.

The wind did not die dowm, it got stronger, and in the middle of the night, it came in bursts so strong it was flattening our tent down on top of us.

and we discovered the magical reason why some tents are shaped like this

instead of the more comfortable, roomier

shape.

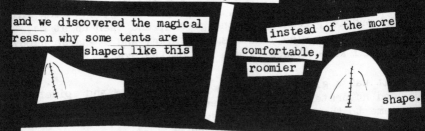

because if the wind is blowing, it goes aerodynamically like this,

but on this style, it goes like this,

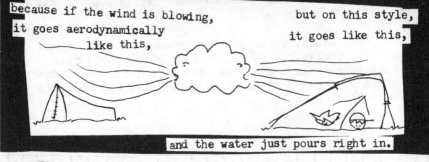

and the water just pours right in.

There was an inch of cold water at our feet, but what could we do? There was nowhere to go. The town was no town at all, just houses, no store, no gas station, no cardboard dumpster, just a beautiful little town with everyone fast asleep, and the rain kept coming and the wind kept blowing and I tried to hold the tent up with my hands and feet while at the same time trying to let my brain sleep, because I was freezing and hopeless and scared and laughing, and trying to believe that it couldn't go on like this forever, trying to pretend it would all be over soon.

The water in the tent just kept rising. We tried to bail it out, using our extra clothes as sponges. We'd soak up the water and squeeze it out, but it was no use. I paniced. I resigned myself. I told Jono we should just ignore it. I curled up small and let my body shiver. I thought warm thoughts, willing warmpth into my limbs, accepting, sleeping.

There are things you shouldn't accept and times when you shouldn't sleep. Like one time, when I lived in Vermont, andI'd just moved in to a new house, part way up a mountain and kind of hard to find, and I was driving home from work, at night, in the freezing rain, with my dog in the backseat, and my car slid into a ditch. I was so tired. It was late. Home was still a ways up the mountain. I was so tired, I thought we could just sleep in the car.

I am from Minnesota andI know better, you just don't do that. When it's freezing out, don't delude yourself into thinking your car will stay warm enough to save you. It won't. It didn't. I woke up and knew I had to move.

The road was ice and the snowbanks were up to my knees, and I walked forever, trying to remember landmarks, slipping and falling. The cold slowed down my brain. I was sure I'd walked too far, so I turned around, then I thought I hadn't gone far enough, so I turned around again. I kept turning, walking a tiny bit, and turning around again. I couldn't trust myself. I was completely disoriented, crying and then numb.

I knew I should just knock on someone's door, but there is something in me that just won't let me ask for help. I'd rather die. It is sad and rediculous. What is my fear? That the door will be slammed in my face? Rejection. That I'll be a burden? That they'll think I'm stupid. I got myself in to whatever mess I'm in, I should be able to get myself out. Some basic, fundamental American individualism bullshit? Some basic fear of strangers? Some feeling inside that I am not worth saving?

I layed down in the road and prayed for hypothermia to take me. At least for it to take me into sleep long enough for the sun to come up and a car to come run me over or save me.

Anna wouldn't let me sleep though. She ran around me barking. She knew there were things you don't accept and times you don't sleep.

Jono knew this too, although he was more articulate about it, listing off our options, bringing me back to life, because I really felt like if I didn't put all my energy into just laying still and focusing on denial, I would start screaming. I know it sounds so weird and overdramatic. It's not like we were actually in some kind of life or death situation, we were just on a little beach in Californa. But I guess if you let yourself, you can die anywhere.

I couldn't stop shivering. It was pitch dark out. We abandon everything we didn't need. I even thought we should just leave the tent there, but it wasn't even ours, so we gathered it together and shoved it into the backpack , and we slid down the bank, finally out of the wind, but still, I couldn't stop shivering, my brain couldn't stop going between panic and numb. I knew what I needed, to get out of these wet clothes and press myself against him. Body heat. We needed real shelter, like hadn't we seen some public bathrooms at the beach access place where we were dropped off? I was sure they'd be locked, but maybe we could break in or something. Or break into someone's car or boat or shed. Maybe there'd be a payphone and we could call someone and give them a million dollars to come get us. Maybe the sun would come up and we could hitchike again, although it seemed like the sun would never come up, and when we reached civilization, the only real option was the bathrooms, which weren't locked, but they were, sad to say, port-a-potties. Huge, handicapped port-a-potties that were magically somehow hardly stinky at all.

It seems really counter-intuitive to lay down on the floor of a portapotty, or to take off your clothes to stay warm, but what could we do? Body heat, four walls and a ceiling.

Sometimes you don't know that all you need is something so little. Something so simple you wouldn't have considered it before. My life felt washed away, my panic easing. Four walls and a ceiling, body heat. Jono held me while I slept, and he waited for the sun to rise, and despite all my doubts, it did rise, and we rung out our clothes as best we could, We walked out to the road, stuck out our thumbs, got a ride.

P is for

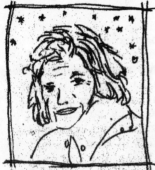

The first time I heard of Grace Paley was at this famous writing center where they had all these 8X10 glossys of all the famous writers who had taught there. All the photos looked so serious, people at desks among stacks of books, looking very serious and smart. Except for one; a woman with wavy white hair, standing in a creek in a sundress, holding up the hem, smiling. She was an Anarchist, an Anti-War activist, feminist, mother.

She was one of the first writers to write about the daily details of women's lives – believing that women's lives matter. She was a New Yorker, and her stories are really New Yorky. She also has a book of speeches called <u>Just As I Thought</u> which is totally inspiring. I met her when I was a young anarchist, full of energy and rage, and Grace was so respectful and sweet to us, talking about the importance of all the different roles people of different ages and temperments had to offer the movement.

Prison Abolition and Prisoner Support

Prison Abolition acknowledges that prisons don't work. It challenges people to envision a world without prisons – where social problems were addressed. I'm always finding out new shitty facts about the prison system – like how tax money is given to towns and cities depending on their population, and prisoners are considered residence of the place they are imprisoned, not the place they are from. And so tax dollars are diverted away from social services in impoverished areas where people are targeted for imprisonment, and diverted into towns that host prisons.

Prison Abolition asks that the legacy of racism be acknowledged – the fact that after slavery was abolished, new democratic institutions to eradicate racism were not created, and so "black people encountered new forms of slavery – from … the convict lease system to segregated and second class education… And this inheritance is not only born by black prisoners, but by poor Latino, Native American, Asians and white prisoners." It asks that we "re-imagine institution, ideas and strategies and create new institutions ideas and strategies that will render prisons obsolete." - Angela Davis, <u>Abolition Democracy</u> p.72-75. also see her book <u>Are Prisons Obsolete,</u> and the book <u>The New Jim Crow</u> (I can't remember the author)

There are lots of great groups working against the prison-industrial-complex. **Critical Resistance** and **All of Us or None** are both really excellent and effective organizations! Check them out!

PUNK GIRL/ SHY GIRL

Someone asked me this question:

what do you think it is to be shy in a scene that asks for punk girls to be strong and bold when some of us are just quiet and self-contained?

THE FIRST REAL PUNKS I HUNG OUT WITH WERE FRIENDS OF MY ROOMMATE MELISSA. and THEY WERE SWEET BUT KIND OF SCARY and I DIDN'T FEEL LIKE THERE WAS A PLACE FOR WEIRD SHY ME IN THEIR WAYS. THEIR LOUD GIRL WAYS.

I DON'T NEED THIS FUCKING ASSHOLE! ALL I NEED IS A FUCKING DILDO!

MELISSA, I FEEL KIND OF WEIRD

BUT THERE WERE OTHER SIDES TO SOME OF THEM and OTHER CIRCLES OF PUNKS WHO MAYBE DIDN'T CALL THEMSELVES PUNKS BUT WHO LISTENED TO PUNK MUSIC and PLAYED IN PUNK BANDS and WROTE ZINES and HUNG OUT and PRIORITIZED FIGURING OUT WAYS TO LIVE FULLY and LIVE TOGETHER and NOT WORK TOO MUCH and FIND THE CRACKS IN THE NUMBING WORLD AND PRY THEM OPEN, TO BE AN EYESORE, A VISIBLE PRESENCE THAT THINGS WERE NOT FUCKING OK IN THIS WORLD, TO BE A DOORWAY INTO RESISTANCE. THERE WAS SOMETHING ABOUT THE WAY THEY TOOK UP PUBLIC SPACE THAT I REALLY LIKED, COMING FROM A WORLD OF PRIVATE PROPERTY + LOCKED DOORS. like the circle A radio interview with from the WIPERS where he says "WE'D JUST SIT AROUND ON THE STEPS OF THE LIBRARY, READING BOOKS, SMOKING CIGERETTES, MAKING THE SCENE."

LIBRARY

I HAD A LOT OF DEMONS I'D BEEN TRAINED TO HIDE AND TO TRY TO IGNORE

but the punks walked hand in hand with theirs usually, sometimes they kicked them.

I WAS SHY + SORT OF SELF POSSESSED, BUT LONELY + WANTED MY ANGER MY HIDEN ANGER OK

AND THERE WAS A PLACE FOR ME. PEOPLE LIKE

WE SET UP TABLES AT SHOWS AND SOLD ZINES OR GAVE THEM AWAY. THERE WAS THIS WAY TO BE PART OF THIS BIGGER THING EVEN THOUGH I DIDN'T SCREAM.

IN ALL THE NOISE MY DEMONS WERE QUIETER

and there were things I could be part of, just on the fringes. no one minded.

AND IN ALL THE FRANTIC ENERGY QUIET

there was the self-containment that I was happy about and the self-containment that was stifling. THEY KNOCKED ON MY WALLS. SOMETIMES I LET THEM DRAG ME OUT

and I could be a confessor a secret teller a holder.

CAN I TELL YOU SOME THING

YES.

WHICH TURNED OUT TO BE BETTER FOR ME THAN I EVER WOULD HAVE KNOWN

♡ THE END

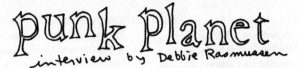

punk Planet

interview by Debbie Rasmussen

You write in *Doris* about growing up surrounded by early politicizing forces but also various kinds of abuse. Can you talk about these early experiences?

My first six years of education were in a school that was very progressive and student-centered. In the '70s, when I was in elementary school, there was funding for alternative education. I wasn't surrounded by issues of materialism, I never learned about gossiping or being cruel, and I learned about movements for social change. But at the same time, my dad was extremely abusive to my mom—physically, emotionally, and sexually. After they divorced, my mom married this guy who was a total alcoholic. She was an alcoholic, too. They were super loving, but total drunks. ¶ In sixth grade, I had to start going to public school. It was a huge, terrible change. I was such an open and loving person and I just did not understand the rules. I started living with my mom and step-dad in eighth grade. There were five kids, and not enough money. My stepbrother was a metal-head, but he started molesting me, and his friends were kind of in on it, too. So joining that group wasn't an option. There were no punks—the people I knew thought punk was dead—but there were about five weirdos, so I hung out with them.

When did you first encounter anarchist or punk politics?

When I was 15, hanging out in downtown Minneapolis, there was some politicizing, but not a ton. I had friends who were in an anti-racist gang and they talked to me a lot about racism. And this anarchist group called Love and Rage was starting. I didn't know that much about them. The first protest I saw was in Uptown—which now is super fancy, but then it was a mix between fancy and scummy—and it was against gentrification. It was 20 punks just marching through Uptown with "Fuck the Rich" signs, and all this media. I was 16. I didn't take part in the protest, I just watched. ¶ When I was 17, I took this women's studies class, and I started retreating from society and dealing with some abuse stuff. During this time there was a lot of US intervention [in Central America], and there were huge protests in Minneapolis, having pretty successful results. I wanted to go, but I was terrified. The second day, the protesters were totally brutalized by the cops. A friend got pepper sprayed directly into her mouth. It was so overwhelming to me, I just cried and felt like everything was totally pointless. I felt like I should be out there, but I also didn't want to be part of all that violence. ¶ Then I went to Vermont—and I still didn't really know what anarchism was or that you could really change anything in the world except through the structures that exist, or changing one person at a time. But I read and talked about anarchism a lot. This is when I started believing in anarchism and thinking that you can change the world and everyone's going to jackhammer up the streets and plant gardens and start making decisions together and create communities. That whole utopian vision was so amazing to me. And I just totally believed and was so excited about things like alternative technology and squatting.

You wrote in one of your zines that realizing that the revolution wasn't going to happen in your lifetime was a turning point for you . . .

At the time, I thought you had to do political organizing pretty much 100 percent of the time, and so I did. It was annoying to always be doing political stuff, but I was so excited about it happening, and there was still so far to go. I also had a bit of a martyr complex. ¶ Partly this realization came because no one else seemed to be working that hard. But also, I asked a friend who was older if she thought the revolution would happen in our lifetime, and she said, "I really hope it doesn't." I was confused because she was more active, more articulate, and stronger than me. But she laid it out and said that if a revolution were to happen right now, it would probably lead to an even more reactionary and authoritarian world, because people's ethics are so fucked up that we don't have any kind of base for an egalitarian society. And it was one of those instances where someone says something and your mind just immediately switches. ¶ I had also recently read *Agents of Oppression*. I hadn't known how much state control there was over political organizing. It was surprising when our phone was tapped, you know? I just didn't understand how much power the state had to come down on political groups.

Can you talk about the beginnings of *Doris*? Where were you then and what was going on?

I started it when I moved to Berkeley, around 1993. I'd always wanted to be a writer, but I wrote mostly fiction. I was in a political collective when I lived in Minneapolis, and we put out a magazine. I tried to write political stuff for that, but I couldn't do it. I still had a lot to learn. When I first saw zines—and I didn't see them until around 1992—I thought they were amazing. *Snarla* blew my mind. She was so pissed off and so crazy but so articulate. I thought it was great that she would write about pissing on her fingers and alienation, and that she was figuring things out in this public way, because I thought that in order to write you had to have it all figured out already. ¶ When I started *Doris*, I was obsessed with secrets. I felt like everything was secret inside of me pretty much. I definitely had concrete secrets about abuse, about family, and about abusive situations I put myself in, and also feeling crazy. I was very afraid of going crazy. I also had secrets about how beautiful I thought things were. A lot of my friends were very tough and thought everything was disgusting capitalism. And I thought, "But look at all this beautiful

stuff just laying around in hidden places," and that was secret too.¶ The main reason I started writing zines was because I was obsessed with how alienated people were. Why did we just talk about music and tattoos, or Foucault? I wanted to break the barriers of what you could talk about. In the beginning I wanted to learn to write about political stuff. And then I stopped caring as much about that.

But to me your zines have always seemed very political, very anarchist. Just not in that hammering-you-over-the-head sort of way.

Maybe that's what I mean. Maybe I thought I had to write about issues, and then I started to see that I didn't. That I could embody it in other ways. That everything inside of me is political, I mean I think about politics all the time. But I didn't have to figure out how to write about politics, it wasn't something separate from my writing, if I was writing what I cared about, because what I care about is changing the world.

What role did writing zines play in your political progression?

It gave me courage to speak politically out loud. I feel like I can articulate when I'm writing. And it's helped my overall self-confidence. I didn't have much before I started. I think the role it's played . . . you know, I started drinking really heavily in 1995, and didn't do anything political, wasn't around people doing political organizing anymore, for probably seven years. But I kept writing. I knew the drinking was temporary, but it lasted a lot longer than I thought it would. So I think writing the zine kept me grounded and reminded me that I still wanted to change the world, and I did still have something to offer, and I could still think if I put my mind to it. I could sober up for a few days or a few weeks and get myself thinking clearly enough to write about something I cared about. So in that way, it kept me alive.

Can you talk more about your experience with drinking? What was going on in your life?

When I started drinking I had a lot of stuff going on. There was so much anger pent up inside of me and I was terrified of it, and so angry that I couldn't find people to be close to. Drinking definitely helped me process that stuff and it definitely helped me be around people who considered each other family in this way. It allowed me to be close to people and to become really angry and to sing, and play punk music, which has been good. And now, I have no problem getting angry when I need to. But I never would've been able to if I hadn't been a drunk for a while. I know other people can, but I don't think I personally could have. ¶ But during this time, I was in a women's health group, and we opened a women and transgender health resource center. And for the first time, I had the power. I knew what needed to get done, I knew how it needed to get done most efficiently, and I didn't have patience for people coming in and not doing what they needed to do. It was very strange for me, because I'd always been the powerless one in groups. I think I was really shitty. I didn't stay in the group very long, because I could see what was happening. Out of all the kinds of organizations, a women's/transgender health project should not have somebody doing that kind of power trip. I think if I hadn't been drinking, I would've been able to handle it better. ¶ So I realized I had to quit drinking, and I moved out to the country, partly just to get away, and partly because I just couldn't take it; I'd been writing a lot about abuse stuff, and people were talking to me about abuse stuff, and it was too much for me.

Is this what *Support* came out of?

One of the reasons I wanted to do [the zine] was because I had called out people who'd been abusive to friends, and I was confronting ex-boyfriends who'd been abusive to me. And everybody really just didn't think they were abusive. Or really didn't mean to be. Or couldn't believe that that's what I experienced. ¶ It became really clear that people just do not know. So I wanted my friends to read about abuse and how it affects us and how not to be abusive. It seemed like I would be a good person to put out a zine about it. I really didn't want to do it. But I felt like that was politically important for me to do, I felt like I was in a position where I could.

Shifting focus a bit, I wanted to talk about the zine you wrote as the DIY guide to depression . . .

[*Laughs.*] When I wrote that, I thought people would think I was completely insane. I just thought, "OK this is what I do, but everyone else will think I'm crazy." But I've gotten the most feedback about that zine than any other.

You've mentioned that depression is an ongoing struggle . . .

Oh yeah. I mean I'm not so suicidal anymore, but I'm still depressed. How could you not be? The world is so fucked up. And I still feel hopeless sometimes, but it's less. I stopped feeling so dramatic about my place in the world, and also, yes, the world is a terrible place, but there have also been incredible changes. Sometimes when I start to feel really hopeless about things, I read about the '60s. It was unbearable then, and the movement was amazing. People thought the whole world was going to change, in a way that was less delusional than how I thought it was going to change. African countries were gaining independence. But at the same time, it was unbearable. Women had so few resources, men were just unbelievable pigs, and that was totally accepted in political circles. So it gives me hope that we've changed so much. And I believe that we're continuing to change in very fundamental ways. Like the trans movement. A few years ago I didn't really even know that trans was an option for people. And it's amazing to me to see this fight to end the gender binary. Just that society's moving in these directions despite all the issues it brings up. There's so much social control, we're losing on so many fronts, especially with state repression, and there's so much materialism, just pushing and pushing, it's so daunting. But there's also some pretty magical stuff going on.

One of the reasons your writing seems to resonate with people is because you use such plain language to communicate complex ideas, particularly around anarchism. How do you define anarchism?

My definition is that people have the capability to live in a world without oppression and without coercive institutions and government, and that we have the ability to self organize. I'm not into this idea that we're going to be free and chaotic. Sometimes what gets called direct democracy is how I envision anarchism—communities organized together, someone can be your representative, but they come back and tell you exactly what was said at this meeting, and if you don't like it they can be recalled. I have this idea how the entire world would be run in an anarchist society, including the postal service, but it's basically the idea that people can self organize, that we can live without coercion, that we can live in an ecologically sustainable way.

How have your politics evolved over the years?

One of the things that's really great now that I'm older, is I'm able to be around different kinds of people, especially older people. My sister is part of this farmers' market, and these people are not anarchists, supposedly. Some of them are old tobacco farmers who are now trying to grow something else, because they're broke. They're people from all different backgrounds, and they might've voted for Bush. But in their farmers' market meetings they can do consensus better than anarchists can. They'll be totally outspoken in their beliefs and disagree with whatever decision is trying to be made in the group. Maybe they want crafts to be sold in the farmers' market and other people don't, and they will go off about crafts and how

they should be there, and when it comes down to the vote, they'll abstain from voting because they see that it would be better for the community. I feel like I have a lot more faith in humanity, I'm much less dogmatic. ¶ I'm also trying to embrace this idea that now that I'm older, I would like to be more of an educator. Often I think that everybody knows what I know. And I'm starting to realize that everybody does not know what I know, because I'm 36 and a lot of people are 15, and I should be conscious about doing some educating, because it would have been useful for me to have zines that explained some history.

You've written a lot about group process and the replication of oppression in radical movements. Do you have any new thoughts on that?

I think when people start doing political organizing, there's this sense of urgency: things need to get done, and there's no time. But when there's a sense of urgency, there's more room for power dynamics, to not make room for people who feel silenced, and not make room for larger discussions. So first of all, I wish people would embrace the basic idea that the ends don't justify the means. And really embrace patience and make enough time for meetings and groups to be efficient but also value the work of empowering people to speak and people learning to be empowered to speak, and formulating ideas together. And knowing that that is a huge revolutionary thing we need to do. And that even if we win a particular issue, we are not going to change the world unless we do this work.

What do you spend your time doing these days?

I've worked for my aunt for a long time as a weaver. I make fancy scarves mostly, for the ultra rich. [Laughs.] When I moved to Berkeley she taught me. It's a great job, but it's just a job. And I'm trying to write a novel. And I'm in two bands. And I'm trying to relax more.

What's the name of your band?

Trouble Trouble Trouble, I sing and play the bass. I was in another punk band before called Astrid Oto. Trouble Trouble Trouble doesn't have any music out, but for the record, my other band did. I just sang in that one. I was also in a band that I just played bass for, no singing, which was called the Blank Fight.

Can you share the storyline of your novel?

[Laughs.] It's ridiculous. Washington DC has had a chemical attack and the central government is in disarray and the economy has gone down the tubes, kind of how it was in the '80s, so there's white flight back to the suburbs and no more gentrification. That's the setting, but it's mostly about these two 15-year-old girls, their friendship. One of them is an anti-racist organizer, kind of a wild ass, but definitely 100 percent for the revolution, and the other is dealing with issues around depression, sexuality, silence and abuse.

You mentioned wanting to get back into political work. Do you know where you're headed?

Yeah, I want to do education about women's health and try to start more of a women's health movement again. Self-care, abortion rights, everything. I'm not really sure if young girls have those resources to learn about their bodies and self-care. I want to teach classes on that and physiology and how our bodies work, and how everything is connected. I want to teach this as a political action. And then hopefully working to make reproductive health clinics better. This whole Supreme Court thing is really frightening. This work is important so that when the time comes, we can take care of things on our own. I also want to do support for a group of Spanish-speaking women in my town who are volunteer translators at our clinic, and who are now helping a group of Latina women to get resources to start their own community health center. I want to be more active in supporting communities of color. ¶ And then eventually I want to be teaching. Not in a regular school, but I want to teach about history and philosophy. I also want to be more involved in street protesting again, and real education about it—giving flyers to strangers on the street. I don't love street protesting, but I think it's important that it's ongoing and not just when major issues that come up. I want to work up to doing all that stuff, helping more counter-institutions, organizing meetings, making sure the meetings have good process. I feel like I'm at that age when that should be my role. ◉

poison ivy

ONCE UPON A TIME I HAD
POISON IVY SO BAD THAT
MY FINGERS WERE PURE
BLISTERS, MY BODY JUST
PURE ITCH. MY PARENTS PUT
GLOVES ON ME AND TIED ME
TO A COT SO I WOULDN'T ITCH.

THEY WERE TRYING SOME KIND OF HOME REMEDY ON IT,
AND IT WASN'T WORKING. THEY WEREN'T TRYING TO BE
TERRIBLE. SOMETIMES I LIKE TO REMEMBER HOW YOUNG
THEY ACTUALLY WERE.

MY DAD SWEARS BY FELSNAPTHA SOAP, AND SO DO
I, EVEN THOUGH I KNOW THE TRICK IS THAT THE
SOAP IS NOT REALLY SOAP, BUT DETERGENT, AND
ANY KIND OF DETERGENT WILL DO.

THE WAY IT WORKS IS, YOU WANT TO GET THE OIL OFF.
YOU WANT TO GET IT OFF YOUR SKIN BEFORE IT GETS THE
CHANCE TO REALLY SINK IN. AND THEN IF YOU DON'T GET
IT OFF IN TIME, AND YOU END UP WITH BLISTERS, YOU
WANT TO MAKE SURE THAT WHEN THE BLISTERS POP, YOU
GET THE OIL OFF THEN. THERE IS OIL IN THE BLISTERS.

ONE TIME I DID
AN EXPERIMENT
WHERE I
SCRATCHED THE
BLISTERS ON
ONE ARM
UNTIL THEY BLED
AND THEN I
POURED BLEACH
ON THEM...

THE OTHER ARM I JUST
LEFT ALONE.

THEY HEALED AT THE
SAME TIME.

WELCOME TO DORIS #24.
FOR ORDERING INFO,
GO TO THE LAST PAGE.
THANKS YOU, ALL

202

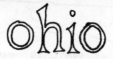

Ohio

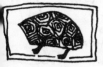

Did you know that on some kinds of turtles
you can read their age by the ridges of their
shells? Each section of shell has concentric
ridges circling in and in and in, and you can
put your fingernail gently there, move it
slowly, read the lines.

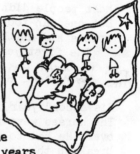

And some turtles, they have a hinge,
like a little door they can pull
their heads into and close themselves
off from the outside world, and then
you can only jab at their feet, you
can't peck out their head. Not that
I wanted to do any pecking.

We were in Ohio. Paul had told me
about the age lines. I was holding the
turtle, counting, thinking about the years
that had marked me. Thinking about this land
we were trying to buy and this chapter in my life, Ohio.

We were walking the perimeter, me and Caty and
Roger and Paul. Paul owned some land nearby. He was our
guide, blazing through the wild roses and the poisonivy,
pouring out information - what trees were hardwood,
what trees were boundry markers, what plants
were invasive, what our priorities should
be to help the land recover and regain
ballance, what we could do to make the wild
animals happy, who owned the surrounding
hillsides, where pasture land had been,
how much the area had been strip-mined,
how much was underpreservation now,
where we could put in a pond, where we
could grow ginseng and goldenseal.

Paul is a New Yorker. He moved to
rural Ohio in the 70's, but he's still
a New Yorker with the quick and certain
way he talks.

He moved to Ohio; 19 years old, long
haired freak. He sat down, he told us, he
just sat down and watched.

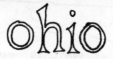

HE WATCHED THE
STUNNING RHYTHM AND
BEAUTY OF THIS FADING WAY
OF LIFE. THE HORSES GETTING
HARNESSED UP, THE CLOMP OF
HOOVES, THE PLOW BEHIND THEM,
THE TURNING OF THE SOIL, THE
NOSES SNORTING AND STEAM EXHALING IN THIS FIRST
~~CLASS OF~~ WARM ENOUGH DAY OF SPRING.

Most people didn't want him there. Outsider. City boy.
But one man took him under his wing, taught him about
horses and anything else he wanted to know.
        The first year was ok. Hard work day and night.

"THIS IS WHAT HAS BEEN LOST IN AMERICA," Paul says
"THE KNOWLEDGE OF HOW TO WORK REALLY HARD."

His second year in Ohio was the coldest on record.
The horses were freezing, the well was freezing
over. He had to wake up three times a night to go
break up the ice so their water-source wouldn't
become a solid block and leave them waterless. He
brought one sick horse in to the house to warm it,
but by the end of winter, he'd lost half his team.
He stuck with it all, and over the years he won his
neighbors grudging respect.

I used to be afraid of rural America.
I thought all the guys out there would
be macho assholes like the ones who yell
at me in grocery store parking lots
about how disgusting I am because of my
mustache, or the ones who tried to fight
me in the bar because I wouldn't say if I was a boy or
a girl. I thought rural america was all ignorant assholes
out looking for fights

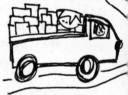

When I moved 3 years ago to the North Carolina country
and I didn't even have a car, just had my friends drop
me off with all my belongings at the last house on the
dead end road in the middle of swithhback roads and
mountains, when they pulled away waving, saying "call
us when your phone gets turned on," I watched them drive
away and I felt overwhelming relief, and home at last,
and fear.

The house came with a 30/30 rifle, and I slept with it loaded next to my bed. I brought it with me to the bathroom when I took a shower. I even brought it with me when I just got up to pee.

I started listening to country music, because that was the only channel I got out there, and it wasn't what I expected. It wasn't "Let's kill all the Iraqi" or even the old standard "I caught my woman with another man so I shot her dead.": The songs were mostly really sweet, about men trying to feel their feelings and remember what is important in life, like family and community and land and helping eachother, and not needing a bunch of materialistic things. Like: "who needs a stupid country club, we just take all our shitty boats down to the swimming hole and tie them together and kick back and we've got ourselves our own redneck yaght club." or "I lost

my job so my wife said she'd get one and I could take care of the kids, which I thought would be vacation, but it is the hardest thing I have ever done. I don't know how she's done it all these years," or "My dad taught me to listen to old people, and he's right, they have a lot of important things to teachuus," or "I caught my wife with another man, so I cried," or "you don't really need a lot of money, as long as you've got a lot of heart," or "that girl is really smart and well traveled and strong minded, but hasn't let it turn her in to a snob and that's hot," or "they say you can't go home again, but they're lieing, because you can and nothing beats real community."

After listening to the music I stopped being so scared.

I thought I would grow flax, a whole field of it, and I would spin it in to thread and weave linen, but I was too shy to ask anyone to plow my field, even though the neighbors told me to let them know if I ever needed anything. Living the way I have, I never learned to ask for help. Or I learned that if I asked, there would be strings attached. and I learned to be afraid of judgement. So I just dug a small plot. Jono helped me. We planted tomatoes, more than I could ever eat. I picked dandilion greens and red clover and dried them for tea.

I pickled greenbeans. I grew Luffas. Did you
know Luffas are a gourd? not a sea creature!?!
It is true. They grow on a vine like a pumpkin.
You dry them out and peal off all the skin and
squashy stuff and turn it inside out and scrape
out all the
                seeds, and you're left with a soft
intricate skelatin. turn it right side in and
dry it slowly until it's done, and there you
have it, a bathtub skin scrubber. Mine has lasted
so far for 2 years.

politics

Yesterday I was reading a book that was talking about
off-road-vehicles, and the author said - how could the
world ever change when people destroy nature just in the
name of recreation. If people will destroy what is
beautiful just because it's fun.

Across the mountian from where I used to live was a group
of people who thought that if you weren't striving to live
like the hunter and gatherers, you didn't really deserve
to live.

I go to the global warming movie, and outside there's a
table of urgent and well meaning ladies selling wholesale
energy conserving lightbulbs, and I think of the amount
of energy I use compared to the gas station down the street
from me that leaves it's millions of lights on full blast
blindingly bright, all night, even when it's closed.

I think of friends who have given up because nothing seems
like enough, or because people let them down and political
projects fell through,   or because they simply don't know
any more what to do.

A lot of people who simply don't know what to do.

I think of the people who say the world is fucked so lets party, and aside from whatever political critique I could give about the privledges and responsibilities we have, giving up like that just seems so boring.

I think about the people who say all you can do is change yourself, and what utter bullshit that is.

I think about the French Resistance, have I mentioned this before? When the Nazis were taking over everything and there was no stopping them, the French Resistance continued to fight with whatever they could. Their motto was:

> We don't need hope to survive or success to perservere.
> Resistance to tyranny is a way of life!

I think about how we should fight for what we love, and how could you not, in some way, love something about this world.

I don't think that tearing up the hillsides with an off-road-vehicle means that you don't care about the land. I don't think eating road kill makes you pure. I don't think my energy conservation measures matter at all. I don't think our lifestyle choices are in and of themselves political. The political part is whether our lifestyle choices help us to become more human. If they help us feel a sense of personal integrity, and if that integrity gives us the power to fight further., to imagine deeper, to want more.

I want to live in a world where kids aren't raped, where no one is. I want there to be about one car for every one-thousand people, for the streets to be torn up and turned into gardens, and for people to form social structures that are not based on domination or manipulation, and where everyone sees that we are part of nature, a really interesting and vital part of nature, and that nature isn't something seperate, not a resource to be used.

I want to win. I want my utopian world, and I'd
even settle for a utopia that I haven't yet
imagined, and I know realistically, that I won't
see it in my lifetime, but I think I could see
somthing better. I think that in our lifetimes
we could make a shift, a huge shift in the way
things are, and that it has to change fundamentally.

And it's not going to change if we give
in to our complacency.

It is hard work that we have to do, but it is
life-giving work.

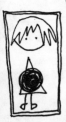

Do you feel a hole inside of you? What do you
do to fill it up? I fed mine with tears and
self-mutilation, suicide thoughts and love
dream delusions, revolution and sex and self-
righteousness, self-hatred and alcohol.

    I was reading a book last week. It was
talking about the difference between subordination
and oppression. What it said is this:

Subordination means you are subjected to the will of
another, but you don't notice or you don't think that
you are being blocked from realizing your full potential.
Like when I was in Jr. High and my biggest dream for
myself was to be a rock-star's girlfriend, and I didn't
see anything wrong with that.

Oppression is when you realize what the hell is going on.

Do words matter? Is some of the hard work we've forgotten
how to do, the hard work of thinking? We are sold into
short attention spans and easy answers.

Do you not see yourself as oppressed?

☆ ☆☆ ☆

What about your thoughts and your actions and who you
love and why you love them, and your dreams and your
goals, and what you've already given up, what about your
desires and the things you talk about, the ways you feel
about yourself, what fills your days, what permeates your
nights: How much of it all is really your own?

Are you realizing your full potential? Your full humanity?
Do you buy into the propaganda that you are to blame for
your unhappiness? You just have to pull up your bootstraps,
think positive? Do you feel meaningful? Do you feel
fulfilled?

♥ i want you to feel happy + full

This is what that one book says:

For social change to happen, people need to come out of
subjegations and see the oppression, and for that shift
in thinking to occur, you need three things.

1. To have access to the tools that will allow you to
   envision a world that lies beyond subordination and
imagine what you could become in that alternative space.

2. Analyze ways you have been caught up and thwarted by
   the relation of subordination

3. Grasp the possibility of collective struggle to
   overthrow the whole subordinating structure

I think a lot of us have a lot of privledge and a
responsibility to use that privledge well, whether it's
waking people up and changing the sturctures of our
worlds, or confronting our own twisted up insides.

or both. we have to be engaged in both.

So what do I do?
Where is the
answer?

I will tell you because
I am tired of people saying
there is no answer.

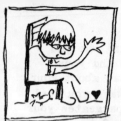

When I was 18, my ancient philosopher friend said that the problem with today's youth-movement was we were too transient. We were obsessed with creating community, but we wouldn't stay put. He said that real, fundamental social change had to be based

in real geographical community, and that we weren't going to be very effective if we didn't stop moving around.

But it was a small town and I was restless, and stuck inside

my self and my fears, and my lack of experience and lack of the physical knowledge of the possibilities - both for myself and for the world.

I needed to find people like me. I needed to find people who would help me feel seen and real. I needed to be around people who were so effected by the insanity of capitalism that they couldn't function in this world, and I needed to experience a world created in the cracks and fissures and forgotten places.

I needed to figure out how to be present in my body and how to say no, how to be able to dance for the fun of it and not because I thought someone might be watching. I needed to learn to feel safe among friends and like I could say what I thought without being judged. I needed to learn my anger and stop turning it inward. I needed to learn to feel good in the woods and fields and among growing things, instead of feeling kind of scared and alienated and like there was something I didn't understand, some missing part of me that was inhuman, or some human part that was cut out and thrown away.

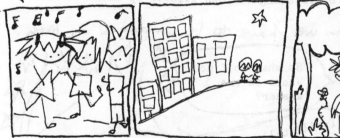

I had to learn to build a small fire out of moss and twigs, hot enough to boil water. I had to learn the difference between numbing myself and relaxing.

Once Upon a Time, my political collective came up with

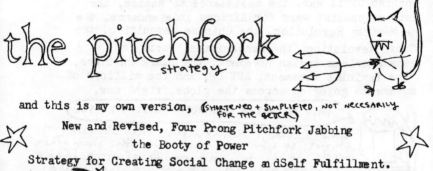

the pitchfork

strategy

and this is my own version, (SHORTENED + SIMPLIFIED, NOT NECESSARILY FOR THE BETTER)

New and Revised, Four Prong Pitchfork Jabbing
the Booty of Power
Strategy for Creating Social Change and Self Fulfillment.

Here are the 4 prongs: (5 PRONGS. I FORGOT COUNTER-INSTITUTIONS!)
-discovery and self education
-affinity groups and political collectives
-direct action, protest, and community education
-internal democracy and coalitions

Ok, so we alredy talked about self-discovery, and of course it is a life-long process, but I do want to say that for a lot of people, there is a really intensive time of exploration, and then it fades out, and a lot of people think that fading out means that they are now sucky grownups who are not excited by the world! NO!! That is not what is happening! Don't give in to that story we've been told! Discovery and self-discovery is not the goal of life. The goal is to become activly engaged in creating a world worth living in!

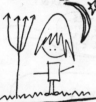

Self Education.

I DON'T THINK YOU CAN SEPERATE THE TWO. ACTIVELY CHANGING THE WORLD CREATES A WHOLE NEW + DEEP KIND OF SELF DISCOVERY and hope ♥

We need to know our revolutionary history. It is our responsibility to educate ourselves about the things we have not been taught. We need to be worthy of the people who have come before us.

I admit that most of my self education has been done alone, but I think study groups are important for a lot of reasons. And I don't mean just studying quirky fun things, I mean taking ourselves seriously and reading books that will challenge us and inspire us and teach us.

I recommend a systematic study of revolutionary movements, like   - the French Revolution, the slave rebellions, the Hatian Revolution, the Russian Revolution, the Spanish Civil War. the Resistance to Nazism, the anti-colonalist wars for African Independence. the the Mexican Revolution, the Chinese Revoultion, the Cuban Revolution, the Sandanistas, Paris '68, the American Indian Movement, the Black Panthers, the feminist movement, ACT UP, and the millions of movements going on across the globe, right now.

THIS IS NOT A COMPLETE LIST AT ALL

and always remember, This learning
is not so you can feel smarter Than other
people. It is to work on developing ideas
and strategies for changing The world.

AND IF YOU DO NOT
LIKE READING, JUST
KEEP AT IT. IT GETS
BETTER OVER TIME

TRY DIFFERENT STYLES.
HISTORY, MEMOIR, FICTION.
READ WITH A CRITICAL
BUT NOT DISMISSIVE EYE

Study Groups

We need to be able to think clearly and deeply. To be passionate about our beliefs. To be able to articulate what we believe and know.

My ancient philosopher said that we need to be able to stand on a soap box in a crowd of 100 people and argue our points succinctly and persuasively, but I also think it is just as important to be able to communicate it all in loving and non-defensive ways.

We need to learn to admit what we don't know, and to reexame our dogmas and the things we hold most dear.

I have found study groups to be especially useful for me when I'm trying to learn about things that are really hard for me to understnad. Like theory and philosophy, and also physiology and how our bodies work. Study group s have been really helpful for me in pushing myself to get over some of my internalized sexism - pushing myself to quiet the voices of self-doubt, and to learn to ask questions instead of just shutting down and thinking l'm stupid. I have also seen study groups be really helpful for people who are full of ego and self-confidence, for them to learn to be quiet and to listen to the ways other peoples life experiences give them different kinds of insights.

AFFINITY GROUPS AND POLITICAL COLLECTIVES

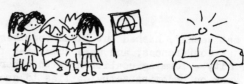

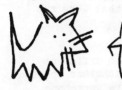

> There is a systematic attack against us. Systematic propaganda that tells us that all we are is consumers, and all we can do to change the world is make good consumer choices.

There are systematic programs of control to keep us depressed and pacified and separated. We need to create systems to fight these attacks. to fight the ambivalence. to not give up.

♡

Affinity groups are formed pretty much around action. They should be made up of friends you trust. You don't have to have total political agreement on all politics, as long as there's a basic common ground, and a lot of trust, especially if you're going to do things that are illegal.

The affinity groups I've been in were just formed for taking part in big protests. We stuck together, watched eachothers backs, did small direct actions. But I really wish I had an ongoing affinity group, and so that is what I'm suggesting to you! I think it would be so helpful! I need to have people watching my back, not just to save me from cops, but also to save me from despair. If I had an affinity group, I think we could do so many more fun political things, like street theater and sabotage and volunteer for things together. I'd feel more a part of something. Less alone.

political Collectives

Political Collectives are more serious and should have more of a long-term strategy and commitment, They don't have to be made up of your best friends, but you should have a strong common politics.

The collective I was a part of was a closed collective, which means it wasn't open for other people to join. I think closed collectives are really good and important. It helped us to form cohesiveness and trust, and allowd us to work on really important internal power dynamics.

We met weekly, hashed out ideas together, planned protests and   conferences, and were committed to becoming part of our city - forming coalitions with other groups and trying to work on becoming actual allies to groups that were run by people of color.

Different people in our group were involved in different things, and in our weekly meetings we kept eachother updated on what was going on. We wrote flyers and gave workshops, and were involved in different campaigns - like working to stop a nuclear waste dump, and working to keep and anti-abortion conference from coming to our town.

of course there are a million different kinds of political collectives, but I would like to see more collectives like that one was.

Direct Action, Protest and Community Education.

Direct Action is an essential part of social movements, but it's often a demonized or glorified part. Property destruction, billboard alteration, sit-ins, walk outs, puke ins, occupations of schools and work-places, strikes and street theater. It is good to think about what the strategic role your direct action is going to play in the larger picture. Whether your action is going to be symbolic or more than that. It is important not to get caught up in the ego-trip of doing illegal things, but it's also important that we have a militant resistance movement.

(protest.)   I've seen protests come and go. times of lots of protesting and then people giving up because their protest didn't stop the war.
    protest is important, even in the shitty give up times. They don't have to always be huge protests, small ones are important to. We need visibility. We need to show that there is resistance. We need to celebrate our resistance.

AND WHEN WE PROTEST, WE NEED TO HAVE REALLY INFOMATIVE FLYERS AND PASS THEM OUT TO PEOPLE ON THE STREET SO THAT THEY KNOW WHAT IS GOING ON!!!

especially if there are ways they can become involved, let them know.

Protest and street theater can be really good places to do community education, so try and make flyers that go really in depth into the issues, and provide people a list of resources so they can find out more on their own or become involved in organizations working on it.

> I wish there were little protests every week. I think it would make people understand that there are real living alternatives to the shitty capitalist way of life.

☆ Community Education ☆

aside from protests and direct actions, there are a million ways to do community education. We used to do a film

series at our library, covered the telephone poles with flyers of info and poetry, handed out radical newspapers to the kids getting out of highschool for the day, organized community forums, For awhile we tried to have people speak on different issues before punk shows, like the history of Yugoslavia, or "how to stay hopeful and

not totally give up (by a 60 year old sortof commie)," and zine tables at shows too.

and doing the hard work of becoming a voice in the larger community. like going to liberal events and being a more radical resource (kind of depressing, but still good to do).

☆ Internal Democracy and Coalitions. ♡

One of the things I like best about the anarchism I believe in, is we are committed to ending all forms of hierarchy and domination, including our own behavior.

Internal democracy means that we are trying to create, in our small groups, the kinds of social dynamics we want in our new world. People who have less traditional power, and are silenced by things like sexism and racism, can't be asked to put aside their needs until after the war is over or after the revolution is won. And people with priviledge have to look at a lot of assumtions they've made.

And we can not be given empowerment, we have to build it up in ourselves, together.

you have to actually care and want this for real. It can't be solved by math or denial.

The committment to this internal work was one of the most hopeful things to me about working in a political collective.

Also, as long as there is patriarchy and racist power structures, there is going to be needs for people of color and women and trans people and a million other marginalized groups, to organize on their own, and we need to learn to be allies. I mean actual consistant and principled allies, willing to look at our own racism (or other ism) and put aside our purist political attitudes and learn about the world and about struggle from people who have different experiences with power, and different ideas with what they want to do about it.

like volunteering is really good. It may take awhile to find a place that works for you, and it may be scary + depressing, but it can also help us get out of our own little bubbles. And if you are able to create a comfortable bubble, then its especially important that you needs to break it, because theres a lot that needs to be done

Counter - Institutions

(I almost forgot this one).

Sometimes I have mixed feelings about counter institutions because I think of the info-shops and community centers that punks and anarchists try and start, and how so often it just takes up all our time and energy and money, and brings out the worst power dynamics, and ends in anger and despair, and it just seems like whats the point. But then I go to the collective cafe my friend is part of, and it feels really good. Like this is a space that is ours, this is people trying to work collectively for real.

And I think of all the very real counter-institutions that were set up that I now take for granted, like rape-crisis centers, and food co-ops (actually, I don't take them for granted, because there's hardly any real worker run co-ops left), community gardens, free clinics, Community Supported Agriculture farms. It is so important that we do this work. That we create functioning alternatives to way we're suppose to live!

that's it! a tiny bit. If you want the full and more eloquent Pitchfork article that AWOL wrote, let me know.

and see resource section at the end of this zine.

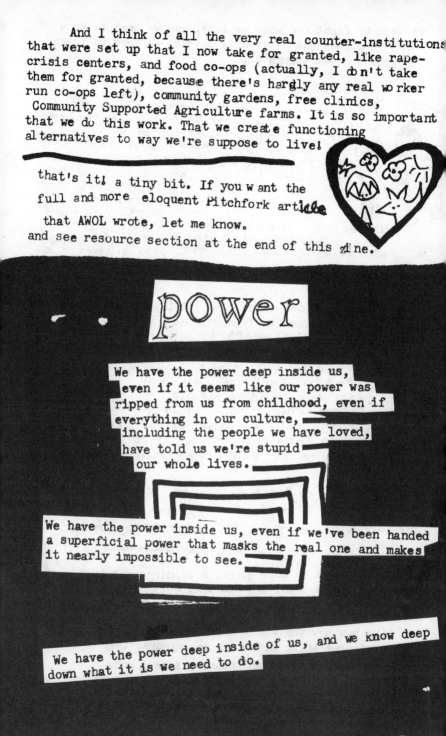

power

We have the power deep inside us, even if it seems like our power was ripped from us from childhood, even if everything in our culture, including the people we have loved, have told us we're stupid our whole lives.

We have the power inside us, even if we've been handed a superficial power that masks the real one and makes it nearly impossible to see.

We have the power deep inside of us, and we know deep down what it is we need to do.

We need to fight for what we love, and we need to know
that sometimes that love will change. We need to learn
to grow and let things go.

I used to love the adrenaline
of fear and the power of
taking back what should
rightfully be ours.
matches and lighter fluid.

I loved spray paint
and cities and
the exposure to
other cultures, learning
about people, how they
thought, what they did, how they
survived, what they dreamed, what
we could create. all the possibilities.

♡ I loved my mom but I could not save her ♡

I tried to learn to love friends,
and maybe I had to get
wasted for years to learn
it. That I could put my
guard down, that I would
be taken care of, that I
could pass out and someone
would carry me home, that I
could scream out all the unforgiving
rage and be forgiven. That strong feelings
were there to be felt, not hidden.

I TRIED TO
LEARN TO
LOVE MYSELF.

THAT CHEESY AND
TOTALLY
NECESSARY THING.
self forgiveness

and I learned to love quiet. A winding road that
no one drives down, and how unexpected things
happen when you ask questions and pay attention.

Like how now the woods and fields aren't just
this strange thing nature to me anymore, they
are particular trees and plants, some I know
the names of, some I don't. And I can walk out
my door in the springtime and there are things
to eat, weeds or things I've planted.

I have learned the difference between relaxing
and numbing myself   most of the time.

And in Ohio, I hold the turtle, count the
ridges, and think of mine. Who would have ever
thought that me, such a city girl, would ever
have ended up loving and needing the shelter
of woods, the fields and wide open spaces.

My ancient philosopher friend said - it is
the role of the youth in revolutionary movements
to be on the front lines, both in body and in
spirit. To demand ways of thinking that we
haven't thought up yet. It is the role of
older people in revolutionary movements to
build institutions that will nurture revolutionary
ideas and practice, through good times and bad,
to hold on to our history and to teach.

Maybe this is true and maybe it isn't, but I
am older now, and thinking - What am I going to
build?

maybe I will build a house, write books and novels,
Maybe I will start an anarchist summer school, like
the Institute for Social Ecology, or a rock and
roll girls camp, or an abortion clinic that is nice
to women. Maybe now I will finally stop moving,
and I will actually know my neighbors.

Chris once told me that a friend of his said
"you can't do everything you dream of. At some
point you need to narrow it down, prioritize."

But you can do everything
That's what I think.
Our lives are long and full and if we love and
work and want, we can do it all.

everything
everything.

even more than we are able to imagine.

219

punk

WHAT KEEPS ME THE MOST IN PUNK IS THE SINGING.
I WANT THE GIRLS TO KNOW THAT THEY CAN SCREAM
TO. I WANT THE FEELING OF VOICE STRAIGHT FROM THE
GUT. THE POWER AND STRENGTH IN MY BODY. I LIKE
BANDS WITH PEOPLE WHO HAVE NEVER BEEN IN BANDS
BEFORE. MUSIC WITH PEOPLE WHO DON'T KNOW HOW TO
PLAY. AND FIGURING IT OUT TOGETHER. SCREAMING
TOGETHER. PLAYING FOR OUR FRIENDS.

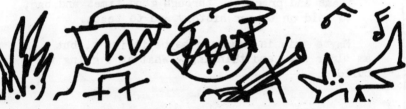

I REMEMBER THE FIRST TIME I TRIED TO SING AND I COULDN'T
GET MY VOICE TO RAISE. I FROZE UP. I FELT SO STUPID.
ME AND AARON HAD BEEN DRIVING ACROSS THE COUNTRY,
PRACTICING SONGS, PLANNING OUR BAND. BUT ONCE WE GOT
TO WHERE WE WERE GOING AND I HAD MUSIC BEHIND ME AND
MICROPHONE IN HAND AND I TRIED TO SCREAM, I COULDN'T.
I TRIED AGAIN. I COULDN'T AGAIN. SO STUPID. SUCH A
STUPID GIRL.

I FELT LIKE I HAD IN THE SELF DEFENSE CLASS WHERE WE
WERE SUPPOSE TO SHOUT "NO" WHEN WE PUNCHED, AND I
COULDN'T. ALL I COULD GET OUT WAS A SQUEEK. ALL THESE
TOUGH WOMEN SHOUTING, AND STUPID, SILENT LITTLE ME.

IT IS HARD WHEN THINGS THAT ARE SUPPOSED TO EMPOWER US
END UP MAKING US FEEL TWICE AS BAD.

IT WAS LIKE IF I SCREAMED NO, THEN I WOULD HAVE TO FEEL
ALL THE TIMES I HADN'T BEEN ABLE TO. IF I COULD SCREAM
NO, THEN WHAT WOULD I DO NEXT TIME I NEEDED TO. IF I
COULDN'T SCREAM THEN, WOULD I BLAME MYSELF EVEN MORE.

/There are things that we keep in our body that are deeper than we can think through. Defenses that are keeping us safe in convoluted ways.

I got in another band a few years later. This time with no strangers, just with people I loved. And the same thing happened. I opened my mouth and out came nothing, and I almost gave up again. But Mike said 'Oh, come on.' and shook me up and made me laugh and said 'It's just us' and said 'I'll sing with you.' And the next time I opened my mouth out came the loudest song, straight from the gut. Straight from this unaccessed place of power.

I think that before I sang, the only time I felt powerful in my body was sometimes when I was having sex. But a lot of times sex made me feel the opposite from powerful. Singing gave me back something about me deep inside. Singing gave me back something that had been stolen.

Even though the songs I sang at first weren't songs I'd written, screaming made me feel like I had a voice that could be heard and maybe mattered. And even though I couldn't always scream when I should have, the power of it seeped in, it changed the way I lived in the world. It changed the way I thought of myself.

And it gave me a place for my anger. It allowed me anger in the rest of my life too. It let me feel a wider range of feelings. It let me scream about things that I need to scream about but don't get the chance to.

There are so many things we need to scream about that eat away at us, bottled up inside.

And so even though I don't drink any more and that can make it hard to be at shows, I still want the screaming. I want the sweet and strange and moody kinds of communications that happen when you have a band. And most of all, I want girls to know that girls are alowed to scream. I want more girls and trannies in bands. I want us up there. I want to remind us that we can. Scream.

scream ♡

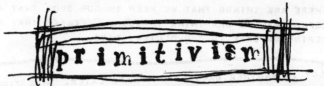

primitivism

Sometimes when my friends have slightly different belief systems than I do, I get afraid to ask them questions, because I am afraid of what their answers will be. But I am trying to unlearn that. I want to learn and talk and learn. So here is my interview/conversation with Chris Somerville. He said a lot of things I really like that made me feel a kind of soundness deep inside of me, like fundamental change was going to happen in a core way, and beautiful.

Cindy What is primitivism?

Chris There are dozens of definitions, like primitivism is a critique of civilization; primitivism is a political movement; primitivism is tanning hides. I consider primitivism to be both the ideology and the act of going back to human roots as hunter gatherers. But I don't think we can find the perfect society and then model what we do after them, and this is one of my breaks with ideological primitivism. A lot of primitivism is concerned with going back in a way like 'let's do that again,' and there are a lot of ways in which we do need to 'go back' but what I want is to build a new culture. I don't want to just reinvent something. I want to live in an egalitarian way and I want to live in a way that's sustainable for the land base.

I think there are a lot of lessons that can be learned from the people who have lived here sustainable for up to 12,000 years. I think it really reflects something important that the Coast Salish ("Coast Salish" is a generalized grouping of lots of different peoples that all lived in the Pacific Northwest) could live here for 12,000 years with the eco-system intact, and this culture -- Western Civilization -- is here for less than 200 years and the place is trashed. I think that says something really powerful about which lifeway is more sustainable. But it's not a choice between the two; you know what I'm saying?

Cindy One of the problems I have with the primitivism I've been exposed to is the romaticization of pre-industrial life, and this idea that if we just became hunter-gatherers again, all other forms of domination would magically disappear. I really don't believe that.

Chris I'm not sure I believe that either. "Hunter-Gatherer" is such an abstraction. It refers to hundreds of thousands of different groups of people over a million years. It's a life way. You can't make these huge generalizations about what "Hunter-Gatherers" did. But there have been anthropological studies of societies that lived a direct return hunter-gatherer life way, which means they did not have any kind of agriculture whatsoever, that have shown that people who lived in that particular way, who had a non-coercive relationship with the land, also had more egalitarian societies.

But there is such a huge spectrum of hunter-gatherer societies, and there's different degrees of egalitarianness, and different degrees of hunter-gathererness. Like for instance, the Coast Salish. A lot of them did do certain kinds of cultivation. They were cultivating a lot of the native plants in this area. They had kind of a hybridized version of agriculture. It wasn't agriculture in that they didn't lay a land base to waste and then sow seed in it, but they were encouraging certain crops to grow that they knew they could use for food. But they also lived hugely on wild food, well, really only on wild food. They lived on salmon and hunted elk and deer, but that gradation from hunter-gatherer to agriculturalist was reflected in their society because a lot of those cultures in the Pacific Northwest had slaves. At the same time, they had an incredible sustainable relationship to their land base. And women were hugely empowered in many of those societies. So there's a different dimensions of egalitarianism and different dimensions of hunter-gathererness. And there's different degrees of sustainability. I don't believe there's even been a society that's 100% egalitarian. And I don't think those kinds of abstractions are very useful anyway.

Cindy Usually when people talk about primitivism, they also talk about being anti-civilization. Can you explain what that means, like how is civilization defined?

Chris: The most comprehensive and accurate definition of civilization I've heard is Derrick Jensens's, which is that civilization is "A culture -- a complex of stories, institutions and artifacts -- that both leads to and emerges from the growth of cities, which cities being defined (to distinguish them from camps, villages, and so on), as people living permanently in one place in densities high enough to require the routine importation of food and other necessities of life."

And while every primitivist is going to say, 'yes, I am anti-civilization,' not everyone who is anti-civilization is going to say they're a primitivist.

Cindy: One of the things I like about cities is that lots of different people with different ethnicities and cultures and ideas are living in the same area and can learn from each other and share. And in my utopian world, if there were hardly any roads and food productions was done where roads had been, and we created a world that wasn't based on consumerism anymore, we could still live in some type of city, just not like any city anyone has ever seen before. Although sometimes when I talk about utopian cities with my sister, I think maybe I am just talking about some villages near each other, and not really cities at all.

Chris: I think what people love about cities, what I love about cities anyway, is that cities are gathering places, that they're places where we get to engage with other humans and see all the glorious, wondrous things that humans can do and make, because we're really amazing animals. But such gathering places existed long before cities did. I don't really think that there can ever be a sustainable city, truthfully, because to me sustainable isn't just something that doesn't damage, but is something that benefits. And cities exist for the sole benefit of one species, which is humans. Everything from what trees are left standing, because they look pretty, to what animals live there, because they're not able to be killed and used by humans. That's the difference between a city and a natural community. In a natural community, everyone thrives or everyone dies. I mean there's always going to be an ebb and flow, getting into balance as far as who's doing ok and who's struggling, and I think that dance is just part of life. But in a natural community if enough species aren't doing ok, the system collapses.

Cindy: So do we just abandon the cities then?

Chris: I don't think it's about just leaving the cities, because there are resources that can be used in cities. And there are lots and lots of people who have their whole lives set up in cities. I've experienced cities in such a way where I've seen areas with a lot of life, especially in cities where there are areas that have been forsaken by industry.

Here's something interesting, did you know that the area surrounding Chernobyl has one of the highest levels of ecological diversity than any other area in all of that region of Russia?

Cindy: You mean since after the nuclear meltdown?

Chris: Yes, after the explosion. And the reason is that no one goes there. Industry has forsaken the place. It's just been left alone and it's just become wild again. So I think there is something to be said for "abandoning" cities, but that kind of abandonment is just not exploiting the land anymore, not trying to suck it dry. So if people were interested in engaging in the actual land base that a city was built upon, and could engage in a process of rewilding with it, where it became more of a natural community, I think that would be hugely beneficial. But then, like we were saying, it sort of ceases to be a city. Because what defines it as a city is it needs to import resources for people to live there, and the population is so large that the land base just can't support it. So I think it's more of abandoning the ideological construct of a city, abandoning industrialism, rather than actually physically clearing out of the entire area.

I do think cities should be laid to waste in a certain way. I want the land to live again. And I want the people to really live again. Those two processes are intimately interwoven, and in cities, the land is not living, and in a lot of ways the people really aren't either.

Cindy: I was talking to a friend of mine about this today, and he was talking about statistics about people in the country use more energy than people in the cities, and there's so many arguments for how to create an ecological society within the framework of capitalism, and I just think we need to start from a totally different framework.

Chris: People talk about how we need to have wind power for our ecotopia, and we need to have solar power, but they're not really thinking about 'what exactly are we powering?' Those things are used to perpetuate industrialism, which is intrinsically destructive to the land base. Sustainability is on a spectrum, like obviously a bicycle is in a lot of ways more sustainable than an SUV, but a bicycle is made out of metal which is mined out of the ground. If we want to recycle the materials that are required to run a metal smelter which are destructive to the land, so bicycles can't truly be sustainable. So it's a question of making choices that are less destructive than others. But I think ultimately what we need to be looking for is what is going to benefit and not just what is going to harm less.

Cindy: I feel like a lot of white activists move to the land to escape from the pain of seeing so much failure in our organizing efforts, and then a lot of us romanticize a rural life as being this pure and politically better way to live. And then we have this lifestyle that may be less destructive, but we are abandoning this whole effort to actively change the world and work with people who don't have as much privilege as we do. That's one of the things I wonder about how to address within myself, and I also wonder how anti-civilization people address this issue.

Chris: I'm really inspired by land projects that are committed to having their community be a service to people who can't afford to live on land, and continually existing as a resource for people who have less privilege. And that's what a lot of people I talk to are interested in doing when we discuss doing land projects. But, a lot of people do just want to get away, and I'm not interested in shaming people for that. I mean, I want to get away!

Cindy: Me too.

Chris: There's a line from this Zounds song, Zounds were an anarcho-punk band who are contemporaries of Crass, they have a song called Demystification there's a line in it that goes "I'm not looking for escapism, I just want to escape," and I think that is totally valid. Why wouldn't you want to escape from this? This way of life is soul squishing and threatening to us on an animal, biological level. Yeah we want to escape. I think honoring that is really important. And I think that once that level of safety is achieved, and once we have a more whole, healthy, integrated existence, it is the natural next step to reach out to other people and to offer the resources we have to others, and to help others. But I don't think we can do that unless we already have a place of safety ourselves. It is SO difficult in the context of civilization to get to a place of safety. When you have a relationship to land it becomes a lot easier to feel more safe, more of the time, it becomes possible to feel sane. And I think that once that level of safety is achieved, and once we have a more healthy, empowered, integrated existence, it is the natural next step to reach out to other people and to offer to share our resources.

Cindy: How do you think that people who are disconnected from the natural world and the nature inside of us can regain that connection?

Chris: People started having coercive, dominating relationships with the land base with the advent of agriculture, and after that came patriarchy, then intensive forms of hierarchy including feudalism and slavery, then capitalism. It just grew and grew and grew and then industrialism came. That whole trajectory began when people stopped having empowered relationships with the land base and started having coercive domination relationships of power. So I think the key is to try, in as many ways as possible, to have relationships that are empowered, and relationships that are mutual, and that are egalitarian with humans and with non-humans. And to listen to the voices that we're not accustomed to listening to - like the voices of the land and of animals and plants and the ocean.

One of the premises of Derrick Jensen's book <u>A Language Older than Words</u> is that non-humans can speak and have always been able to speak and historically, humans could listen, but we don't anymore. Our culture has conditioned us to not listen anymore. When I read that book, and I started orienting more toward that view of reality, it just started happening everywhere. I couldn't get away from it. I was communicating up a storm with everyone. I stopped referring to plants and animals as "everything" and started referring to them as "everyone". Like I'd walk into a forest and I'd be this noisy human crashing around, and I'd stop and feel like, oh, wow, everyone's listening to me. And it was true. And I started interacting with non humans in really profound and interesting ways.

I asked Derrick at a talk once, what would be a conceivable role for humans in a sustainable natural community, and he just sort of narrowed his eyes and looked at me and said, 'Damn you.' He didn't really have an answer. He turned the question over to the audience first, and there was a very stock looking primitivist kid in buckskins, and he said 'I think may be eating berries and pooping them out.' Which is true of course, but I was looking for something a little deeper, so then Derrick said, 'I think may be singing... yeah, singing, try that.'

So then I started walking in the woods and just singing. I went down through one forest to the Puget Sound and there was a row of trees behind me and I sang this song for an animal that was swimming around, and then I listened and I could feel the trees behind me wanting more songs, so I turned around and sang a song to them. I felt purposeful. And I could feel the way that those creatures were communicating. Its how the energy changes and how I feel in my own body. Just that we are engaged in relationship.

Cindy: I remember when my sister started talking herbalism classes, and we were pretty punk, and she said that we had to thank the plats that we picked. She said it might seem kind of stupid, but we had to start doing it. So we did. And at first it did feel pretty stupid, but after about the fourth time, it just felt totally normal, like of course you would do that, like it would be weird not to. And it made me feel better. Not like I felt like I had to thank the plant for its sacrifice, not in some heavy spiritual way, but just in acknowledging our relationship. It's nice to feel that. And it makes it easier to pay attention to what's around me.

Chris: You brought up a really interesting thing right then, which is that it started to feel normal. And I think that's really our task in a lot of ways, is to start normalizing those experiences. Because it shouldn't feel abnormal. It shouldn't feel abnormal to have empowered relationships with non-humans, and I think that in this context, in this culture, it is. And that's something that has to change in a fundamental way.

Cindy: I think some people are introduced to primitivist ideas and they don't know how to bring it into their lives aside from becoming a hunter-gatherer in modern society, so I'm wondering if you can give some examples of other ways people can work toward social change, while embodying the ideals of primitivism.

Chris: The tactic that's rallied around the most in publications like Green Anarchy, which honestly, I wish didn't set the standard for anti-civilization thought, there are so many outlooks and analyses in that publication that I find so intensely problematic, and so racist and so disturbing. But unfortunately, at least in anarchist subculture, I think that's where a lot of people get their ideas about what it means to be anti-civilization. The tactic that's supported the most in Green Anarchy is insurrection. I do think insurrection is really important. I think it's really obvious that the power structures of this culture need to be dismantled, and unfortunately, the closest we ever see to this is Earth Liberation Front and Animal Liberation Front stuff. I think it is important to support that work, especially for those of us who have made the decision not to do that ourselves, but it's certainly not the only thing. And unfortunately, a lot of green anarchists act like it is.

I think another important example of anti-civilization political work is to support Indigenous resistance. These are the people who are still actively engaged in combat with civilization. These are the cultures that are actively being erased. Every indigenous language, every place-based language that dies, it's a battle that civilization won.

I recently was involved in a project helping some local indigenous women start a pirate radio station on their reservation, which is going to program almost exclusively in Lushootseed, their native language of which there are only a handful of fluent speakers left. That's an amazing project that I feel honored to have been asked to support. That's a vivid example of anti-civilization political work. Being an ally to indigenous struggle provides an opportunity to do really powerful anti-racist work, especially for white people, although I think honestly that people of all races have been exposed by civilization to some really destructive and fucked up ideas about indigenous folks.

There's the Earth Bound gathering in the Twin Cities (Minneapolis/St.Paul, MN) that is a free conference that's organized every year which is all about coalition building between native and non-native people. It's organized by anti-civilization folks in Mpls, who want to have empowered relationships with indigenous folks and who want to do earth-based organizing with them. The conference is based around discussions of cultural appropriation, racism, looking at examples of coalitions that have worked in the past, environmental defense, and primitive skills.

I think the work Derrick Jensen and Ward Churchill are doing is really powerful and is radicalizing thousands of people. Also, Twig Wheeler's Western Civilization Recovery work is really amazing. It explores the traumatizing nature of the dominant culture and offers tools for trauma reintegration (healing) to radical people.

As far as primitivism, talking again about the split between primitivism and the anti-civilization critique, one of my favorite things about primitivism is that it isn't really political. The practice of doing primitive skills is just the practice of learning to be human again.

Cindy: That's how I feel about it too. Sometimes I hear people glorifying these things, and I'm just like - that's just being human.

Chris: Exactly, which is something that ought to be glorified, really. Especially since we live in a culture that doesn't let us be human in so many ways. I remember the first time I butchered a deer, the person that was guiding me through the process said, "It looks like this is going to be an important part of you learning to be human again." Those words resonated with me so strongly, and I had this feeling inside when I was taking it apart, specifically when I was taking off one of its forelimbs, there's this way that you flick the knife into the armpit, and the flesh just separates in this way that's really fluid and really... really beautiful is the only way I can describe it. I did that and I had this feeling like I had done that thousands of time before, even though I was doing it for the first time.

I believe I have the genetic, ancestral memory of having quartered a deer. Humans and deer have had a predator/prey relationship for probably a million years, and feeling that in my body was so powerful.

I think that any practices that allow us to feel connected in that way are good things, and should be explored, and can be empowering on a deeper level than just feeling good. I think they can do a lot to help us reinterpret our ideas of community and communication and relationships.

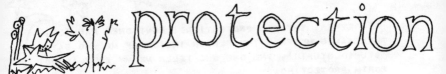

protection

THERE ARE PROTECTIONS THAT HAVE BUILT UP INSIDE OF
ME, VOICES THAT SOMETIMES FEEL LIKE OTHER PEOPLE ALL
TOGETHER. AND SOMETIMES SELF PROTECTION BECOMES
SELF DESTRUCTION. I NEVER GOT TO JUST HOLD HANDS, I
NEVER GOT TO JUST BE FRIENDS. ACTUALLY, THAT'S NOT
TRUE. ONCE I DID. JUST ONCE. WE WERE 14, AND WE
HELD HANDS, AND WHAT WAS GOING THROUGH HIS MIND IS
"THIS IS NICE. WE ARE HOLDING HANDS", AND WHAT WAS
GOING THROUGH MY MIND WAS "HOW AM I GOING TO TELL HIM
ABOUT MY FAMILY, HOW AM I GOING TO TELL HIM ABOUT
MY ABUSE, HOW AM I GOING TO TELL HIM ABOUT HOW I WANT
TO KILL MYSELF. DOES HE EVEN WANT TO KNOW? WHEN WILL
IT EVER BE THE RIGHT TIME? WHY DOESN'T HE ASK ALREADY?
CAN'T HE SEE? DOESN'T HE CARE?"

ONCE UPON A TIME I BUILT UP A PROTECTION INSIDE OF
ME THAT LET ME FINALLY FEEL MY BODY, LET ME FEEL
PLEASURE, LET ME FEEL STRONG. SHE WAS BRASSY AND
CYNICAL, SLUTTY AND SWEET. SHE FLIRTED AND PUT PEOPLE
AT EASE. SHE HAD CONTROL. SHE MADE ROOM FOR ANOTHER
PART TO COME OUT. THE PART THAT WANTED TOUCH. THE
PART THAT WANTED CLOSENESS AND PURE FEELING. THAT
WANTED TOUCH THAT WANTED LOVE AND CALLED THEM THE
SAME THING. THE PART THAT LOVED EVERY FLAW. THAT CRIED
FROM THE SHEER BEAUTY. TOGETHER THESE TWO SAVED ME.

♡   ♡   ♡   ♡   ♡   ♡

I NEEDED LOVE LIKE OXYGEN. I NEEDED ARMS AROUND
ME TO HOLD ME TOGETHER. I NEEDED SOMEONE TO SLEEP
NEXT TO SO I WOULDN'T BE SO SCARED. I NEEDED SOMEONE
TO THINK ABOUT TO TAKE ME OUTSIDE MY OWN FUCKING
HEAD. I NEEDED SOMEONE TO REMIND ME TO LAUGH. MOSTLY
I NEEDED SOMONE TO GIVE TO. SOMEONE WHO WOULD ACCEPT
THE LOVE I NEEDED TO GIVE, OR AT LEAST SORT OF
ACCEPT IT. I HAVE ALWAYS BEEN BETTER AT GIVING.
I AM MORE COMFORTABLE THERE. FEEL SAFER THERE. STUPID
STUPID.

Together, the two protections I mentioned earlier, they saved me from the person inside of me who says 'stupid stupid', the one who tells me my body is not worth protecting.

When I lived in Vermont, I felt like it was holding my hand. There were fields and trees and we tapped the sugar maples and boiled down the syrup to sugar. There were people doing all the right things, all the healthy things. And I felt like Vermont was holding my hand and it was saying 'this is nice' and I was thinking, "When are you going to ask me about why I cry every night, when are you going to notice that sometimes I fuck when I don't want to? Is it true that the world is so corrupted that we would go to war for oil? And how can everyone live their lives like nothing is happening, and what about all the people who have had way worse things happen than whats happened to me? And how am I ever going to change? How am I ever going to learn to have just one feeling instead of a million conflicting feelings all the time? When am I going to get the voices to shut up?

There were ideas about how to go about life. One idea was that you had to fix yourself before you could fix the world. One idea was that the world was going to shit so fast there was no time for internal work, just revolution now. One idea was that the two things informed eachother. That part of our inside problems were because of a lack of meaningful social change engagement. I went with that one.

What I liked about city was the spray-paint and anger, the promise of the empty lots. The ways people found ways to make meaning, the examples of neighbor-hoods where people actually lived as neighbors.

I LIKED BEING CHALLENGED TO WORK ON MY RACISM.
I HAD ALWAYS LIVED AROUND WHITE PEOPLE, AND ALTHOUGH
I DIDN'T LIVE AROUND PEOPLE WHO TALKED IN RACIST WAYS,
I WAS AMAZED AT HOW MUCH RACISM HAD SEEPED IN ANYWAY.

IN THE WOODS I HAD FELT LIKE MY PROBLEMS WERE MY OWN
AND THAT THEY WOULD GO AWAY IF I COULD ONLY ALLOW THE
NURTURE. IN THE CITY I COULD SEE THAT MY PROBLEMS HAD
A LONG AND COMPLEX HISTORY THAT WAS TIED TO ALL THE
INSANITY AROUND ME.

WHAT I LOVED ABOUT CITY WAS THE PUNK GIRLS. THE
SCREAMING ON STAGE IN A TORN PROM DRESS, THE SMELL OF
BODIES NOT PERFUME. I LOVED THE WAY THEY TOOK UP
PUBLIC SPACE, SITTING ON STREET CURBS, SITTING ON
NEWSPAPER STANDS, DRINKING IN ALLEYS AND AT RAILROAD
TRACKS. PEEING BETWEEN CARS WITH ONE GIRL AS LOOKOUT,
NAPPING IN PARKS, CURLED TOGETHER, DOG NEARBY. LOYALTY.

DRINKING WAS USEFUL FOR AWHILE. IT WAS A PROTECTION
THAT GAVE ME NEW THINGS. IT LET ME SIT CLOSE TO PEOPLE
AND QUIETED THE OTHER VOICES. IT LET ME TALK AND TALK,
AND IT LET ME FINALLY SCREAM. BUT WHEN IT WAS TIME TO
QUIT, I COULDN'T.

I DON'T THINK YOU HAVE TO CHOSE BETWEEN CITY
AND NATURE. YOU CAN BE AN URBAN ACTIVIST AND STILL
LEARN TO DEVELOP EMPOWERED RELATIONSHIPS WITH THE
LAND, WITH HUMANS AND NONHUMANS. AND WHEN YOU
MAKE THE DECISION TO DO THAT, EVERYTHING CHANGES.

WHEN I DECIDED TO QUIT DRINKING, IT WAS IMPOSSIBLE
FOR ME TO DO ALONE. AND IMPOSSIBLE FOR ME TO LOSE THAT
PROTECTION WITHOUT ADDRESSING THE OTHER PEOPLE INSIDE OF
ME TOO. I AM GRATEFUL TO THE CITY FOR OUR GOOD LOCAL
RAPE CRISIS CENTER AND THE GREAT COUNCILING THEY HAVE
THERE. AND I AM GRATEFUL TO THE COUNTRY FOR BEING THERE
STILL, WHEN I WAS FINALLY READY. BECAUSE IT IS TRUE.

IT WILL NURTURE YOU. IT WILL HELP YOU BECOME HUMAN
AGAIN. THE DIRT. THE BIRDS, THE WEEDS THAT ARE FOOD,
THE SECRETS THAT COME TO YOU IN YOUR DREAMS, THE SILENCE
AND THE QUIET CREEKING NOISES. THE FEELING THAT YOU
WILL NOT FREEZE OR STARVE. THE FEELING A PART OF. NOT
SEPERATE.

I MADE FRIENDS WITH MY PROTECTIONS. THE VOICES INSIDE OF ME QUIETED. AND THEN ONE LEFT. SHE LEFT ALL TOGETHER. AND TO THINK OF IT MAKES ME CRY. SHE WAS THE ONE WHO NEGOTIATED HUMAN TOUCH. THE BRASSY ONE WHO HELPED ME STAY INSIDE MY BODY. AND I KNOW IT IS GOOD, BUT FOR NOW I FEEL LIKE I WILL NEVER BE ABLE TO LET ANYONE TOUCH ME EVER AGAIN. IF SOMEONE TRIES TO HOLD ME, ALL I CAN DO IS CRY OR TRY NOT TO. CRY OR TRY NOT TO.

THAT'S WHAT I THOUGHT ANYWAY. BUT THEN LAST WEEKEND I WAS IN A DIFFERENT TOWN, WATCHING JESS MIX TOGETHER VEGAN CUPCAKES. HER TINY GRINDER GRINDING UP THE FLAX SEEDS, POURING IN THE BAKINGPOWDER, LAUGHING.

THERE ARE SOME PEOPLE WHO REMIND ME OF SOME WAY I WAS ONCE. SOME PEOPLE WHO HAVE RESOURCES INSIDE OF THEMSELVES THAT I WISH I HAD HAD. THERE ARE SOME PEOPLE WHO FOR WHATEVER REASON, EVERYTHING FEELS CLEAR WITH. IN THE PAST I COULD NOT TRUST THAT FEELING OF CLEARITY, BUT NOW I CAN. AND WHEN SHE WAS LOCKED OUT OF HER PLACE SHE CAME AND SLEPT BESIDE ME, CURLED UP TOGETHER, SIMPLY. THIS SIMPLE THING I THOUGHT I WOULD NEVER HAVE.

punk women
over 30

this is an interview I did for a zine Quinn was putting together about punk women over 30 . The first question was something about identity, but I can't remember exactly the question.

Cindy Crabb. 37 years old. I identify as a woman, but sometimes I pass as a guy. I am white, with sort of a Finish and Minnesota upbringing. I'm an anarchist, feminist, punk, queer, writer, singer, survivor.

Tell me a little about your identification with radical and/or DIY culture. How did your radicalization come about?

There are a lot of things from childhood that helped form my politics. To really talk about how my radicalization came about, I'd have to write a book. First I was just a kid who loved people and loved nature and the world, and didn't want the world to end in nuclear war. When I was a pre-teen I didn't fit in at all, as a teenager I became a freak, a vegetarian, a poseur (that's what the punks called us), an atheist. I was introduced to feminism when I was 17, and it was when black women and other women of color were talking about how the white liberal feminism didn't speak of their experiences, and I loved a lot of those theorists - Angela Davis, Bell Hooks, Audre Lorde. Then when I was 18 I found out about anarchism, and soon after that, started studying about revolutionary movements and social ecology. Years later I became a punk.

I love punk and diy, but it's not where my politics come from. I fell in love with punk, in the early 90's, for a few reasons - it was the only place I saw girls who were just really not going along with what girls were suppose to be. There were punk girls who wore the most fucked up ugly stuff and were fucked up and not hiding anymore. There were punk girls screaming on stage and playing music. There were punk girls who were writing theory and craziness all at once. And girls who danced for their own rage and friendship. Punk was the only place I saw that allowed women to be angry, and angry together, and find strength in anger.

Also, I fell in love with punk because I needed family, and acceptance, and I liked the way some punks stuck together, and didn't expect each other to be perfect. It felt real. I never had any delusion that punk was some pure thing that would fix the world, or that punk was a cohesive identity. My politics came from somewhere else, and I never saw punk as a very effective place to do the kind of politics I am interested in. But a lot of the people who did the kinds of political organizing I liked, didn't live in ways that made sense to me, and had much more hidden and corrupted emotions.

I grew up with belief in people, a basic understanding that people had to fight for what they believed in - like I grew up during the Anti-Apartheid movement, and the Central American solidarity movement, and our church was part of the sanctuary movement, and harbored El Salvadorian refugees. Our minister went to jail for harboring refugees.

I grew up in a violent household, and was sexually abused when I was a pre-teen, and I grew up knowing that people could be very good people, and do very terrible things. I learned the ability to see different sides of people and to always be struggling to understand what would turn good people into monsters, and what could bring them back.

I bought into a lot of sexist crap and self-hatred and suicide and girl-hatred and the constant need for male approval. The "Courage to Heal" came out, around the same time that I was starting to learn about radical feminism, and I started looking at my abuse and how and why it had been ignored and how it affected me.

One of the things that really inspired me about anarchism was the way it talked about changing every aspect of humanity, including the ways we viewed friendship, work, leisure, sanity and action. I liked the revolutionary call to make every minute of the day useful, and to have real conversations with people instead of just time-wasting conversations. I liked the challenge to try and get to the heart of people and things. I liked the promise that we might be able to rid ourselves of neurosis. I felt a reason to live when I found out that it was possible to struggle for fundamental change and not just reform, because the world was just too terrible for me to feel like reform was enough.

I started working at the Institute for Social Ecology, and was part of the Youth Greens, and the protests against Wall Street and the first Gulf War. But mostly I was terribly shy and thought I was stupid. I read a lot though, and dedicated myself to learning as much as possible.

Can you describe your current community? How has that changed over time?

I'm not sure what my current community is. It has changed a lot over time. Lately, I'm feeling a real need for a solid geographical community. But I do love the punk community, and it was pretty nice to be able to go just about anywhere in the country and find the punks and have somewhere to stay probably, and people who were possibly interested in similar things, or at least who I felt like I knew what to expect from, and knew how to communicate with a little bit. A common language.

I've lived in Asheville for 11 years now, and defiantly have a community of friends there. They are people I like and who support me in many ways, and who would probably take care of me if something terrible happened, but I'm not 100% sure of that, really, I'm not even 75% sure. No one's ever really been there for me in total times of need, except my sister. I am not the greatest at letting people close to me, but I know there are a lot of people who care about me in Asheville, and that feels good.

I also defiantly have some community of sorts with people who read my zine and write me letters.

Mainly though, I am really looking forward to working on building a community of people who are just my neighbors and people I live around - not cultural community. I think both are important.

In what ways does your community sustain you? In what ways do you see room for growth?

My community sustains me by being nice to me, and loving me, and helping me remember to not isolate myself, reminding me that relaxing is important. And by sometimes working on projects that are inspiring and pushing me to think in new directions, and challenging me to work harder in different ways. I wish more people were doing more inspiring things. There is too much lethargy and not enough passion and hard work and critical thinking. Too much drinking and hanging out.

Also, I do usually feel like I could fall off the face of the earth and no one would notice for a long time. I don't know if that's their fault or mine, but it's probably mine, mostly.

What is your experience with visibility/ invisibility, as you have gotten older?

I love getting older. It is by far the best thing that has ever happened to me. I feel much more visible. I used to feel objectified all the time. I also put out a lot of sexual energy. I didn't really feel safe being friends with people. I remember one day, when I was about 33, I decided to make stronger boundaries, stand further away from people, not flirt, and there was a huge shift in the way people dealt with me, and a frightening loss of power, but it also felt so amazingly great.

Also, I feel kind of smart now. When I was young, I always felt stupid and inexperienced, and like I had to pretend to know things, and like I didn't know anything. Now I actually do know a lot about a lot of things, and it's funny and nice. It's still hard to believe sometimes. I have finally had the time to work thought a lot of family stuff, a lot of abuse stuff, a lot of self-hate stuff, a lot of a lot of stuff, and I don't want to kill myself, and it doesn't feel so helpless, and I feel like I really have things to offer the world, and not like I am just trying to make sense of things and break silences so I don't go crazy.

Getting older has taught me to become calmer, more centered, stronger, more efficient and more balanced. I trust myself. These are all huge things that I thought would never happen to me.

How has your experience with health, sex and sexuality changed as you have gotten older?

I have been really lucky with health, although my body is defiantly more sore and creaky. As far as sex and sexuality. Sex was a huge part of my life, like really huge, and sexuality was confusing and dramatic. When I tried to come out when I was a teenager, you pretty much had to be straight or gay. If you were bisexual, then you "had one foot in the door of heterosexual privilege" or you were just a "fence sitter" or just experimenting. I did not feel welcome at gay events. I wasn't able to give up my need for relationship, since I got so much of my feeling of self-worth from being loved, and I was scared about being no good at sex with girls. It was really confusing.

I pretty much dated men my whole life, I had a couple girlfriends and a couple one-night stands with girls, but it was mostly guys. I always hoped some day I would be brave enough to just date girls.

Now, I'm at this place in my abuse healing, and in my life, where I just really don't want to have sex, and don't feel weird about it, and am just so glad to not have to think about it all the time. It makes me feel so much more at ease in the world, and I am excited about it.

Would you talk a little about "compromise?" What it means to you, and to what degree you are making them in your life?

The political tradition I come from doesn't have a rigid dogma about how we're suppose to live, it is not a lifestyle politics, and it is focused on how we need to have a multiplicity of tactics and we need people with access to all different tools and specialties to be doing revolutionary politics and to be bringing revolutionary ideals into all different areas of our society. So I don't really feel the feeling of compromise, like some people I know do who built their political identity around lifestyle and personal choices. I've had a certain amount of privilege (I didn't grow up rich, I started working when I was 13, and didn't get to go to much college, but I did luck into a pretty good and flexible job), and have been able to structure my life in a way that allows me integrity.

I don't work a whole lot. I've lowered my standard of living so I don't need as much money as some people do. I think I make about $8,000 a year. I would like to own a house, and am at the point in my life where I might try and actually work more so I can do that. Sometimes I think about trying to go back to school now, and become a therapist or something, and that feels

a tiny bit like compromise, because it's not my first choice of what I would want to do, but I think it's important work, and so I'd feel ok with it.

I think it is really depressing when I see a lot of older punks and activists, white men especially, who are very purist in what they will involve themselves with, and who see anything outside of our subculture as compromise. I think they are selfish and not dealing with the realities of their privilege.

How are the compromises you are making related to your level of privilege?

I don't feel like I'm making compromises. I am still totally dedicated to social change, and my privilege helps me because it gives me more time to do this.

What are your relationships with older women in your life? How about with younger women?

I didn't have hardly any older women in my life until pretty recently. I didn't really have my family in my life until last year, and it's been nice getting to know my grandparents and one of my aunts. It's good. They have traditional expectations of me, but it's nice to talk with them about history and about grief and things like that, and also to get an insight into "normal america".

I also have started going to women's AA meetings, and the main one I go to is almost all older women, and it is just so great to see older women. To be in a room and get to really look at older women when they're talking, and see the wrinkles, and the ways faces change, and the things that are supposed to be covered up, the things that are supposed to be ugly, and just really looking and finding these women so beautiful. I mean, there is just so much there in the faces, and in their experiences. I really wish I'd been around more older women earlier in my life!

I am mostly around younger women, so I'm not really sure how to sum up my relationships with them. I suppose I try and really meet everyone on a level ground. Like, just because I have been around longer doesn't mean I know more. I know more about some things, but younger women have a lot to teach me too. I like it. I like the exchange. Sometimes young people make me nervous because there is so much pent in energy a lot of times, and because I want to make everything better, or they have really strong opinions that I don't always totally agree with, but I give people space to make their own discoveries. I don't try and push my point of view. I just sometimes say what my experience has been, or I just leave it alone.

Do you have children? Do you want children or to help parent children? In what ways does your community support/ not support that?

I would like to have children I think. I never did before, but recently I've been thinking about how much my mom liked raising us when we were really little, and I've been thinking that I might really like it too. But I'm not sure if I will actually have children. I am about to move in with my sister and her partner, and so for the first time it seems possible, because I know they will always be there for me, and they would want to help me raise kids.

I think my community is supportive of children, but not in a really consistent way. I actually really don't know if they are or not.

What role models have you, or do you currently have?

My sister, my mom (before she started drinking really heavily), some of the women who were involved in the underground women's health and abortion movement of the early 70s, Emma Goldman, Grace Paley, Audre Lorde, women writers around the world.

Were you ever someone who traveled or relocated a lot? How has that changed over time?

I don't feel like I was much of a traveler, but I did live in a lot of places, and drove around the country a few times. I also used to get restless and hitchhike places. I had a 90-pound German Shepherd, and I stopped hitchhiking when she got too old. I've always wanted to find one place to settle down, and then to be able to go and live in different places for a few months at a time, but still have a home to go back to. This is still what I want. Now that I've been all over, I don't feel the need to explore so much, but it is still nice to go other places, get out of ruts, and get new perspectives.

What are your feelings on "home?" How do you envision that for your future?

I have a funny relationship to "home". Since I have moved around so much, I call home anywhere where I've stayed more than one night. It's ridiculous. But, I am planning on moving to rural Ohio with my sister and her partner this year, and buy land, build a house. What I want is a place to never have to move from again. A place where I can work to make dreams possible. To plant and to still be there to see the plants come to fruition. I want to have a place where I can start an Anarchist Summer School if I want to. And a place that can be a sanctuary for my friends, especially when they're in times of need.

How do you make a living or sustain yourself?

I'm a weaver. I work for my aunt who is a fashion designer for very rich people, and I weave fabric and scarves for her. It is not a profession I would do if I had to market it. I hate marketing. Sometimes there isn't enough work, and I do something else, like wash dishes. Also, I have a little side business sewing skirts. I try and volunteer on farms, and get some plants or food from the people whose farm I help out on. I sometimes dumpster food, and get clothes out of free boxes. I do a little construction work every once and awhile.

What projects do you work on?

I write a zine called Doris and also edit a zine called Support. I'm in a women's health group, and also in a punk band. Those are my main projects.

Do these two things intertwine? Are they kept separate on purpose, or are you trying to meld them?

I do keep them separate on purpose. I like weaving, and it's sort of meditative. I really hate trying to figure out ways to make money, and sucking up to store owners. I think it's great if people can make money from doing things that are politically fulfilling, but that's just not what I do. I've considered trying to write for money, but it never really appeals to me when it gets right down to it. I feel like there's only so much writing time in me, and if I'm doing it for money, I probably won't write the things that really mean the most to me. I have a friend who writes for money, and it helps her to write more in general, so I know it's different for everyone.

Do you have a spiritual practice?

I never did until recently. I was in therapy a few years ago, after my mom died and I was drinking like crazy and also a lot of abuse stuff was coming up. I have always thought I was crazy, and a lot of times thought maybe I had some kind of multiple personality thing going on. My therapist worked with me a lot on all these different voices inside of me, and it sort of developed into a weird type of spirituality I guess. I talk to these parts - and I don't know if they are parts of me, or if they are some kind of collective conscious, or spirits or gods or what, but mostly they feel like parts of me. I talk with them every morning, telling them thanks for all the ways they have protected me throughout my life and asking for help in getting though the day. If I'm having a really crazy feeling day, I sit at my alter of special things, and try to get grounded and talk with whatever inner person is having a hard time. It's a lot about learning to be embodied, listening to the voices instead of pushing them away, comforting the parts of me that need comforting, and reassuring the parts that are harsh and mean, and telling them they don't need to be so hard. I also take a lot from dreams. Sometimes I ask my inner teenage boy to visit me in my dreams (it's not really always my inner teenage boy, sometimes it's embodied in different ways, but it's the feeling of wholeness, the feeling of being loved). Every night I thank them for helping me. If that is a spiritual practice, than I guess it is.

Can you talk a little about how your spiritual practice is or is not supported by your community?

I don't talk about it all that much, but when I do, people are pretty interested. I think it is an especially useful for people who are healing from trauma, or have been split off in different ways because of abuse.

What brings you satisfaction? What do you feel passionately about?

Writing, walking around, real conversations, cooking, women's health, supporting abuse survivors, abortion, girls and trans people screaming their heads off and finding their anger and power and strength, breaking silences, thinking deeply about how to organize and change the world, learning, creating underground cultures of resistance.

What are your fears? Also, what are your fears about the future?

I've had a lot of people die, and I don't want anyone else to die who's close to me. Sometimes I worry we won't have the money to get by in the world. And I worry that all the people from NY will move to Ohio when global warming wipes out the east coast, and then the water supply in Ohio will be over taxed and there'll be riots, but I try not to worry about that too much. I worry lately that I won't be able to figure out how to have a baby. But mostly for the first time in my life, I don't worry too much. I feel pretty solid.

What do you hope for the future? What do you want to create? In your daydreams, what do your 50's, 60's, 80's look like?

I want to have a permanent home, and maybe a couple kids. I want to have time to write a few books, and to become a public speaker. I've always wanted to have a school sort of like the Institute for Social Ecology, which was a summer program that taught anarchism, feminism, appropriate technology, community health, theory, alternative agriculture, etc. Sometimes I think I would still like to do that, but in a way that would be more accessible to poor people. But maybe I'll have just a writing retreat, or a summer teenage girl and trans rock and roll camp. Or maybe I'll figure out some ways I can be effectively active in anti-racist work. And sometimes I think I'll work on starting an abortion and women's health clinic in my new town. I just know that I want to work really hard, and be around people working really hard, and that's pretty much my dream for the rest of my life.

How do you feel like your community is preparing for old age? How could we?

I don't know. I know some people are getting better jobs, and working on getting health care. One of my friends is going into social work so she can start a nursing home for gay and queer and trans folks. My sister has become an herbalist to help people with their health issues.

Mostly I don't know anyone who's preparing very much. I do think that when we have a larger community, and a lot of friends, that we'll all be able to help each other as we grow older. I think one of the big problems with getting older in america is the isolation, and families not wanting to help their older people.

I think ideally, some of us would have land and houses, and have knowledge to offer to younger people, and younger people would come to our places for sanctuary and learning, and they'd help out with things we couldn't do as much any more. I think we have to really commit ourselves to stay connected to a larger community of people of all ages as we grow older. We have to build lives based on mutual aid. We have to not become bitter and crotchety. That's my advice.

q is for

QVILTS

one of the most beautiful art forms + almost impossible to ever actually finish! I have so many little tiny cut out squares, log-cabin, star pattern, crazy quilt. bags of fabric old favorite shirts, a bag of silk ties, my dead moms old clothes, scraps I've forgotten the meaning of, all hauled from house to house, collecting mold, getting washed + aired out, cut a few squares and pack it all up again for another few years.

the one quilt I did finish is what I recommend for new quilters. cut pretty big squares, like 10 inches. sew them in strips. you can use them as curtains until you get enough for a whole quilt. It will be beautiful

Quinoa

Weird magic grain, kind of shaped like mini-UFO's. I think it's really great and am not just putting it in here because it's one of the only things that starts with Q.

To cook quinoa, first rinse it thoroughly to remove a sort of bitter outside flavor.

Boil 2 cups of water, add one cup quinoa + a little salt. Bring it back up to a boil, turn it down to a low simmer, cover and then cook for 15 minutes.

Eat it with sauteed veggies on top, like in place of rice or couscous.

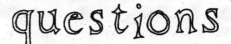

questions

1. WHAT DO YOU WANT TO DO MOST?

I want to sing at the top of my lungs
in a rainstorm. catch hail in buckets
and roll stones on my tongue. I want to
whisper soft songs of encouragement in
your ear, songs that will unravel the
tightly wound strings that mess it all
up in there.

I want to pull down the world of desks
and yawns, exhaust and celebrity gossip,
forced numbness, forced boredom, forced
meaningless nothing what's the point -
I'll tell you the point. there is beauty
inside of you, in your scars, in your
heart, in your wrinkles, in your protection,
in your disguises, in your honesty, in
your truth. You are capable of things
you haven't even imagined.

and it is true. we can change it all.

I want a new puppy. I want shoes that
don't stink. I want fingers soft from the
hot water of canning the tomatoes you grew.
I want fingers strong from typing, strong
from pulling burrs out of kimbas fur.

I want to watch meteor showers holding
hands, to overcome my fears, let them go
with a sweet goodbye. I want to see
dinosaur bones, eat blackberries right off
the vine, cut my lip, scrape my knee, pull
out splinters, kiss you.

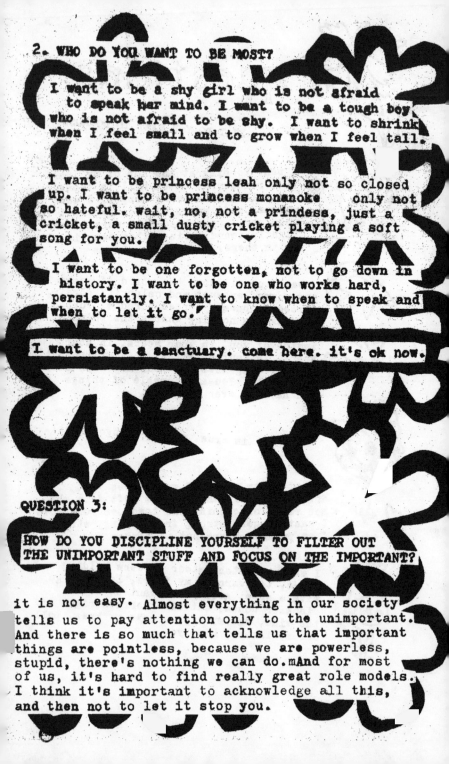

2. WHO DO YOU WANT TO BE MOST?

I want to be a shy girl who is not afraid
to speak her mind. I want to be a tough boy
who is not afraid to be shy. I want to shrink
when I feel small and to grow when I feel tall.

I want to be princess leah only not so closed
up. I want to be princess mononoke   only not
so hateful. wait, no, not a prindess, just a
cricket, a small dusty cricket playing a soft
song for you.

I want to be one forgotten, not to go down in
history. I want to be one who works hard,
persistantly. I want to know when to speak and
when to let it go.

I want to be a sanctuary. come here. it's ok now.

QUESTION 3:

HOW DO YOU DISCIPLINE YOURSELF TO FILTER OUT
THE UNIMPORTANT STUFF AND FOCUS ON THE IMPORTANT?

it is not easy. Almost everything in our society
tells us to pay attention only to the unimportant.
And there is so much that tells us that important
things are pointless, because we are powerless,
stupid, there's nothing we can do.mAnd for most
of us, it's hard to find really great role models.
I think it's important to acknowledge all this,
and then not to let it stop you.

If we take ourselves seriously and we examine our lives with attention and care, we become more focused and our lives become more vibrant, full and satisfying. It's true.

I remember reading the autobiographies of revolutionary women to try and see how they did it - like Assata, Angela Davis and Elaine Brown.

I read interviews with writers and tried to copy their habits, but everyone works differently and everyone needs different things.

For me, part of what I needed to do was to look at what I'd learned to survive. and what things were still useful and which parts did I want to change. It is a slow change, the unlearning of a lifetime, but worth it. I promise.

Part of the filtering out of the unimportant stuff has been the slow filtering out of the voices. The voices that say I'm worthless, that all I'm good for is my body. and the deadness inside me that says 'what's there to be curious about?' conform. don't ask questions.

Part of becoming focused was first allowing myself to dream, and to believe that my dreams were real,

reachable

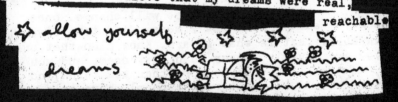

✫ allow yourself
dreams

Allow yourself to dream. What would you do if you could do anything? without fear to stop you. Part of dismantling capitalism racism and patriarchy is learning to let ourselves dream.

so here is what I do. Make a list of everything you wnat to do in your life, even if you know you can't do it all. It can be a long list or a short one. Even if it seems impossible, write it down.

like
learn Spanish, Mandarin and Russian, open an old
dog retirement home, open an abortion clinic that

treats women with care and respect, have twin babies
learn about gardening, solar panels, composting
toilets, learn to talk about politics without getting

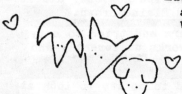

muddled or defensive, open an
anarchist summer school,
write books, go to that city
that has waterways instead
of roads, hold tight to
the people I love, learn
to form close friendships,
pass as femme, become a
public speaker,   write zines until I die, start
a publishing company, get a printing press, learn to
make paper, learn to dye yarn with natural dyes,
make my lungs stronger, stretch more,
make a new punk yoga video, learn to
play the guitar, become a therapist,
become a teacher, open a writing retreat

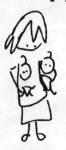

center, build a tree house, build a
brick oven, learn about local organizing
learn about canning and food preservation
form a dance troupe, dance more, write
a rock opera, learn to do a head spin,
talk to strangers, live.

know that your list will change. once
mine maybe said - sail the 7 seas, find true love -
changable. that is what we are. Know also that our
lives are usually longer than they seem, and you
can do more than you think, no
matter what people have told you.

ok.

so put that list somewhere you
won't see it. hide it somewhere.
hide it from yourself. or hang
it on the wall, whichever.

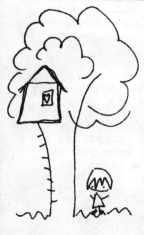

then make yourself a plan for the
next 5 years. The five year plan
can be magical dreaming, like -
escape my hometown, move to the
ocean, with crashing cliffs and
crashing waves, dig clay and
become a potter.

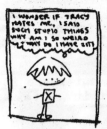

the five year plan can be vague, like - travel a lot and see what there is to see.

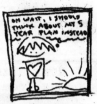

it can be concrete, like create a cooperative child-care center in my community.

it is good to have something to think about that is far away, and a long range goal to work towards.

I am good at dreaming, but sometimes it is the daily life that is hard. My mom once told me "fake it til you make it" and it sounded terrible then, but truthfully, that's sort of what I do. my sister has the same strategy too. We work on the little stuff, the practical stuff. She plants seeds and when the plants come up, there's that feeling of hope. she makes medicine and helps people heal. i write this little zine, type it out to you. this daily stuff that keeps us engaged, keeps us involved, keeps us thinking, keeps us fighting for a whole new world.

so even when I have no motivation and no hope, I just look at my 5 year plan and try and figure out what the fuck to do next.

When my motivation is really sucking, and my head is full of distractions, I make a list every night before I go to bed. The list says what I should do the next day. This way, when I wake up, I already know what to do. I try not to make it too complicated, or too much. just enough so that when I start to get distracted I can look at the list and do one of the things.

also I swear by getting out of The house first Thing in The morning and going for a walk to clear your head and keep focused

I think it is important to read books that are challenging or educational so when the unimportant thought come up, you can redirect your brain to think about new ideas instead.

sometimes...

sometimes the obsessive, seemingly unimortant
thoughts are really trying to tell us something.
Maybe it is a fear we're afraid of facing, or a
loss we're afraid of mourning.

sit down with it, speak to it, find out where it's
coming from, be gentle with it, let it go.

I make one year plans too - with small projects
that I can achieve - like put this zine out twice
a year - and if I only manage to do one, I try not
to beat myself up about it.

also on the one year plan there's some inside things
to work on. This year it's learn to slow down. learn
to stop caretaking.   they are hard things.

In the past there has been inside lists like-
work on jealousy, work on self-nurture, stop
gossiping, stop apologizing for being alive,
learn to raise my voice, learn to value women's
friendships, work on setting boundries.

and some things maybe I'll never be able to fix,
like no matter how I try, it seems like I'll
probably never be able to say No. but I can
work on the things around it - prevention and
self-forgiveness, and may bæ I can figure out ways
ways to keep myself safe despite my limitations.

it is important to push yourself,
but go easy on yourself too.

Know that whatever it is you have been doing to survive deserves recognition and honoring, even if you don't particularly like it or if it's

not serving you well any more. Know that if you are alive right now, you have been practicing self-defense. you have pathways in your psyche that have kept you in some ways safe, and they deserve thanks. also, it is hard to change all at once, so take what you can from how you've been surviving so far, put it in your pocket for reference.

and sometimes it seem like a spiral to me. sometimes it seems like I repeat the same mistakes over and over, relive the same bullshit and never learn a thing, and if I think about it that way it becomes so hopeless,

but if I think about it in this other way, it makes more sense and I think it's truer - that there's a spiral like a spring that is the pathway out of entrenched ways of being, and you travel up the

spring and you hit sections that are similar to what happened on the spiral below, but hopefully you have more tools each time, and at some point you just fly by without even noticing or getting stuck.

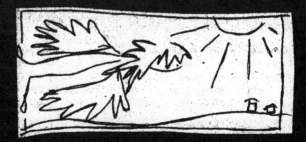

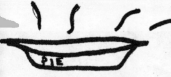

WHAT IS YOUR FAVORITE COMFORT FOOD?

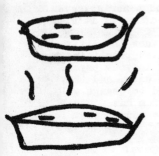

my mom's famous pumpkin pie,
honey buns, and something else
I'll tell you at the end of the
story.

When I was little, my mom
was a gourmet cook. Not at
a restaurant but just in
our own home. I mostly liked
grilled cheese sandwiches,
so I didn't appreciate it all that much,
except that she did make some good sweets.

On special occasions she'd make Honey Buns
for breakfest. She sing some sort of edited
down version of a song from the musical
South Pacific, and she'd say, "ugh, I know
it's terrible, but when you make the HoneyBuns,
you have to sing the HoneyBun song."

They were not gourmet. I think it was melted
butter, melted up with honey and powdered sugar
and may be vanilla, and then Pilsbury crescent
rolls cut into slices instead of peeled apart
and rolled. You put the honey sugar concoction
into muffin tins, put the Pilsbury dough on
top, bake itup, flip it over, eat it up, freak
out and bounce off the walls.

Once, one of the times when we didn't have
enough money and we weren't allowed to answer
the phone because of bill collectors, mom
decided to start a catering business. All us
kids helped her, cutting tiny slivers of
vegetables, turning radishes into beautiful
roses, baking sheet after sheet of pastries.

We worked a few parties for this lady who
was the cousin of Dear Abby. Us girl children
were all dressed up in maid costumes, and we

brought around the hors d'oeuvres, politely
lifting the platters up to little huddles of
finedressed adults who were either sweet to us
or pretended like they didn't even see us,
which was a signal that they didn't want any.
Rich people. It felt like a privelege to be
invited into this world, even if it was just
to serve them.

We worked for other, less exciting people,
but I remeber the Dear Abby lady the best.
and my mom was always very forthcoming with
recipes. she stored them in her head and
wrote them down for anyone who wanted. All
except for her famous pumpkin pie. She
would never share the secret of that.

Until I moved away. One time I got ahold of
her on the phone and she said to me
"You know that pumpkin pie? The secret is
that it's just the recipe on the back of
cans of Libby's pumpkin." Just buy a frozen
pie crust, she said. they're actually really
good.

I hardly ever remember to make pie, and I
can't always find the paper with the honeybun
recipe, and sometimes what I think will be
comforting is macaroni and cheese, and it's
true, it's not too bad. Ice cream can't hurt
either. but my secret comfort food these
days is something I never thought would
happen. It's greens, cooked up boiled untill
they're melt in your mouth done, add a
little vinegar, a bit of sesame oil, and
some tamari, and sesame seeds. A big bowl
of that, sitting wrapped up in blankets in
my warm bed. It makes me feel the best of all.

WHAT DO YOU REMEMBER MOST ABOUT YOUR MOTHER?

I wish I could lie and say some sweet memory.
something about her commit ment to alternative
education, and what a good teacher she was in
those years when she taught. how she believed
so strongly in the goodness of all the bad kids,
and how they became so well behaved with her.
you could see their faces and the way they held
their bodies so tense, and under her gaze, they
soften. love.

but like anyone else who was close to me who died,
my strongest memories are the ones of the last
time I saw her. not the hospital times, because
those are mostly blocked out and fuzzy, but I mean
the last time I saw her, which was maybe a year
before that, and she was finally happy, after a
decade of suicidalness, but even happy, there was
such brokenness in the way she moved. I remember
the liquor smell of her, and the careful way she
stood, the stilted steps of walking across the
street to the beach. When I wake up after a hard
day of work and my joints hurt, I remember this
vision of her.

she looked like a hurt bird.

something I wanted to hold gently in the palm
of my hand, but everyone had said I couldn't save
her. which I suppose was true.   not on my own
anyway.   not just me and my sister.

There were so many messed up feelings
after she died. so many things I'd
never gotten to say, so much unresolved
shit. I felt like how would I ever be
able to find resolution.

this has been the biggest surprise, ·
after these 7 years, and all this
hard work, suddenly I mostly feel her
with me, without the memories. and it
feels sweet, and a little bit sad.
but mostly resolved somehow, in ways we
never could have figured out in lifetime.

#6:
DO YOU HAVE ANY SECRET HABITS?

when I feel especially ugly I like to wear my tiara. when I feel especially lonely I put on a purple or yellow prom gown. when I feel especially bad at everything I get out the chain saw and cut shit up. I mean, only if there's a wood stove somewhere that needs firewood.

I like to chop the wood and make a nice tall wood pile.

it feels like such an acomplishment and so useful.

when no one is around, I listen to new country music.

when I can't get out of bed in the morning, I lay there + play with my collapsible flower toy

sometimes I prune back my mustache so it's not quite so big

I kinda like hello kitty band-aids

I like to put on my new hat leslie made me and pretend I'm a bear

I download cheesy books from my library + listen to them when I'm working

I guess my biggest secret habit is that I pray. Not to any all knowing God and not to any culture I've stolen. just to something, to some part inside me or to whatever force gives me ESP with my sister

249

books

QUESTION 7:

What have you read that makes your heart swell up the way doris does for me?

★ _Cruddy_, and _Freddy Stories_, by Lynda Barry

Annie John and _At the Bottom of the River_,
by Jamaica Kincaid

♡ _The House on Mango Street_ by Sandra Cisneros

The Bean Trees and _Animal Dreams_ by Barbara Kingsolver

The Gangster We Are All Looking For,
by Lê Thi Diem Thúy

Enormous Changes at the Last Minute, + ♡
Just As I Thought, by Grace Paley

Firebird: A Memoir, and _My Alexandria_, by Mark Doty

Zami: A New Spelling of My Name, and _Sister Outsider_
by Audre Lorde

Trash, _Bastard Out of Carolina_, and _Skin_
by Dorothy Allison

The Girl. by Meridel Le Seur

Stone Butch Blues, by Leslie Feinberg

"How To Have No Fear", by Euh-ha Paek

Assada: An Autobiography, by Assada Shakur

Last Standing Woman, by Winona Laduke

China Men and _The Woman Warrior_, by Maxine Hong Kingston

Papa, You're Crazy, by William Saroyan

Love Medicine, and _The Last Report on the Miracles at Little No Horse_, by Louise Erdrich

Housekeeping, by marilynne robinson

Betsey Brown, by Ntozake Shangé.

Ceremony, by Leslie Marmon Silko

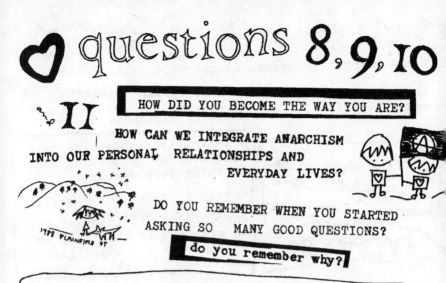

♡ questions 8, 9, 10

II

| HOW DID YOU BECOME THE WAY YOU ARE? |

HOW CAN WE INTEGRATE ANARCHISM
INTO OUR PERSONAL RELATIONSHIPS AND
EVERYDAY LIVES?

DO YOU REMEMBER WHEN YOU STARTED
ASKING SO MANY GOOD QUESTIONS?

1998 PLAINFIELD VT

do you remember why?

Before I found anarchism, I asked myself a lot of
questions, but not always the most useful ones.
I asked myself Why couldn't I get my mom to stop
drinking and what was wrong with me, why did no
body love me, and why couldn't I get my dad to
stop being so angry. Why couldn't I fix it all.

BOOKS!
i read a lot

I ran across ideas like atheism and
vegetarianism and how fucked up war
was and how fucked up beauty standards
were. I asked myself what was Fair and
what was Right, what was Good and what
was Bad.

Some of the questions were good. Like, why did
the suburbs suck so bad, why did people live like
this? Why did everyone just do all the normal,
boring, robotic things when there was a whole
world out there full of something, somewhere,
there had to be something worth living for.
And why were people so shallow? Why were they so
mean? What were they looking for or not looking
for? What did we need?

I had no real framework to put my questions into.

they floated around between self-righteousness and self-hate.

mostly self-hate.

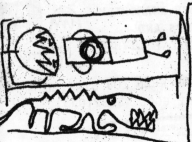

a protective, defensive hate that kept me from being able to think very deeply.

mostly I looked for a savior, a soulmate, someone to complete me, to distract me, to give a shit about me, to reaffirm what I knew, that I was no good at all.

I found feminism first. I took a Woman's studies class, and it helped me to start to see my life within a political context. Like I wasn't Bad because I wanted male approval - that was a normal response to all the bullshit that had been drilled into me since childhood. That was part of what patriarchy was about.

and the extreme isolation and silence kept most of us from being able to find ways to effectively resist.

Feminism gave me the first inklings of a new world, and a new self I could be in that world. but may be because most of the feminism I saw outside the books was a mainstream reformist feminism that didn't really speak to me - the voting campaigns and Take Back The Night rallies - I took feminism into my personal life, but didn't see the possibility of living in a non-patriarchal world.

but that is when I started to ask myself better questions.

Like, what did I want? and where did that desire come from? and why did I think in terms of good and bad. I looked back at the

lessons I learned from childhood - the stories I read and the lives I saw around me, and I started looking critically at the messages I was bombarded with from movies and billboards and wondering how would I feel if I wasn't bombarded day and night with all that shit.

I started asking myself what was it I hated about women and being a woman, and where did that come from, and how did it kill me and how did it keep this sick culture running smooth, and what would happen if I looked to my girlfriends for

the support and self assurance and comfort that I tried to get from sex. I started asking about the effects of abuse and why didn't my mom protect me, and those questions led me into an inquiry into the life she lived instead of just blaming her for it. I started looking at how the world had changed in the last few generations, how she had been silenced, how she'd had her spirit killed. and what did it mean politically that I was able to name my abuse when a generation before me it was an unspoken secret.

I started asking these questions because the only other option I could really see was suicide.

I learned about the courage of the people who had
come before me, and I asked myself how could I
help create a world where the fight against

silence could go beyond naming. How could I help
create a world where everything was different?
How could I start to tell the truth about my life?
I studied and learned that change is possible,
despite the deadly repression, despite the heroic
failures, change is still possible.

Not all these questions came at once. I was
so tangled up. It was like a crack in the
surface, the beginnings of being able to think
instead of just go. For me, feminism was the
beginnings of integrating anarchism into my life-

because I think real feminism is anarchism at
its best.

and that part of making change is asking
questions. all the time questions. good
questions. finding the right questions is
half of it.

Anarchism showed me a vision of a world I hadn't
been able to imagine. One where true equality
and freedom could be real, and ways we could get
there, and why it was possible and even if I
wouldn't see an anarchist utopia in my lifetime
working along anarchist principles was the most
ethical and most fulfilling way to live.
Anarchism showed me that there were people out
there willing to risk it all, willing to try and
live a true life rather than the fake lives we
are forcefed.

so how to integrate it? may be first you have to
define it. What does freedom mean? Free from
someone telling you what to do? or free from the
bonds that have been pounded into us. How do
you unpound something so insidious? How do you
start to make cracks?

You need to **live with intention.** take yourself
seriously but know that you are not always right.

a lot of times there is no right or wrong. Learn
empathy. If you are too empathetic, learn to not
be a doormat. These are both hard things to learn.

If you jump to conclusions and **always** have
something to say, **take a breath** first, think about
what the other person has said and what it might
feel like to be them and if you have any questions
that could clarify or draw them out.   If you
don't talk much because you are afraid, take a
breath, know that not talking won't save you, and
blurt it out. If you are friends with people,
talk about the changes you are trying to make in
yourself. See if they want to help you learn these
things, and if there's anything they want help
with.

Friendship should not be a way to
pass the time, a way to kill time,
a distraction. Friendship should
be a beginning place for the
revolution.

Prioritize friendship. don't get sucked into the
isolation of just being a couple or wanting just
truloveonepersontoreallyunderstandyou. don't force
someone to be monogamous, don't force someone to
be non-monogamous. If your loved one is sick or
hurting so, bad, prioritize them. Know the
difference between self-righteous politics and
a politic of compassion and love. But prioritize
friendships. Talk to your friends about your **hopes**
and dreams and fears and secrets that you usually
save for your lover. Let them close to you. Commit
yourself to them. Move to maintain friendships,
not just to maintain relationships.

Don't let yourself become bored. If you are bored,
there are things that need doing. If you involve
yourself in projects - even volunteering with
unperfect organizations, you at least keep your

foot in the door that is trying to
slam shut on a life worth living.
Keep doing things. Don't let the
dogmatic anarchopolice get you down.
Don't argue with people who aren't
interested in real dialogue unless
you like that kind of arguing.

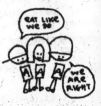

Try to find people who are real and ready and not
so scared as all of that. (but also know that so
many of us are so hurt and we need to know how and
why to trust).

If you can't find people, keep looking. Know that
they can appear in strange places under unexpected
guises.

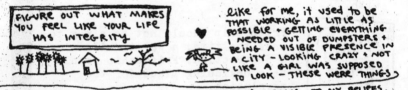

FIGURE OUT WHAT MAKES
YOU FEEL LIKE YOUR LIFE
HAS INTEGRITY

like for me, it used to be
THAT WORKING AS LITTLE AS
POSSIBLE + GETTING EVERYTHING
I NEEDED OUT OF DUMPSTERS +
BEING A VISIBLE PRESENCE IN
A CITY - LOOKING CRAZY + NOT
LIKE A GIRL WAS SUPPOSED
TO LOOK - THESE WERE THINGS
THAT MADE ME FEEL LIKE I WAS LIVING ACCORDING TO MY BELIEFS.
IT MADE ME FEEL MORE TRUE TO MYSELF, WHICH MADE ME MORE
CAPABLE OF WORKING ON THE OTHER PROJECTS - LIKE WRITING +
ORGANIZING.   I STILL DO THOSE THINGS, BUT NOT AS ADAMANTLY.
NOW I LIKE TO HAVE A COMPOST PILE THAT'S ACTUALLY DECOMPOSING
+ NOT JUST ROTTING, AND I LIKE TO TRY + CONNECT WITH
PEOPLE OUTSIDE THE PUNK SCENE TOO. THESE THINGS GIVE ME
THE ENERGY + GROUNDEDNESS + INSPIRATION TO KEEP FIGHTING +
WORKING   ♡ ♡ ♡

don't let other people's
dogmatic politics influence you too much. Don't
do things because you think that's what you
have to do to be accepted (but if you do, forgive
yourself. It is what we all want, acceptance).
Learn to trust yourself. Ask for help. Reach
out. Let people in. Set boundries.

Try not to over commit yourself. Do what you
say you're gonna do.

Learning to work in groups can be totally
challenging and is totally essential.
There is so much we are forced to confront
inside ourselves when we try and work with
people collectively.

and when we do the work, and everything comes
together and your group moves like one amazing
creature - you feel the feeling of what a new
world could feel like, and once you've felt that
feeling, you can never truely give up.

so...

Start groups. study groups, bands, community
groups, potluck groups, childcare groups
(even if you are not one with children, most
parents need some breaks), health groups, men's
groups, self-defense groups, anti-racist action
or education groups, queer groups, dance troupes,
art collectives, political theater groups,
political theory groups, prisoner support groups,
Don't expect everything to last forever. Don't
expect groups to be easy. Honor the good things
and learn from the crap. Have a written down
set of beliefs and guidelines for your more
serious groups so you can hold people accountable
who are being unethical - I mean so you can kick
out disruptive authoritarian shit-bags. And if
people are shit-bags, don't give up on anarchism
itself. there is just a lot of sickness and a
lot of brokenness out there. Keep looking for
good. Keep fighting.

Forget the difference between work and leasure.
This is how we have learned to section up our
lives. work time, leasure time, work time,
forgetting time. oblivion. Find things that are
political but fun too to do when you aren't
working for the money or doing more difficult
political work. Make political or beautiful art
and walk around the neighborhoods with your
friends putting it up. Help build community radio
stations, help a farmer with their harvest, learn
to can food. Learn to share. Talk to strangers.
You have nothing to prove. Spend time with people
who are older than you or younger than you. Spend
time alone. Read books.

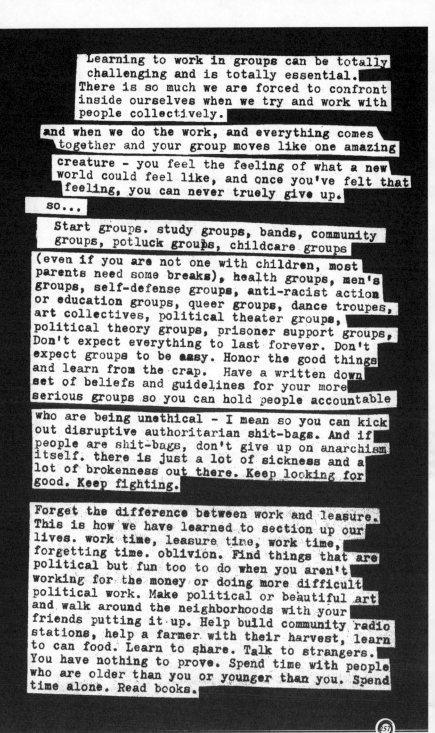

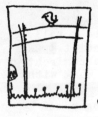

and every day.......

write down at least one beautiful thing
you have seen or felt or heard. and tell
someone. even if it's just someone
inside yourself.

♡ ──────────────────────────── ♡

definition of anarchism, written by Kropotkin
for the 1905 Encyclopaedia Britannica:

"...the name given to a principle or theory of
life and conduct under which society is conceived
without government - harmony in such a society
being obtained, not by submission to law, or by
obedience to any authority, but by free agreements
concluded between the various groups, territorial
and professional, freely constituted for the sake
of production and consumption, as also for the
satisfaction of the infinate variety of needs and
aspirations of a civilised being."

Living My Life, by Emma Goldman

The Free, by m gilliland

anarchist books
I have loved ♥

Anarchism: A Very Short Introduction, + *Anarchy in Action,*
by Colin Ward

Anarchy: A Graphic Guide, by Clifford Harper

*Anarchism, Marxism, and the Future of
the Left,* by Murray Bookchin

Woman On The Edge of Time, by Marge Piercy

Anarchism,
by Daniel Guerin   *The Dispossessed,* by Ursula LeGuin

Free Women of Spain, by Martha Ackelsberg

Ya Basta: Ten Years of the Zapatista Uprising, by Marcos

*The Modern School Movement: Anarchism and Education
in the US,* by Paul Avrich

quitting

quitting drinking was the hardest thing I've
ever done. I had no idea it would be so impossible.
it was kind of embarrassing, kind of humiliating. It
seemed like once i decided to quit i should just be
able to do it. it was hard to see why it should be so
hard.

I never really heard anyone talk about it. like maybe
i'd heard people say -"i quit drinking for a month and
now i feel so much better and now i'm gonna get wasted.'
and i'd heard people say -"i used to drink a lot and
now i just drink a little." and i'd seen people try to
quit and fail and i'd seen people leave the punk scene
to quit and i never saw them again. but i never heard
any one talk about the way i was feeling - like i
wanted to just drink a little but most of the time
ended up drinking forever. and i was tired of the
person i'd become. i was sick of being a shitty friend
and saying mean things to the person i loved and
not being able to move forward in any way because i
was so stuck in the cycle of picking up the peices.
i never heard people talk about having every intention
of not drinking, but then not knowing what else to do
when a feeling came up - good or bad feelings. not
knowing how to be around people at nighttime without
drinking. not having any friends who didn't drink,
and how patronizing it felt when they would offer to
not drink around me but how i couldnt be around them
if they were drinking. and the total humiliation of
months of swearing -"this is the last time. never
again." and then a week later there was another last time
promise. and then what's the point of even trying i
obviously cant do it. and what's the point of living
because i dont want to keep living like this.

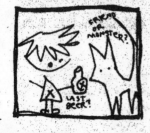

i doubted myself and my intentions
i couldnt get out of bed half
the mornings and i couldnt get
my writing done. everything took
forever. i'd given up on a lot of
my dreams because there wasn't time
becasue so much time was taken up
with drinking and hangovers.
i didnt trust myself any more.

i didnt start drinking until my mid 20s. which i
realize now is kind of weird. it didnt seem that
weird at the time, because even though a lot of
my friends drank and a lot of them did heroin,
i was also friends with some sweet little straight-
edgers. it was before straight-edge turned crazy and
anti-choice and violent jock style holier-than thou
jerks. at least it hadnt turned that way in my hometown.
so not drinking was weird, but not unheard of, and i
knew about alcoholism and what it did to you.

    i knew my mom was alcoholic and i knew i didnt want
to be like her - the way it made her happy at first
but then so crazy and so needey and so needing me to
take care of her instead of the other way around.

the way i didnt feel like i could trust her. the way
i didnt feel like i could count on her. the way it
took the vibrant sweetness of her and turned it into mush.

and i'd read that as a child of an alcoholic i'd turn
into one the minute i drank. and i didn't want anything
to do with drugs because my step-brother said he didn't
remember doing what he did to us - the incest stuff -
because he was too fucked up on drugs to remember.
later when he was in treatment he wrote to tell me
that wasn't true. he did remember. he was sorry. but
it didnt end up keeping him from doing it again. i
think i still wanted to believe in some way. i still
blamed it on the drugs.   growing up in a house of
denial i gained some pretty weird coping skills.
like just thinking everyone was crazy and strange and
not really recognizing drunk or high unless people
were falling down. so i didnt really drink, just a
couple times - uneventful times - except actually the
first two times i enjoyed sex after a year of doing
it i was a little bit drunk both times. i didnt
really make the connection then. i thought it was
magical connection and love.

i started drinking for reasons. i was tired of feeling
so cut off from everyone - so separate from other
humans. and i watched drunks and punk/expunk drunks
in the bayareacalifornia and they had
something i   wanted.

they hung out in a group all the
time like community like family. the
girls were crazy looking and angry
sometimes and they could loose control
and still be safe. there was a group to
hold them up and carry them home.
i wantd that. i practiced drinking
alone in my garage or with my sweet
friend Ulla who i wish i had just
confessed my love to instead of
talking crazy boycraziness, because i
had learned a true fact which was
gay girls hated semi-gay girls who made passes at them.
which wasnt true at all and now just sounds rediculous.
i will confess it to you now. ulla, you were the best
of anyone i met and you still inspire me and i loved you
then and istill love you. forgive me for being such an
idiot.

i started drinking for reasons

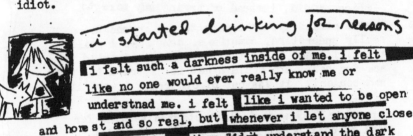

i felt such a darkness inside of me. i felt
like no one would ever really know me or
understnad me. i felt like i wanted to be open
and honest and so real, but whenever i let anyone close
to me they didnt get it. they didnt understand the dark
parts the hell parts the hurt parts. at least not in the way
i needed them to understand. i needed the darkness to be
seen and not just talked about once and then pushed away.
all the time when i was laughing i felt like i was faking.
i falt like all over the place were people living these
seemingly happy existences, and how could they not see
the deamons eating away our insides. the drunks seemed to
be well aware of the deamons. not in denial. feeding
them the only way they knew how. i needed that.
i needed to stop pretending. i needed those parts
of myself seen and recognised and not
pushed away. i needed those parts of myself
brought to the surface,
normalized, celebrated.

and they were.

there were i think 4 years of drinking sometimes and not sometimes. where it wasn't a big deal but getting bigger. 2 years of giving into it entirely. learning acceptance. accepting the fucked up things i did half the time when i was drunk.

i learned to be angry. i learned to be not so hyper-self-critical. i learned to be a shitty friend. sometimes. sometimes a good one.

i learned to sing. i learned to dance for my own self. i learned the feeling of being in it together- the feeling of family, of community.

i learned new kinds of self-loathing. i learned defensive shame. i learned to start using my history of abuse as an excuse for the shitty things i did, instead of trying any more to

behave ethically, or trying to get anyone to really understand. sometimes. sometimes i still tried. i tried to quit and i couldn't. i tried to ask for help, and couldn't get it. i tried to quit and couldn't. it was out of control. i was. it was.

i remeber 1999 when i first started wanting for real to quit or at least cut way back. and i came up with crazy ways to try and do it. like trying to count how many beers it took before i blacked out - because maybe if i just didn't black out things wouldnt be so bad. but of course, no matter what kind of scheme i had for counting, it didn't work. duh. funny

and then the plan was - wake up at 6 or 7 pm, when everyone else is starting to drink, because i never liked drinking in the mornings. so if i woke up then, i could get a bunch of things done, and then b y

the time i really wanted to drink, the stores would be closed, and then they didnt open until 6, so that

only gave me 3 hours to drink before bedtime.

plus   it was hard to find people to drink with at 6 am.

usually

it was kind of a funny game, but not really so funny.
because the truth was, i couldn't fucking stop. i had
no control over it. i could make fun of myself and
i could embrace it, but i couldn't quit. and i did
a lot of things i regretted. there were a lot of things
i wanted to change. like #I, i didn't want to have
sex anymore when i didn't want to, or with people i
didn't want to.

so for 7 years i tried everything. i won't bore you with

the litany. and there were periods of time, whole years
even, when i gave up   trying to quit. but it
was always on my mind. my failure. the knowledge that
i couldn't do it alone and i couldn't find the kind of
support i needed. i didn't know what i needed.

i knew about alcoholism, but i thought it
should be different for me.

its ok now
monster

i went to an amazing therapist for 3 years
but i lied to her about my drinking. so we
never talked about that. but we talked about
other things. and she taught me to make friends
with the darkness feeling inside myself. she
taught me to find a name for it. to ask it what
it needed instead of trying to erase it. she
taught me to forgive myself - not just in my

brain, but with my whole body. to forgive myself for
the ways id protected myself.   and for everything.

she taught me that even though the weight i felt on
me was put there by other people, that no one else was
going to be able to take it off. no one or nothing.
i was going to have to let it go - to remove it myself.

she taught me about the mean voice in my head, the
self destructive voice. the one that made me do things
that i didnt really want to. she said it was a
protector that had gotten kind of twisted up. like
the no face monster in the movie Spirited Away.

i had to talk to it gently and explain to it calmly
that i knew it was trying to help, but that i didnt
want those strategies any more, and could we try
something else instead.

i moved to a dry county.
i didnt have a car.
as long as i didnt go to town,
i didnt drink. as long as i
wasnt around people, i was fine.
maybe i could have
lived like that forever,
but it wasnt the life i wanted

in the end. after i had tried everything to quit and
still couldnt and still couldn't get out of the traps i
was in, ‾   there was a straw that broke my back.
something terrible i said. it was no more terrible than
things i'd said before. no that's not true. it was truely
terrible. and i knew that i would be this way forever
stuck. shitty. sometimes funny, but forever? this same
stupid shit? in the end i went to aa.

i know. you are probably sighing. not this. fuck not
this. that's what i thought too. fuck. not this.
and there are things i like about aa and things i dont
like, and sometimes it is terrible and intollerable,
and sometimes it is totally inspiring. but the truth
is, nothing else worked. without it i don't think i
ever would have gotten sober.

what i like about it is being around older women who
have been sober for a long time, and hearing about how
they did it, how they keep doing it. and hearing the
stories again and again of people who were sober for
a long time and then one drink one drink more and a
year or a lifetime of drinking floors them. i need
this reminder.

because i know that is how it would be for me too, even
though i try to trick myself otherwise.

and i like the model. how you pick a
woman who has a bit of sobriety and who
has something you want   some way of
being you want to strive towards, and
you ask her to mentor you. i like
mentorship. i think it should happen
more often in all different kinds of ways

WILL YOU
HELP ME?

and i like the mixed gender meetings too.
the way it is one of the only places i
have heard men honestly and humbly turning
to other men for help. and thanking each-

asking for help =
almost impossibly
hard thing
for me to do

other without any weirdness. and thetruth of the feelings.

and the ways that even when people don't like eachother,
they can work in groups together without their personal
bullshit getting in the way.

and theway so many of these people, all these normal people
they talk about thefeeling of darkness inside themselves.
the hole inside that needs feeding andcan't be filled. the
feeling of never feeling ok. neverfeeling real.

at first i hated it mostly. i thought most of the people
were neurotic and stupid, and i couldnt do all the things
they told me, and talking about drinking made me want to
drink more, i drank and lied about it, and i thought this
was my last hope and it wasn't working. give up give up.
but i kept trying.

i keep trying. it has been a year a a half now. and
at first it was pure hell. but already it is so much
better. the clear way my mind feels, the solidness i
feel inside. the way i know what i need and what is
not so good for me. and how i can actually be there
for my sister instead of empty promises. how i can
actually be there for myself.

and the dreams i'd given up on are coming back to me.
and are realizable. the dreams are real. and i know
how to make them come true.

r is for raccoons

Right to the City

Right to the City is a great organization that works to fight gentrification and to "halt the displacement of low-income people, LGBTQ, and youths of color from their historic urban neighborhoods." Members are "committed to doing political education and leadership development with their membership bases; and engaging in place-based struggles that protect low income communities of color." They are an alliance of groups in various cities – including Boston, Los Angeles, DC, New York City, San Francisco, Providence, and Miami. They are an excellent organization to get involved with and to support!

ONCE WE HAD A PET RACCOON WHICH WAS THE COOLEST THING EVER + IT WAS SO WEIRD TO SEE WHAT IT KNEW INSTINCTUALLY AND WHAT IT LEARNED BY WATCHING + WHAT IT HAD TO BE TAUGHT. IT KNEW ON ITS OWN TO CLIMB TREES, GET NUTS, CRACK THE NUTS OPEN TO GET INSIDE. IT WATCHED US OPEN DOORS + IT FIGURED OUT HOW TO CLIMB UP ON THINGS + THEN LAUNCH ITSELF OVER TO THE KNOB TO GET IT TO TURN. IT KNEW TO HUNT GRASSHOPPERS IN THE TALL GRASS DOWN BY THE HIGHWAY. BUT IT WAS TOTALLY UNINTERESTED IN WATER. ME AND MY SISTERS WOULD GO SWIMMING BUT OUR RACCOON WOULD JUST STAY ON THE SHORE, FAR FROM THE EDGE OF THE WATER. NO AMOUNT OF COAXING WOULD BRING HIM DOWN. WE HAD TO DRAG HIM IN, OVER + OVER UNTIL HE REALIZED HOW GREAT IT WAS + AFTER THAT HE'D JUMP IN EVERY CHANCE HE GOT ♡

Rubyfruit Jungle

I think this was the first lesbian, working class novel ever. I know it was the first one I ever read and it was so funny and mindblowing. Rita Mae Brown now writes cat mysteries, co-authored with her cat, but back in the Rubyfruit Jungle times, she was part of one of the first radical-feminist collectives.

I love reading about late 60's early 70's feminism, and recommend Daring to Be Bad: Radical Feminism in America 1967 - 1975, by Alice Echols. It's so inspiring and also just really bizarre the amount of shit they had to deal with both from the outside world and each-other as they struggled to change the world and to figure out what it meant to be a revolutionary and to be a human being.

Sometimes I think me and Robin speak two different languages. She says "Do you think people will ever voluntarily change and start living sustainably?" In her voice is accusation. Her voice says I am an idiot if I answer anything other than no. No I don't think people will change,
but I think Yes.

Maybe we are talking about two different things. May be she is thinking about the tiny percentage who own the media and own the government and have the power to shape our collective imaginations and our visions of what is real, and the power to command guns against any resistance. I don't really think they'll give it up either.

But I am thinking about my neighbors in Laurel, one of the most economically depressed rural areas in America, and how one of the daughters left and came back with a grant to try and help turn things around. She was hosting a series of workshops in the community center about how to bring sustainability to the area now that the family run tobacco farms were failing. The workshop I went to was on raising oyster mushrooms.

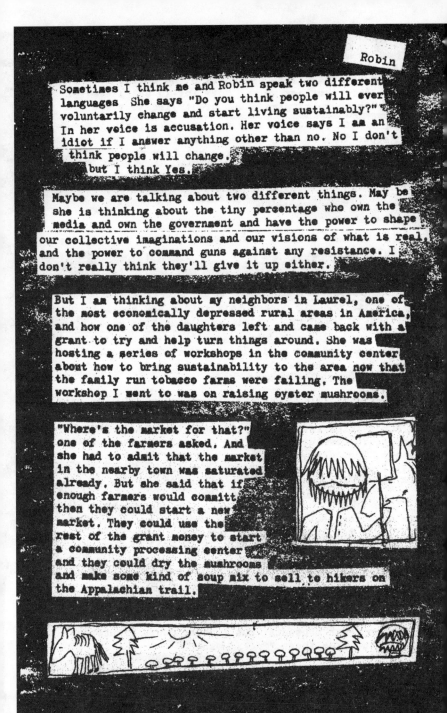

"Where's the market for that?" one of the farmers asked. And she had to admit that the market in the nearby town was saturated already. But she said that if enough farmers would committ then they could start a new market. They could use the rest of the grant money to start a community processing center and they could dry the mushrooms and make some kind of soup mix to sell to hikers on the Appalachian trail.

Most of the farmers faces were a mix of sadness and disgust and anger and scepticism. -- Where's the honest work in that? Is this the best we can hope for in our lives? catering to these strangers who are trying to prove how strong or how conscious they are by walking along the ridgetops that we have called home. These do-gooders who buy locally made soup mixes but look down paternalistically on the people in the world who make everything. Catering to that?

Is this the best dream and the best solution we can come up with?

There was anger and there was resignation and desire for something different. an answer to an unarticulated question. and despite the big screen televisions and the all-terrain vehicles, I think most people want something else. but if the solutions just stay within the capitalist framework, and the radicals are so full of dogma they don't know how to relate or how to be real, then what.

Dora Maria, from the Nicaraguan revolution said

"I don't think revolutions are made by totally ordinary people. We revolutionaries are visionaries to a certain extent. That analysis might not be very formal, nor very political, but it's true."

I believe that most people want. They laugh too loud, they buy too much, they hate what they're told to hate. they want to be part of something but they don't know how to get there, or even if there's a there worth getting to.

like the guy sitting next to me on the plane who was on his way to a new job interview. He said "I went to a few anti-war protests, but I never could figure out what to do from there."

Like when the snow falls three feet overnight
in Minneapolis, and everything's shut down
except people's faces, which are bright and
happy, looking eachother in the eyes, shoveling
eachother out. Meaningful work. helping.
finally some meaningful work.

I think people are dieing for meaningful
work. I think people are desperate for
meaning. and the lengths the ruling class
has to go to in order to keep us passified is
a testiment to our continuing desire for
true freedom.

Dora Maria says "The process of the revolution
itself created the conditions that made it
possible to break with the past."

Yes. I tell Robin Yes, I think people will
voluntarily change.

Robin says "I don't think you should fly out
here. Do you know what a big carbon imprint
planes make?" and I say "How about if I off
a businessman first. Those fuckers fly every
week."

and when I get to her after car, plane, bus,
ferry, bus. I climb into her truck and match
my hand to hers. lips on ear. lips on throat.
"I'm glad you're here," she says.
this language we share.

Robin says "this is not political," as she
touches my ribs and I grab her in handfuls
and we crawl together into nest-warmth-heat-feeling.
political. yes. political I say, because this is
what it feels like to be alive full in the body
    heart beat to heart beat alive beyond hope.
    I want everyone to feel this much,
    this sweet.

"Hope," she says, "Hope is nothing but denial."

but I think hope is like a crush.
not the resigned hope, like - i hope things
get better --- but the hope that feels like
suspended disbelief. where spaces open up
and everything is possible again, and
you're pushed to adventure, pushed out of
your regular boxes, pushed to show off,
to be the person you want to be the most,
working hard to show your best sides, your
secret scars, your hidden dreams.

hope is like a crush, making things as
beautiful as possible even knowing you'll
get hurt.

it won't sustain you, not like the hard
work of love will, but it pushes you
beyond what you thought you were capable of.

i am not optimistic, but hope, yes, hope.

S is for

sloths

Me and Dan Herman used to talk about sloths a lot. We liked to talk about animals that had weird symbiotic relationships with each other, like how some kinds of moss grew on the sloths fur that helped the sloth by keeping it camouflaged. We also liked how it lived in the trees and never came down, except about once a week to take a dump. We lived in a warehouse down by the river. My mom had just died Dan was inventing windmills out of dumpstered wood and dumpstered motors. We didn't go out much. It was late fall. An old friend of mine was going on speaking tour, talking about mental health stuff. I thought it might be nice to go along. There were good things about it and not so good things. I drank too much and gave myself a stick and poke tattoo that said "never give up," except I had twisted my arm around while I was doing it, so when I look now, the part I see says "ER GIVE UP." I really have to crane to see the NEV part. In Philly we were supposed to stay at this long time squat. The charismatic pirate radio dude there was a guy I knew from a long time ago who had raped a friend of mine and I was sworn to keep confidence. I called a pen pal who I referred to as my benefactor, since he had sent me $75 dollars a couple times, which to me was a fortune. He came and rescued me. I was so freaked out by everything. I was freaked out by the way he could buy gas with a card in the gas machine and never have to even have human contact with an attendant or anything. I was freaked out by the movie we watched about privileged kids who have graduated from college and don't have any motivation or direction. I was freaked out by how nice he was and not sleazy at all. I was not used to someone offering me safety. In the morning we went on a walk. It was freezing out, the first snow of the season. We walked through a cemetery and across the street was the Philadelphia zoo. I know zoos are fucked up, but I wanted to go. It was just a small thing, so out of place. I wanted to be around animals. For the longest time I stood at the sloths. I had never actually seen one before. Two huge creatures, holding upside-down to a strong tree limb, so close together. One of them would move its hand forward. It would take about 5 minutes just to lift and place it back on the limb. The way they moved was the slowest, most beautiful thing I had ever seen. The sloth. My hero.

s is also for These amazing authors + books STONEWALL, SURVIVORS GUIDE TO SEX, SANDRA CISNEROS

"Nearly all the survivors I have worked with report having had sex when they didn't want to. It's almost as if this were taken for granted; unwanted sex becomes such a given for survivors that many hardly notice it any more."

"Sometimes there are a number of seemingly contradictory feeling happening in your body at once. You may feel sexually turned on in your hops and vulva, and feel pulled away in your chest.... What do you do then?

Actually, experiencing contradictory feelings is familiar territory for most survivors. Consent then becomes a matter of distinguishing what sensations are what." -The Survivors Guide to Sex (consent and boundaries chapter)

"Survivors are not alone in needing to heal sexually. Our culture leaves little room for people to develop healthy, integrated sexuality. Almost from birth, girls are given mixed messages about their sexuality. They are alternately told to hide it, deny it, repress it, use it, or give it away. The media flaunt sex constantly as a means of power, seduction, and exchange. As a result, most women grow up with conflicts around sex. For women who were abused, these problems are compounded." - Courage to Heal (the chapter in changing patterns: sex)

 SC8 etc.

Talking about sex can be really hard - when we were ever taught to talk about it? What language do we use? How do we not feel embarrassed? But really, it is our bodies, it is our lives, it is something that's supposed to be cool and fun and amazing, and why shouldn't we talk about it?

It shouldn't be the responsibility of the person who was abused to initiate conversations about sex.

Spacing out and flashbacks: talking can help. if she looks like she's not present, ask. you could ask her to open her eyes, (don't demand it. just something like "I wish I could see your eyes," or "are you here?") sometimes just a voice can bring us back. sometimes not. it is good to stop or slow down if you are not sure where she is. sometimes you can come up with a code word, like "ghosts" because some people cannot say stop and cannot express what's going on. please don't overreact. don't press her for information. don't feel inadequate. what is appropriate will vary. Sometimes she may want you to leave her alone. sometimes she may want to stay with the flashback and open it up so she can gain information about the past. sometime she will want to be in the present.

You can talk about what, if any, kind of help she might need to stay present. Maybe she needs to say out loud that she wants to be in the present. maybe she needs you to say her name or to tell her who you are or maybe to tell her a story of something simple and nice, not sex related, that you've done together lately. The spiral down can make us forget that there were even nice simple times or any feelings other than fear and helplessness.

When things come up, it can be really important to talk about them again when you're not in bed. You can say "I know you couldn't talk about what was making you so scared and sad last night, but I do really care and really want to know. do you think you can talk about it now?" maybe she'll say yes, maybe she'll say no.

you can say, "It was confusing when I asked if you were ok and you said "I'm fine" but you didn't really sound fine and I didn't know what to do. What should I do when that happens?" maybe she'll say - yeah, she actually was fine, just trying to bring herself back into the present and she was glad you didn't stop and that you trusted her; - maybe she'll say, - yeah, actually, she was saying fine to be cynical, and she's glad you noticed, glad you stopped.

you can say "Do you like it when I _____? I can't tell." maybe she'll say - I want to like it but it makes me feel weird. - maybe she'll say - it's triggering, but I'm trying to work through that trigger. - maybe she'll say - I don't really like that, I just didn't know how to say anything.

If you are courting someone, sleeping with someone, thinking of getting in a relationship with someone, always assume that they could have been sexually abused. Know that for many sexual abuse survivors, even ones who love sex and are aggressively sexual; there will very likely be a period of time when they don't want to have sex. Think about whether you are willing or able to be in a relationship that isn't sexual. It is totally sucky to be an abuse survivor, be emotionally dependent on someone, be having a time of serious abuse triggers, try to set boundaries, try to say you don't want to have sex for awhile, and then have that person freak out or threaten to leave.

If you are willing to be in a relationship that isn't always sexual, (even if you love sex) then it could be a good thing to remind the one you love that if they ever don't want to have sex, it's totally ok.

Every abuse survivor has different needs. They may want to touch you but not be touched. They may want to be touched but not touch you. They may want to have really wild sex. They may want to start over as if they were a teenager and learn to just make out without going all the way. And everything may change at any given moment.

"Your experience of sex can change within a single relationship as well. With a new lover, there's often a passionate rush that obscures problems. But as the relationship settles, sexual issues may need attention again. As you risk more emotional intimacy, you may start to shut down sexually. Or you may find that as your trust grows and deepens, you heal on a deep body level, surpassing even your own expectations.

Because it takes a long time to heal sexually, you may wonder whether you're making progress. But even though the process has ups and downs, you are headed in the right direction. If you are putting steady, consistent effort into developing a fulfilling sexuality, have patience, accept where you are, and trust your capacity to heal." - Courage to Heal

terrible. What happen

The first time I ever told the truth about the abuse I experienced, I put all these qualifiers first - saying it wasn't rape or anything, wasn't as bad as what had happened to other people, it was just being touched while I was asleep, and watched while showering and things like that.

The person I was telling it to said "Never compare it. Everyone I've ever met tries to invalidate what happened to them by saying it was worse for someone else. What happened to you was real. What happened to you was terrible. What happened to you counts. Don't belittle it."

This struck me so strongly. I had never believed that I deserved to feel as fucked up as I did about what had happened. That night I practiced writing in my diary, just writing what had happened without any qualifiers, just writing it over and over and finally letting it carry the weight and the pain that it actually did.

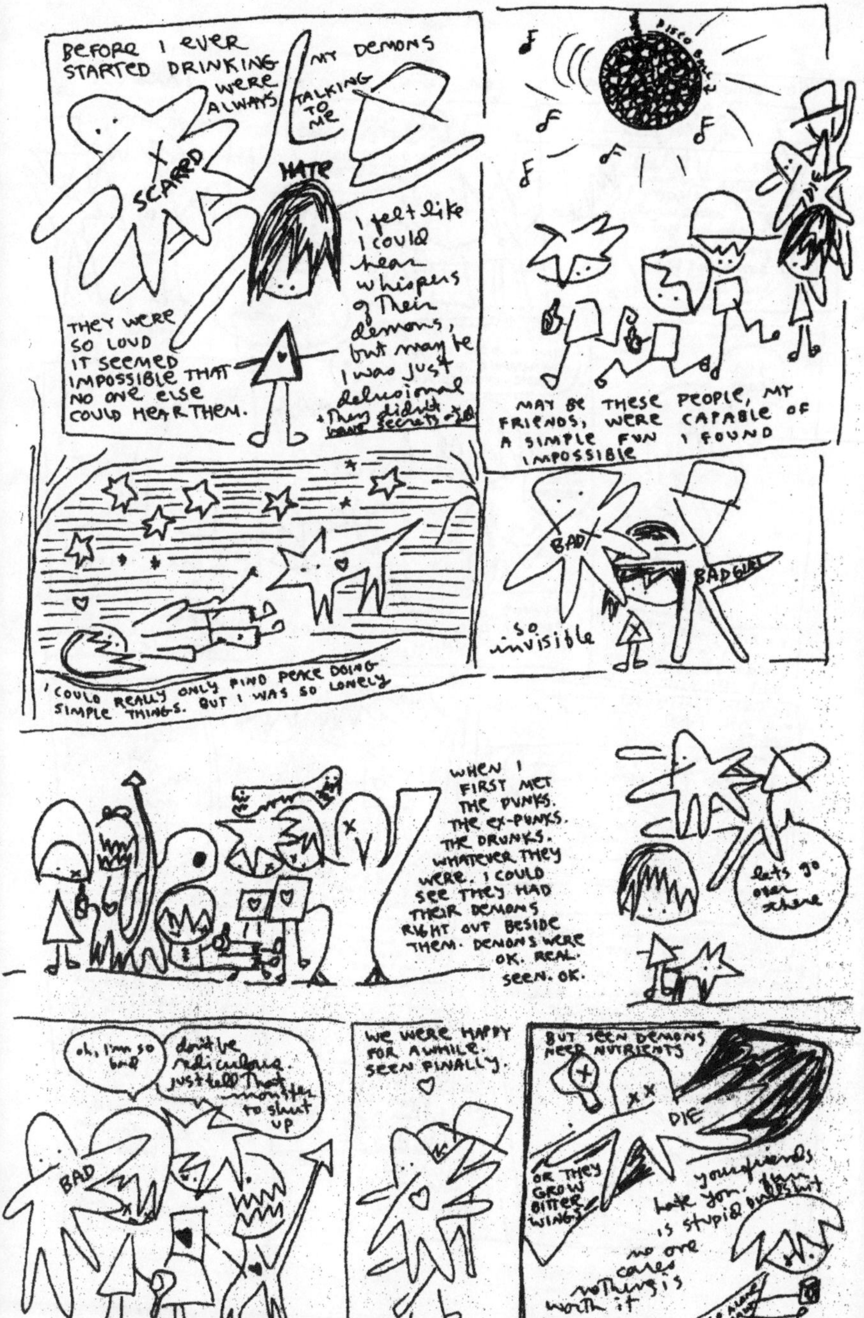

BEFORE I EVER STARTED DRINKING MY DEMONS WERE ALWAYS TALKING TO ME
SCARRED
HATE
I felt like I could hear whispers of Their demons, but maybe I was just delusional
+ They didn't have secrets
THEY WERE SO LOUD IT SEEMED IMPOSSIBLE THAT NO ONE ELSE COULD HEAR THEM.
DISCO BALL
DIE
MAYBE THESE PEOPLE, MY FRIENDS, WERE CAPABLE OF A SIMPLE FUN I FOUND IMPOSSIBLE
I COULD REALLY ONLY FIND PEACE DOING SIMPLE THINGS. BUT I WAS SO LONELY
BAD
BAD GIRL
SO invisible
WHEN I FIRST MET THE PUNKS. THE EX-PUNKS. THE DRUNKS. WHATEVER THEY WERE. I COULD SEE THEY HAD THEIR DEMONS RIGHT OUT BESIDE THEM. DEMONS WERE OK. REAL. SEEN. OK.
lets go over there
oh, i'm so bad
don't be ridiculous. just tell That monster to shut up
BAD
WE WERE HAPPY FOR AWHILE. SEEN FINALLY.
BUT SEEN DEMONS NEED NUTRIENTS
DIE
OR THEY GROW BITTER WINGS
your friends hate you. this is stupid bullshit
no one cares
nothing is worth it

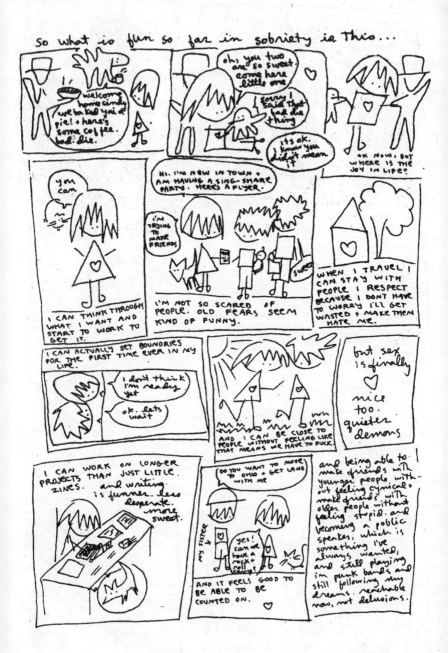

Self Defense

A few years ago I was part of a small women's health group – it was 3 friends of mine and me and we were slowly, awkwardly, learning how to learn things together. We were all pretty shy and pretty self conscious and we talked about how cool it would be to someday be able to teach or facilitate classes on things like physiology, self defense, nutrition, herbs, self exam, stds, birth-control; things like that. There were a million things to learn, and it would be so nice to learn and then to share what we'd been learning in ways that would empower women instead of making them feel judged or lectured to.

We were talking about this one day at our meeting; how we wanted to teach, but God, who could even begin to imagine getting up in front of people. We'd been talking about wanting to teach a self defense class, because it was the one thing we really did know something about, and there were no self defense classes taught by women in our town. The class that was recommended by our rape crisis center (which was otherwise a really great, feminist organization) was taught in a way we had serious problems with. The instructor taught important moves and skill, but didn't acknowledge the emotion that went along with learning self-defense. The assistance were all pretty strong men, and we had to line up, get choked, and practice choke releases; line up, get in a "potential rape position" (that is actually how they worded it, as if we needed reminding) and practice throwing the man off, rolling out from under him, running away. They never acknowledged that any of this could be triggering and traumatizing, and they didn't really give us a way out – it was just "line up" never, "you can sit out this one if you want to."

It was a particularly bad time in our town. There was a serial rapist who was targeting women who worked at downtown bars, and my friends and I went directly from our health group meeting to a community meeting about the situation. Maybe the meeting was helpful to some people, but to us it felt like a nightmare; a room packed with fear and tension and anger, and there were no real answers. We were lectured to about how important it was for us to report to the cops if we were raped, because how can they do their job if we won't let them. (our fault). The cop read off a bunch of statistics about how little crime there actually was (we are blowing it out of proportion. we are hysterical). And then he said some statistics about how downtown was more scary because homeless people were statistically more violent. "That's just their lifestyle," he said.

I am a shy person, but when I snap; I snap. I stood up and yelled, "That is a lie!" He explained with statistics and antic dotes. I yelled some more words, but this wasn't the place for this and I was shaky, wanted to flee, was trapped in this packed room with no escape. When the rape-crisis center person got up and started recommending that instructor I mentioned earlier, my friends started whispering. – Let's just do it—How? —We'll have to just figure it out – ok – ok. So one of us got up and said "We're offering a self defense class and skill share too. We passed around our contact information and set a tentative date and place. Shy and awkward as we are, we planned a six week course and we did it. We made our own hand held punching bags out of vinyl from the fabric store, stuffed with foam from the back of carpets that the carpet store was throwing away.

We shared stories. We talked about how wide a spectrum self defense really is; how if you are alive, you've probably been practicing it. We talked about the social political reasons women are denied their voices, denied the right to defend themselves, denied their own bodies. We talked about honoring all forms of self defense; from punching and screaming, to disassociation – leaving your body. We practiced kicks and releases; practiced different techniques that can be used in different situation. But in ways that are hard to explain, it was even so much more than that.

There is something so fundamental about women learning self defense together – or women and trannies, or trannies only, or sissy boys, trannies and women – whichever feels right, or is most needed. There is something so fundamental about self-defense. It can open us up, bring us together, make us stronger, both physically and emotionally. It can make our friendships stronger. It can help us fight our own internalized sexism. It can help us really value ourselves and each other. So many things; such importance, I wish everyone would form their own little self-defense group!

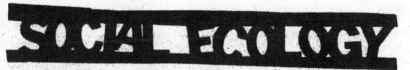

SOCIAL ECOLOGY

"We desperately need coherence... not dogma.
(We need) a structure of ideas that places
philosophy, anthropology, history, ethics, a new
rationality and utopian visions in the service of
freedom."

WHAT DREW ME TO SOCIAL ECOLOGY
WAS THE PROMISE TO THE END OF
MY CRAZINESS - MY ALIENATION AND
FEAR NOT JUST MY OWN. EVERYONE.
COULD IT BE THAT WHAT I THOUGHT
WAS ONLY ME ONLY CRAZY ME
WAS ACTUALLY THINGS EVERYONE
FELT - SOCIETY NOT PERSONAL.
AND IF THERE WAS A WAY IN TO
THIS SUCKINESS, SHOULDN'T THERE
BE A WAY OUT? I LOVED MANIFESTOS
I LOVED THE SQUATS. I LOVED US
ALL IN BLACK WITH CONTAINERS
OF GASOLINE
AND MATCHES.
I LOVED MUSIC
AND GARDENS
BUT IT FELT
LIKE STRAWS. IT
FELT LIKE
GRASPING. SOCIAL
ECOLOGY PROMISED
A SOLID GROUND TO
STAND ON. AN
ANALYSIS OF TIME
SINCE THE BEGINNING
AND WHOLE LAYERS+
LAYERS OF STRATEGY FOR HOW
TO CREATE REVOLUTIONARY
SOCIAL CHANGE

but now I have a hard
time getting through
the language, even
though I know this is
what informed my most
basic beliefs - and I
think that having this
strong + comprehensive
belief system is what
has allowed me to
stay committed to changing
the world when a lot
of my friends have given
up.

"IN A VERY REAL SENSE, THEN,
WE ARE STILL UNFINISHED AS
HUMAN BEINGS, BECAUSE WE
HAVE NOT AS YET FULFILLED OUR
POTENTIALITY FOR COOPERATION,
UNDERSTANDING, AND RATIONAL
BEHAVIOR."

Social Ecology is a philosophy and system of
thought that says the domination of human
over human came first, before the domination
of nature. and so to solve the ecological crisis
we also have to solve the social crisis. We cant
reform our way out. we have to end all forms of
domination and hierarchy.

it is the belief that dedicated people can create
revolutionary fundamental social change, and that

when "insurrectionary people take... power from...
the elites who oppressed them and begin to
restructure society along radically populist lines
(they) grow aware of latent powers within
themselves that nourish their previously
suppressed creativity, sense of self-worth, and
solidarity. They learn that society... is

malleable and subject... to change according to
human will and desire." [2]

social ecology calls on us to learn our
revolutionary history. It says we don't need
the traps of acadamia. We can form our own study
groups. we can find our own mentors. we can build
our own self-discipline. Part of the revolutionary
project is learning committment,
    working together,
  communicating our ideas,
      learning together.

    Like many nature philosophies, social ecology
draws inspiration from tribal and pre-capitalist
societies.

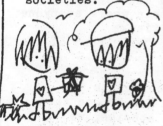

It talks about how many of
these societies were based on
cooperation, public service,
mutual aid, interdependence,
and giving - not accumulating
a bunch of crap, not trading
one thing for another, but
gift. giving.

it talks about how a lot
of tribal societies
didn't have words for
ownership, and there
was a belief that
everyone was entitled
to the means of life
no matter what their
contribution was.

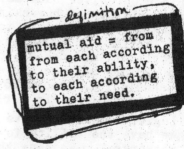

definition

mutual aid = from
from each according
to their ability,
to each according
to their need.

The basis for society was respect and people
saw themselves as part of nature. These are
all things we need to reclaim.

But while some nature philosophies believe we need to destroy civilization and return to tribal societies, social ecology places the beginnings of hierarchy within tribal society itself. It talks about the slow development of hierarchy within tribes - with the elders and then the shamans misuse of power and how most tribes were based on blood ties and family and feared or hated outsiders.

it talks about how most societies grew along non hierarchical, classless ways, using customs to curtail and discourage competitiveness, but if there was just

one tribe in an area that became a class based, warrier community, it forced the others around it to respond and change.

Social ecology believes that while there was a lot of amazing shit about tribal societies, they were mostly closed societies concerned with their own preservation and self-interests, and that cities were part of a growing toward an understanding of humankind working to create a world where everyone belonged, regardless of kinship ties.

I'm totally simplifying, but that's part of it.

part of the project of social ecology is to place ourselves back in nature, and to see the potentiality of humankind. As a species, we developed the ability to use logic, to use self-reflection, to organize in systematic ways. To create art and dance. to create written languages. to explore science and math. to create technological innovations that, yes, have been used to destroy the world, but because we have

logic, because we have self-reflection, because we have the ability fo form organizations and networks, we have the ability to end the destruction of the world and of ourselves.

We have to use our collective wisdom, we

have to use our creativity, we have to use our ability to envision the true potentiality of human kind, and to work towards recovering, reclaiming, and fighting for it.

Hierarchy, in all it's forms, must be confronted,

"The earth can no longer be owned, it must be shared. Its fruits, including those produced by technology and labour, can no longer be expropriated by the few; they must be (made) available to all on the basis of need. Power... must be freed from the control of the elites; it must be redistributed in a form that renders its use participatory." ;

"The move from here to there will not be a sudden explosion of change without a long period of intellectual and ethical preparation. The world has to be educated as fully as possible if people are to change their lives, not merely have it changed for them my self-anointed (activists) who will eventually become (corrupted by power). Sensibility, ethics, ways of viewing reality and selfhood have to be changed by educational means, by a politics of reasoned discourse, experimentation, and the expectation of repeated failures from which we have to learn, if humanity is to achieve the self-consciousness it needs to finally engage in self-management. "

it is the belief that humans have the ability to look at their community and the problems it faces and to find creative solutions. It is the belief in a democracy that is locally based, where representatives are directly accountable to the people they represent and can be fired at

at any time. And that we can create local governments , where the people actually have the the power, and these local governments can confederate with eachother and we can build a real democracy rather than the corrupted, authoritarian, oppressive bullshit we have now.

To get there we need organization and examples, and projects to inspire us and to make us feel like there is some reason to pull ourselves out of our isolations, and to inspire other people

out of their isolations too. Like free clinics and child-care
co-ops. tangible things.

Caty was telling me about one of the original models for
community supported agriculture farms; which went like
this -

the farmer would make an estimate about how much
money would be needed to buy the seed and run the farm for
the year, and the community would get together and put in money
and if it wasn't enough, then people would put in more until
there was enough to run the farm and support the farmers
and then once a week everyone would get a share of the crops
and if they had more food than they needed, they could
give away the extras, and people could volunteer on the
farm and feel what it felt like to plant and grow and
harvest. and the farmer could focus on the land and the
crops and not have to worry and spend time on selling.

maybe that seems idealistic, but what I have seen is
that most people, if they feel like their decisions and their
contributions matter in their lives, and if they are part
of a community that is actually trying to work together and
provide for one another, people usually want to contribute
what they can.

What social ecology asks of us is to think about community
and how to build it in whatever aspects of the struggle we
are involved. It asks us to make the connections between things
- like food production and alternative technologies and childhood education and community health and protest struggles and
community organizing; to make the connections between them
all and to build on them, and to push toward a more radical
analysis, and to work towards community control, community
empowerment, and a vision of fundamental change, not just
better consumer choices under capitalism.

One of the things I love about social ecology is is deals
with the beauty and complexities of humans; like the
ballance between individualism and collectivity. It talks
about how communism has proven that it does no good to try
and deny our individualities for a perceived greater
collective good - and that when people are forced into
that, it leads to apathy, sabotage, corruption and
rebellion. And people find ways to assert their
individuality no matter what the cost.

But pure individualism - doing what we want when we want to - doesn't really work and isn't really freedom.either. It doesn't help us fulfill our greatest potentialities. We are social creatures. Our biologies and the ways our brains work make us that way. We form societies and no society can be organized by pure individualism. And plus, being in community helps us discover our individual potentials.

Personally, I like spending a lot of time alone, and I'm glad my beliefs push me to keep working with other people, and keep my goals focused on trying to figure out ways to become more engaged in collective education and collective action. and to find my place, to find my grounding, to find my voice.   I like being alone, and a lot of times I find people pretty frustrating, but when we do stuff together and it works and I can see us all growing and changing, that feels better.

"Every people has its own libertarian background... and its own libertarian dreams, however much they may be confused with media-generated propaganda..."

"...Every revolutionary project rests on the hopes that the people will develop a new consciousness if they are exposed to thoughtful ideas that... meet their needs and if objective reality (shows the need for change)... Without the organized means to advance it publicly, there will be no long-range change. Every revolutionary project is above all, and educational one. The rest must come from the real world in which people live and the changes that occur in it.

An educational process that does not retain contact with that real world, its traditions as well as everyday realities, will perform only part of its task."

✶ anarchism, Marxism + The Future of The Left, bookchin ✶

footnotes: 1. MURRAY BOOKCHIN, Remaking Society, I can't remember what page. 3 + 4s were from the same book p. 172 + 189.197
2. M. BOOKCHIN, THE THIRD REVOLUTION: Popular Movements in The Revolutionary Era v:1

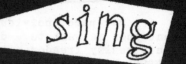

sing

I had tried to sing before, and it just came out
like a croak or a squeek. stupid. scared like a
girl. that self hate and hate for all of us.
can't do anything, can't even sing. I stood in
the corner, facing away from the band, like some
well of self-confidence would come forward if I
couldn't see the boys waiting to play the music.
pitying me. no songs, just try and scream and
not cry.

never again, I swore. never again.

When do girls learn to raise their voices? Some do.
I know. some do. But we stood on the playground
in our 4 square boxes, chanting. Some of us
fastened capes out of old sheets and ran around
together, superheros. protect and save. stop evil
before it begins.

I could see it in my dad's eyes sometimes. Too long
of a day. too much coffee. too much of all this
no happiness and life going by. "Let's wrestle.
Come on Dad, look at me! Look at what I can do!"
I tried to distract. tried to take his mind off
where it was headed, with his raised voice and
hands against my mother. And eventually when she
left, the voice fell on me.

Worthless, worthless, don't talk back. I kept the
peace. I stopped evil before it happened. I could
take it. stay quiet and save the family. I can
protect them. stay quiet, I can take it, take it in.
I am stronger than them as long as I keep it in,
hold it inside, stay quiet. As long as I hold it
close to the gut and covered.

It is systemic. sneaks in through all channels. I know this, but I wish I could pinpoint the blame. Blame it on my dad's voice. My step-brother's hands. I know it's this culture, this fucked up world that teaches some girls that the only option is to try and stay safe. try and figure out what it

is that other people want you to do, and then do it before they even think of it themselves. And do this so often that it becomes second nature, a part of you, all of you. and you don't even have your own wants and desires any more. You have them but they are held so close to the gut, kept so hidden, that all you feel them but don't

know them. One more thing that makes you feel stupid.

When I tried to sing, I felt all that in me. the tightness and everything holding it down. and to raise voice meant to break through all of that. too dangerous. too much.

but once, years later, in the basement of the resturant Mike Pack said "babygirl, just sing it like you feel it." and this time, I was safe among friends. it was ok. I was ready. I screamed and sang. It was fine. It was good.

sick

Fifteen years ago, the person I love the most got sick. I was living in a punk house, she was in school. At first it was emergency mode, of course. Get her away from the family. Figure out what these drugs were the doctor gave her. She came out to live with me and we poured over medical books and drug books, trying to decifer the insane medical language.

I think I had an idea that we could fix it. I thought the problems were enviornmental, that the doctors were crazy. It thought we could fix it by diet and may be enviornment. In the beginning, it seemed to take up my life, but the truth was, I don't think I spent that much time actually doing anything. I mean, we must have only spent a few hours a few times trying to decifer the books, and I don't remember cooking that much in the stupid house we lived in. It is that trap of emergency mode. You feel like you're doing a lot when it's really your body stress and brain crazy.

I remember then, feeling angry. Angry that there was nothing I could do. Angry at the world for making this happen to her, and angry at all the old angers too - the angers about having to take care of my mom and my dad, of never getting to have an easy time, of no one ever taking care of me, of the stupid fucks and stupid jobs and no community. We were in a new town, we didn't have much in the way of friends. The anger and helplessness made me self absorbed. I thought about her all the time, I was absorbed by how I felt about her, but I was not there for her. We've talked about it and she's said that even if I wasn't there, actually, she still knew I was there for her in my heart, but I am still ashamed by it. And I think this is something that happens a lot. I have seen it in other places. And I think it's important to talk about and recognize and maybe then it can be avoided.

I see the crisis/anger thing happen a lot - like when my friend Hanna's boyfriend got in an accident and had bleeding in his brain and was in the hospital for weeks and all the friends came and swarmed the place. Crisis. Would he live? Would he be permanently damaged? Everyone was there, trying to give support, freaking out. But it was too much, and Hanna just wanted some quiet, she didn't want to have to deal with everyone else's shit, everyone else's memories and drunkeness and fear. - Go away, go away - she said - I'm going to be the one taking care of him.

And the friends got pissed. At her, may be at their own things too. Blame, self blame. And when the bleeding finally stopped and he had to relearn movement and speach in the rehab hospital for months, the friends were mostly so angry or alienated they didn't come to help much. Burned out. But that was when it was really needed, and really mattered.

Caregiving is something about pacing. And I don't mean "take care of yourself first." I think that is bullshit. but it is about learning to caregive yourself while learning to caregive others. It is about getting out of savior mode into something that is workable, and recognizing that this is long term and needs will change: my needs and hers. Sometimes I'll find something that seems workable like I'll decide to cook breakfest for her every morning, and then it becomes unworkable. it starts to feel like a burden, and then I get resentful, but the truth is, she doesn't care one way or the other if I cook her breakfest every morning. And one of the big problems with the whole burden/resent thing is that if I'm already feeling burdened by things she's not even asking me to do, then there's not as much of a chance that she's going to ask me for the things she really needs. Plus, feeling like a burden sucks. I know. So it's being aware of things like that, and being flexable. Finding the small things that actually do matter and that are doable, and then being flexable with the extra stuff. And knowing that some weeks I'll be more present and capable than other weeks. For me, a big thing has been to stop promising to do things I won't be able to do.

One thing I had to do was to learn to recognize her new body language. Her face sometimes looks like it's saying "get the hell away from me," when it is really saying "I feel like I'm going to puke." The pain movements sometimes look like "leave me alone" when it's really just hurt. I've had to learn to not take things so personally. I've had to accept that she is in pain and sick, and to take that in to consideration not just in my mind but in my body too. to feel the weight of it and the sadness of it and breathe and move forward. I have to cry. I have to have other people to talk with. I have to mourn. I have to be angry at the world and the people who have hurt us, and the lack of support and the lack of community and the invisibility of illness, people's quickness to forget, their easy to slip into denial. I have to walk and sing and write and plan for a future where we'll be able to do the things we want to do, despite everything, and to work as hard as possible to reach those goals. We were always big dreamers, and even scaled back dreams are more than most people think possible.

I think one of the biggest problems I had, and it's a problem I see a lot particularly in punk/acitivst circles, is I survived on crisis all my life. I didn't know how to slow down or sit with my feelings. But in order to be a good friend to this person I loved, and in order to be able to be who I wanted to be, I eventually I had to learn to stop running. At one point, I had repeated the same mistakes so many times, that I had to make change a priority in my life. I had to learn to be still and present. I had to quit drinking. I had to look at the way I deal with stress and sadness and fear, and I had to feel it, process it, learn new ways of coping and living. I had to learn to be grounded and in my body. I'm still learning, and it's hard, but it's making everything much better, and I can actually do more and do it in more sustainable ways if I'm not doing it all out of panic, guilt or fear.

t is for

My first tour was just me and my best friend in my
truck, driving across the country, going to old places
he knew, looking for old friends he'd lost touch with.
This was before cell phones or facebook so if your
friends had moved out of their house and had their
phone shut off, the only way to find them was to go
look. Mostly we didn't find the people we were looking
for, but it was so amazing to learn that I could just
go anywhere, sleep in the truck. to need so little.
and I still love sleeping back there - knowing home
is where ever I am.

The thing I like about touring with bands is that the
days are so simple. you just wake up and eat, go to the
next place, figure out how to eat again, play music,
watch bands, hang out and sleep. I like being in new
places and seeing the projects people are working on-
being inspired by new lives and experience. and I also
just like the break from my real life - where I have to
constantly figure out how to organize my days and how
to make them meaningful.

My favorite tour I ever went on was with 6 people,
two bands, middle of the summer in the South. It was
unbearably hot, and the shows were pretty crappy, but
it was so nice because every day we figured out how
to go swimming, and instead of hanging out at the
bar, getting drunk and waiting for show time, we just
hung out at the ocean or a creek and at the very last
minute, jumped into the van and drove into whatever
town was next.

THIS BRIDGE CALLED
MY BACK: WRITINGS BY
RADICAL WOMEN OF
COLOR, ed MORAGA +
ANZALDÚA

THIS BOOK
HAS INFLUENCED
+ INSPIRED
ME MORE
THAN ANY
OTHER BOOK
EVER

here
kitty kitty
tiger

THAT'S REVOLTING!
QUEER STRATEGIES FOR
RESISTING ASSIMILATION
ed MATILDA BERNSTEIN SYCAMORE

excellent book!
please read!

truth

I was not a pretty girl. I was skinny like a
toothpick, the kind of girl that got made fun
of, all arms and knees. I'd blow away in the
wind, you couldn't see me if I turned sideways,
I looked like a signpost, like a scarecrow.
I had my hair cut short. I hated to brush it.
My sister didn't mind, she wore hers long,
tucked behind her ears.

We were girls who climbed trees, rolled in
leaves, played in the mud. We lived on quiet
streets. I liked to pick up garbage from the
park as a self imposed do good project. We
were best friends with two other sisters who
lived up the street. They were both figure
skaters and they were both very good. We'd
ride bikes together to go buy candy or icecream
on Saturdays when we got our allowance, and we'd
ride forever, across the big roads where you
actually had to look for cars no matter
what time of day, not just in the
mornings or evenings when the
Dad's were leaving or coming home
late from the office. Those were
the middleclass days.

I was not a pretty girl.
Hair cut short and too skinny,
scabbed knees. It didn't matter.
It made me cry when
waitresses called me son.
I got my ears peirced
but no one noticed and my ears
turned puss around the little
fake amethyst studs.
I needed gold posts only,
but realistically, how
many gold earings did I
expect them to buy?

My Grandpa was in charge of building shoppingmalls.
He'd explin it like this: "It was just useless
land out there, just useless land. Just farms.
There was nothing out there. We took it and
bought it and turned it into a place for people
to congragate."

He loved malls. He loved to talk about the ones
that were planned well and the ones that were
planned poorly. They held a vision for him that
I can't quite explain. His eyes shine for them
in the same way my eyes shine when I talk about
my own vision of utopia.

a utopia where we don't repeat all the mistakes
of the past.

I would hide in meadows. Not that there was
anyone looking for me. but I was learning
to hide. learning to take my body where
it matched my insides. In the tall meadow
grasses I would look for matted down areas.
Have I told you this before? I would look for
deer beds, or what I hoped might be deer beds.
I would lay down and cry for my mother. my
mother deer that I dreamed would come and find
me and walk me quietly quietly into the woods.

I told this to Rath and Indigo at the Cafe
Bodega when I was waiting for my grilled-
cheese sandwich, not long after getting off
the phone with the sweetest boy who I dated
twenty years ago. Rath said "You were a real
weirdo." Indigo said, "I did something like
that too."

I love Indigo already, and Rath is growing on me
in this new town where I am trying to learn how
to make friends and keep them.

I was walking with Megan and her sweet dog with the sweetest ears, in the 100 acre woods behind my house. We were talking about Grace Paley, who is her favorite author too. I was telling her a story about this thing that Grace said to us. We were young. She was quite old even then. She said there was a place for all of us. this is what we needed to know—what we needed to remember.

This was back in the days of the first Gulf War. Grace said that her and her friends had been doing a weekly picket against nuclear power and whatever else needed picketing, like for instance, this war. They'd been standing this picket once a week for longer than some of us had been alive. "You would probably find it really boring," she said."That's why there are places for all of us. We like it" she said. "Our bodies are tired. We get out of the house, see eachother, if someone's not there we notice, say 'Where's Dorthy?' Later we call her up and see if she needs anything. We pass out information get honked at. We let the world know that we're still here, these are still issues, we're not going away. But you,"she said, "you are just discovering. may be. May be some of you are already old beyond your age.

But you are the ones whose idealism hasn't gotten as muddied up as ours has, hopefully. And your place is not just to be on the frontlines with your bodies, but also with your thoughts, pushing us, us oldies to rethink things and grow again."

the arrogance of youth, they call it. I'm glad there were elders around who recognized the gift or it, and who treated us with patience and respect.

when I
was walking
with Megan and
telling her this
story, I was trying
to remember if it was a
true story or a make-believe.
I've been telling it to myself for so many
years now. I can see her wrinkled face, hear
her voice, but I can't fill in the background,
and there's something of a kernal of a lie. like
it was someone else who said it, but once long ago
I told the story this way, and this is the way the
story stuck.

stuck stories.

Like the story I always told myself about that
sweet boy I dated when I was 17. I always said

that he was too nice to me, I couldn't handle
it and so I broke up. I remember myself being
just a miserable person, just a big black pit
of hell. but when I asked him he said 'You were
actually really fun to be around.' and I start
to remember that. The way I was a spazzy girl,
full of desire. wanting life lived fully.
wanting exploration.

the true story is: I went downtown
in a horrible self-destructive
mood telling myself I was
just going to find someone
and pick them up
who-fucking cares.

if they were going
to use me like that,
I'd do it right
back.

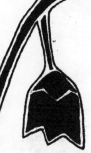

But this motorcycle boy turned out really
different from the others. He treated me
like a human. He treated me with respect.

He rode me out to the country one time so I could
meet his sister. He snuck me into the basement
of the art gallery where he worked so I could use
the spray paint machine to paint these huge things
of cotten I needed red for a performance art class
thing I was making. red cotton batting.

I'd been reading The Courage to Heal, and
recognizing myself in these survivors stories.
In the middle of my performance art peice I
realized that was what it was about. It was telling
me that the abuse I went through was real. And
that's why I broke up with the sweet boy. Because
I wanted to deal with this and I thought I had
to do it alone. . . it could be that his niceness
was part of what brought me there - that he helped
me see I was worth fighting for.

so why did I tell the story the way I did? That he
was too nice and I wanted someone mean? May be
because it is a simple, traditional story,   and
easy to tell. It is a self-hating story and I did
hate myself back then. And may be I've told it
that way because for me there are usually a number
   of contradictory stories playing themselves out
inside of me all at the same time. and most people
want to push away the hurtest part, and so
sometimes that's the part that takes over,
demanding their story be heard.

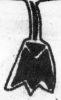

but the problem with
telling my story that
way is I start to
believe it myself.

so instead of seeing myself as someone who is
generally good to the people I care about and
who prioritizes taking care of myself when that
is what needs to be done, I start to see myself
as someone who, when confronted with goodness,
pushes it away.

and so when I see niceness, my brain goes 'oh,
here is this again, what do we do with this? We
push it away.'

I've been practicing telling the truth and
remembering not just the bad parts and not
just the good, but all the parts inbetween.
I've been practicing a funny kind of openness
here in this new town. I live with my sister,
half an hour from anyone, and I work at home
so at first it was impossibly lonely. At first

I wanted love. I wanted someone to come and fix
my loneliness. Then I decided to make friends
instead. I started going downtown and talking to
anyone who I'd ever been slightly introduced to.
When people asked me what I was up to, I'd say

"I just moved here and I'm trying to figure out
how to make some friends. It's lonely down in
Meig's county." Then I'd laugh, like that was a
pretty embarrassing thing to say,
and sometimes they'd laugh too.

and my own laughter says to me "let go fear, it's
it's ok now." it says, "come close, I won't
cling too tightly and I won't push you away."

u is for

Umbrellas

When I was in high school, it seemed like everything was telling me that I couldn't stay full of hope. Like, you couldn't stay human and live. It was in the books I read: the female characters that were symbols of innocence or truth always died. Like <u>Fahrenheight 451</u>, where the TV's covered the walls and talked to you and the firefighters burned houses and books; there was the girl who just reveled in the small beauties of the world, and felt the sadness and emptiness too, instead of numbing herself. She tipped her head back to taste the rain. It tastes like wine she said.

The death of innocence was symbolized by the death of girls like me. Also the poets I found - the women poets who wrote about life and pain and love and want like I felt it, Anne Sexton and Sylvia Plath: suicides.
I didn't want to grow bitter and numb. I wanted to kill myself, but not actually, not if there were better choices.
When I was 18 I was trying not to let the world define me. I was trying to find better choices, trying to let myself write, trying to make sense of the politics of the world, trying to create my own family. It was a sweltering hot muggy summer in Minneapolis, and everything was falling apart. I didn't have the courage to take to the streets and get beat up by cops. I was broke and working and going to school. My new family that I thought would last forever was starting to bore me, they didn't get me. I thought, may be this is it. May be the world was right after all. You can not live and be human. I sat in front of my fan, sweating. And the sky cracked open. The pent up rain came pouring. I went out with my umbrella and folded it up, lifted my head to the rain, let it wash over me, and then I ran. Drenched though, running down the streets and in the puddles until I could feel the life deep inside me, the undying life, the celebration, human, alive.

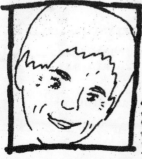

♡ URSULA LE GUIN ♡

ANARCHIST, FEMINIST, SCIENCE-FICTION WRITER. I love her book THE DISPOSSESSED + a lot of her young adult fiction + her books of speeches + essays. WHEN I WAS REALLY WANTING TO HAVE KIDS I WAS RELIEVED TO READ HER ESSAY ABOUT HOW PEOPLE SAY YOU HAVE TO CHOOSE BETWEEN BEING A WRITER + A MOTHER, BUT THATS NOT TRUE AT ALL, SHE SAID. YOU JUST FIGURE IT OUT.

under it all

Once upon a time I moved to the city of rain,
the city of roses. It wasn't bravery so much as
desperation.

Some people think of me as a great adventuress.
I just want to clear the record.

I had gotten accepted to Reed college. It was
my way out, my excuse to leave behind my suicidal
mom who I'd been trying to save and couldn't.
One day I was driving her to the mental ward to
have her locked up, and arguing with her about
why she should stay alive. She kept saying,
"I'm so tired. Why would it be so bad?" and I
finally broke. I didn't say it outloud, but I
thought, "May be she's right. May be it's
selfish of me. May be she would be better off
dead. Who am I to force her to stay alive."
But I couldn't just leave. I needed an excuse.

And to be completely honest, I was trying to
leave my sweet surface love too. He made me
laugh every day, but he didn't understand the
deep, deep sorrow. I think he didn't have any
reference point for it. Either that, or he was
just too scared to go there. He was my love
and my only real friend,
but those of us who have
roots that go deep into
the marshes, need at
least some people
around us who are
mucked in too. or
who know how to
dredge. or who know
how to build bridges. We need
people who know. We get exhausted trying to explain.

I didn't have the strength to make other friends,
and I didn't have the language to explain why I
had to go.

so that is the beginning of this true story.

But it also true that we are born with certain strengths, or we learn them so early they become part of our cells and our skin. Other strengths we have to work for.

and may be I was born with adventure somewhere in my spirit, but I was also really scared. There was always a pull both ways. Mostly I did what my older sister showed me. I didn't stray outside the blocks I knew. She was the one who wanted to go further.

I had empathy and the desire to please, the need to fix things, the ability to love strongly. I was not distrustful or bitter. I learned early on to see the good in people and to want to draw that out. I responded to care, any tiny bit of care. I did not let go easy.

and I was scared of things. I didn't like to go places where I wasn't wanted, and I didn't know where I was wanted. I was scared of doing things wrong and I was scared of rejection. When I was 15, I rode the city bus to then end of the line because I was scared to ask the driver to tell me where my stop was.

I thought that everyone knew more than I did, like there was a secret language to the world that everyone had learned but me. I cried when I was put on the spot.

When I moved to Portland, I was trying to get there in time to meet up with my little sister. She had been on a road trip and I'd given her my dog for protection. I drove straight across the country without stopping except for gas. The Dakotas were more beautiful than I knew, with fields of sunflowers turning to the sun. In Montana a storm blew through the mountains like a judgement: stop here. go no further.

but I drove because I was scared of everything, and if I stopped, the fear could catch up to me. I was scared of what I was leaving and what I was going to, and scared of rest areas and scared of small towns. Scared I'd get lost or if I slept in my car someone would break in and hurt me or I'd get arrested for vagrancy, and if I left my car to go sleep in the woods, may be all my belongings would be stolen. I drove until I started to hallucinate, and then I kept driving.

I'd seen hollywood movies and read the bestseller books and the fashion magazines and I was not immune to their messages. I knew what I was worth as a girl and a woman. I had not learned to defend myself yet. I had engrained deep inside of me the fear of everything and the fear of rape. I wanted to fight those fears but hadn't really figured out how.

There were other strong messages too. They went like this: people who don't numb themselves to the world can not live. love without violence or manipulation is nieve. strong idealistic belief is childish innocence. You have to grow up and leave behind childish things. If you hold on to wonder, belief, love, you will end up killing yourself or murdered or in some other way dead. especially if you were a girl.

I promised myself I would prove that shit wrong. I would live. I would always lift my face to the rain and taste it like wine. I would prove them wrong. I would stay alive.

It is hard to keep promises to yourself, and it's
true that at one point I did try and kill myself.
but I lived.

Have you ever seen the movie Wings of Desire? It
was a German movie about after WWII, East Germany.
In the beginning, everything is grey and black and
white and devastated.   There are these two
angels, they are just plain looking angels, and
what they do is they observe life. They meet
up with eachother at the end of the day, usually
in the library, and they report back what they
noticed —a

a woman folds up her umbrella is The
pouring rain + lets herself be drenched.
a man reads to a child and The child
listens without blinking.

I was friends with people who worked at the art
theater when it came out, so I used to go a few
times a day and watch just the beginning, just that
part. "That is what I will do," I said to myself.
and it is. still.

When I got to Portland, I went to the campus and I
had a total panic attack. Everyone looked so healthy
and they scurried around like they knew just where
they were going. I felt crazy. I was scared I
wouldn't be able to find the right room. In highschool I sometimes sat through whole wrong classes
just because I'd walked in to the wrong room and
was too embarrassed and ashamed to admit it.

At the college financial aid office they said it
didn't matter how many years I'd been on my own,
I wasn't considered independent until I was 24. I
knew I wouldn't be able to get my dad to fill out
my financial aid forms even though he didn't have
much money anymore. and my mom, I didn't want to
bother her with anything. So that was the end of
that.

I rented the first room I could find. I couldn't relate to or talk with my roommates. I couldn't find a job. I had a little jewelry making business that brought in just enough money to get by. I budgeted it out and after food and bills and rent

I could only spend $5 a day. I sat in coffee shops and watched people and wrote, but I got really depressed and lonely. There was so little meaning in my life. I finally found a flyer for Food Not Bombs, and I went there.

Food Not Bombs was still a new organization back then. In Minneapolis, my political collective had been asked to help start a chapter, but we didn't because it was decided that even if it had revolutionary intentions, it was still basically just charity. I didn't have anything to say about it because I still didn't trust myself enough to voice my own political questions or opinions.

FOOD NOT BOMBS BELIEVES THAT PEOPLE HAVE THE RIGHT TO FEED EACHOTHER. WE HAVE THE RIGHT TO GET FOOD OUT OF THE GARBAGE THE RIGHT TO COOK IN OUR OWN KITCHENS + TO SERVE FOOD IN PUBLIC PARKS TO THE HUNGRY + TO WHOEVER WANTS IT. AND ANYONE WHO WANTS CAN COME AND COOK WITH US. THERE ARE NO PERMITS TO SIGN + NO GOD TO BOW DOWN TO.

So in Portland, I went to the Food Not Bombs house, more hoping to meet people than expecting to change the world, but even so, I was terrified they would reject me. Was it bravery or desperation that got me to walk through that door? I hadn't talked to another human in weeks.

it didn'tcome naturally. the friendships didn't blossom out of nowhere. I felt uncomfortable for awhile. I came each week and cooked and peeled and chopped, and eventually I felt normal there, and eventually I made friends.

I had studied a lot, even though I hadn't gone to much college, and I knew what I thought about some things, like what bullshit private property was and how here in America we are always trying to buy things to fill the void in our lives, when really the void could only be filled with meaningful social and political engagement, active citizenship, work that had tangible benefits for myself and the people around me. What is it called? alienated labor? no more alienated labor! I believed in creating rest that was restful and not just pure escape. I knew I shouldn't hate my body and I should value women's friendships at least as much as I valued men. I knew these things, but I didn't know exactly how to fit them into my life. There is only so far you can get alone, reading. Eventually you have to live some of it.

In the rain, with my new friends, I started to confront some of my fears.

Leila, who was only 9 years old then, took me through the alleys to pick fruit. I said "but aren't these other people's trees?" She said "The trees don't belong to anyone. If the people yell at us, we can just yell right back." I learned to stop buying much of anything at all. We made eachother presents. What we made was more beautiful than anything we could buy. When there was real life to live, there was less of a void to fill. I got over my fear of admitting poverty and I went to the damn foodstamp office.

I moved in to the Food Not Bombs house, and living there with a bunch of people, I got to think and rethink, andfeel and refeel, what it means to live and have grown up in an individualistic society and to try and live collectively. When do you call people on their crap and when do you accept them for who they are. when do you struggle for more cohesiveness and when do you let it go.

The girls in the house helped me start to learn to
stop hating my body. First we just talked together
about the ways we felt and the messages we were
always getting from magazines
and our families and the whole
world around us. Then we got
out our sewing machines and
made cloth pads, which I
thought was kind of stupid
and also disgusting
because I didn't want
to touch all that blood
and what was wrong
with that? But I did it
and honestly, it really
did begin to change the
way I felt about my body
and my self. Plus my

cramps weren't so bad anymore and I didn't
bleed nearly half as much after I stopped
putting chlorine up inside of me, or whatever
it is about tampons that fucks you up, I
can't even remember any more.

but I became less afraid and less afraid of myself.

Travelers came through the Food Not Bombs house,
and they talked about places I'd never seen,
freight trains and cities and cops and going hungry
and desolate nowhere and the strange people who
would come to their rescue. It was pure adventure
and part of me wanted it - a freedom with nothing
to tie me down. But I also believed in staying put
and fighting and building where you are. and finding
adventure in the life you are living.

I promised myself I would live. I would not box
myself in, no matter how tempting. I would confront
my fears, little by little, and I would live a
life of intention and passion and hopefully that
would save me.   and it did.

v is for

Vandana Shiva

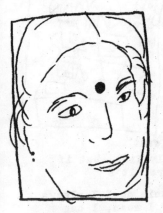

Activist, feminist, writer and total badass! Check out her book <u>Soil Not Oil</u> and everything else she's written, plus she has a great website. My sister saw her speak on a panel at a Seeds For Change conference which was actually organized by a company that was patenting seeds (going into countries and finding plants that have been used forever for medicine or food and then being like 'the seeds from this plant belong to me now and if you want to harvest them or save them for next years planting, you are breaking a law! You have to buy them from me now!') Crazy but true!

On the speakers panel with Vandana Shiva was Bill Molsten (the Permaculture guy who is a total sexist) and a bunch of other respected, professional dudes who are used to being in charge and heard, having their opinions believed and acted upon. Vandana Shiva just blew them out of the water. Not by being mean or argumentative, but just by telling the truth and not trying to manipulate anyone or anything. Just the passionate, articulate truth. All these guys who are used to being in the spot-light, and have probably never been at a loss for words, she just blew them out of the water. They were speechless.

VIRGINA WOOLF

writing so beautiful it hurts and you have to let go of holding on to story + line + let yourself be carried along by her river. <u>Orlando</u> where the main character lives for generations + switches gender back + forth. <u>Mrs Dalloway</u> the story of one day in a womans life. I even love the movie "The Hours". I cried all the way through. Oh Virginia! I wish I had been there for you!

voice

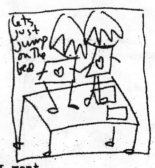

I have never been able to
figure out a way to talk
comfortably about consent.

I think I am pretty good about
asking other people, but figuring
out a way to explain whether or
not I want to be doing something
is pretty impossible. I mean, if I want
to be doing something, it's usually fine, but if
I don't, or especially if I'm unsure, it's

impossible. If someone asks, "is this ok," I always
say "yes."   Everything is "ok" I mean, I can
survive anything, right? So even the best of
intentions don't usually work for me,   and just the
words like : "do you like this?" or "do you want me
to be doing this?" they are triggering, or even if
they're not specifically triggering, they make me
doubt myself - like "Oh, I thought I wanted this,
but do I? What if I don't? shit. How do I know for
sure?" So generally when people ask me for consent
it not only ruins the mood I'm working so hard to
maintain, but it triggers me, then I have to try
and navigate wheter or not I'm going to be able to
get out of the trigger, stop thinking so much and
get back to just feeling good.   And if they notice
me flinching or withdrawing for a second and they
stop and want to tqlk about it, then it is just
over, and may be I don't want it to be over, I
just want to be able to work through it myself and
forget.

So I've never really known what to do.
There are some things that have worked
- like talking beforehand about what
I need - like being held after sex. And
asking them not to ask me things like
"how was it for you". There are just too
many words and sentances that are
triggering for me. But I love sex and
want to be able to do it. I want

to be able to be asked for consent and to give
consent. If people don't even try, then that's
frustrating too.

So, talking beforehand, and also trying to figure
out ways to talk about what's happened during sex,
but later. like when we are not in bed. and trying
to figure out ways for them to not get freaked out
if l admit to faking it or having a flashback or
just not wanting to do something. lt's important
for me to be able to talk about it later, because
l can't usually talk about it at the time, but
that usually makes people feel like shit and feel
guilty and then question every move they make, and
they feel like they can't get anything right and
l have to take all initiative and give so much
reasurance, and that makes me never feel like
doin' it, and that sucks too.

One of the things that happens a lot is that I
am really sexual in the beginnings of relationships
but when they get more serious or when they have
been going on for awhile more things start to come
up. my last partner came up with an idea. l have
to say that the fact that he came up with an idea
instead of me having to do it, helped so much! He
came up with a number system He would ask me 1-6
We worked together to come up with what the numbers
stood for.

1. I feel like being held. No sex. Nothing. Not
    even sexual energy.
2. I want kissing but nothing past that. No
    moving against me in a sexual way.
3. I want to kiss and might be open to other stuff
    too.
4. I want to do stuff, but check back in a lot
    as we go.
5. I want to do stuff, and don't want much checking
    in, just check in before doing anything with the
    downthere parts and check in if you feel like I
    might be feeling weird.
6. Let's do it!

  Something about the number system took the
  weight off things. It made it more easy and a
  little bit funny. I was totally able to say 2,
  where as I would never say "I want to kiss right
  now but nothing else". Saying those words would
  make me feel totally guilty where as saying "two"
  just felt like fact.
  It didn't always work perfectly, but it was way
  easier for both of us.

vamoose

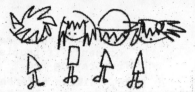

ONCE UPON A TIME... OK JUST KIDDING. THIS IS ACTUALLY ABOUT TOUR. THE BEST TOUR I'VE EVER BEEN ON! MY SISTER IS FINALLY IN A BAND WITH ME! I CAN'T BELIEVE IT! SHE SAID "WHY WOULD I WANT TO SING IN A BAND? IT'S THE TWO THINGS I HATE THE MOST, BEING IN FRONT OF PEOPLE AND PEOPLE HEARING ME SING!"

I WISH I HAD AN INTERCOM SO I COULD ASK HER IF THAT WAS A PROPER QUOTE. WE USED TO HAVE ROOMS RIGHT NEXT TO EACHOTHER WHICH WAS PERFECT BECAUSE WE HAD PRIVACY BUT COULD ALSO SIT IN OUR SEPERATE ROOMS AND THEN YELL AT EACHOTHER WHENEVER WE THOUGHT OF SOMETHING FUNNY OR WHENEVER WE HAD A QUESTION OR IDEA. NOW I HAVE TO GET UP AND WALK ACROSS THE HOUSE AND SHOUT UP THE STAIRWAY OF OUR NEW HOUSE. WE BOUGHT A HOUSE! THIS IS THE BIG NEWS. ASIDE FROM TOUR.

OK. HOLD ON.

(hey cats!)

knock knock

what?

OK. I'M BACK. SHE SAYS THAT WAS PRETTY MUCH A DIRECT QUOTE. "BEING THE CENTER OF ATTENTION. I HATE THAT!" SO I ASKED HER HOW SHE LIKES SINGING IN A BAND NOW AND SHE SAYS "IT'S STILL SCARY, BUT IT'S EXCITING TO BE AFRAID OF SOMETHING AND THEN JUST SAY 'FUCK IT' AND DO IT ANYWAY. I THINK IT'S GOOD FOR ME." THE OTHER THINGS SHE SAID SHE LIKES ABOUT IT IS THAT SHE GETS TO LEARN TO USE HER VOICE IN NEW WAYS, AND SHE LIKES STARTING TO UNDERSTAND MORE ABOUT HOW MUSIC WORKS. "MAYBE I'LL WRITE MY OWN SONGS" SHE JUST SAID! THAT IS THE BEST NEWS I'VE HEARD ALL DAY! OF COURSE I HAVEN'T HEARD MUCH NEWS TODAY BECAUSE I SPENT THE DAY

RAKING LEAVES OUT OF THE CREEK THAT OUR GREYWATER RUNS INTO, AND SAWING UP A BIG OAK TREE THAT FELL DOWN, AND REPLACING OUR MAILBOX WITH ONE THAT HAS A FLAG SO OUR MAIL LADY WILL START PICKING UP OUR OUTGOING MAIL HOPEFULLY. BUT EVEN IF I'D HAD A DAY FULL OF GREAT NEWS, THIS WOULD STILL BE THE BEST NEWS EVER!

Our band is called SNARLAS. It is me and my sister and Miguel and his sister Tessa. A few months ago we went on tour, and this is what it was like:

Pittsburgh Pittsburgh! When did it get so good in Pittsburgh? It is a city on the decline, so the punks and expunks have been buying houses and fixing them up in that way that punks do, salvaging scraps and creating something new. One of the houses had salvaged so much hardwood flooring, they ended up using it on the walls too. There were hand-printed posters everywhere and art covering every inch of everything. This is one of the things I love about punk - how the aesthetics of our lives show our resistance to the - commodification of everything. The world says "Buy this, buy that, want this, it'll make you happy," and we say "Fuck that! We want you out of our heads! We will live our own lives! We want some kind of meaning, we want some kind of culture, and we will build it with whatever we can find. We don't want your mass produced products. We are not your consumers or your target audience, we are humans."

And I love it when our resistance is brought into our homes and turned into a history and a testiment and a nest. A nest of color you can curl up inside and breathe.

In Pittsburgh we had a zine reading first. Well, first there was a potluck with lots of good food, then there was a zine reading with lots of good stories, then there was the show. Also Lasers played, who I loved. Then Bad Daughtors, who I loved even more. Bad Daughtors was a 3 decade band: one woman in her 20's, one in her 30's and one in her 40's, all of them amazing women, Simone, Artnoose and Alisa.

Last time I saw Alisa she gave me a little zine she'd made. It was for Leanne's "Fun a Day" project. "Fun a Day" is something Leanne came up with to help people get through the dreary month of February. How it works is, everyone picks something they like to do, and then they do it every day, and they document it, and then at the end of the month there is an art show so everyone can see what everyone did.

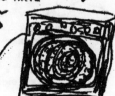

CAIT PLANTED A SEED EVERY DAY AND HAD A SHELF FULL OF DELICATE SEEDLINGS. LEANNE SENT A LETTER TO A DIFFERENT FRIEND OR ACQUAINTANCE EVERY DAY, AND INSIDE EACH LETTER WAS A POSTAGE PAID POSTCARD SO PEOPLE COULD WRITE A STORY OR DRAW A PICTURE OR JUST WRITE BACK, AND THESE POSTCARDS WENT UP FOR HER DISPLAY. ALISA FOUND A SLANG WORD EACH DAY THAT WASN'T REALLY USED ANY MORE. LIKE "FLUFF IT!" WHICH MEANS GO AWAY! AND "SWANNING" WHICH IS "GOING PURPOSELY ANYWHERE WITHOUT A PURPOSE."

WHAT ABOUT "VAMOOSE!" IT'S ONE MY MOM USED TO SAY. IT MEANS "TO LEAVE HURRIEDLY" BUT SHE'S SORT OF USE IT MORE LIKE "SHOO SHOO. COME ON KIDS, GET YOUR COATS ON AND GET OUT THE DOOR! VAMOOSE!".

IN PITTSBURGH, CATY AND TESSA SLEPT AT ARTNOOSE'S HOUSE, IN THE ROOM ABOVE THE ROOM WITH THE PRINTING PRESS. I HAVE ALWAYS LOVED THESE KINDS OF PRINTING PRESSES, THE KIND WHERE YOU HAVE TO TAKE EACH LETTER AND PLACE IT IN PLACE. FOR SOME REASON WE HAD ONE OF THESE PRESSES IN MY JR. HIGH AND IT WAS REDICULOUS HOW LONG IT TOOK JUST TO PEICE TOGETHER A FEW SENTENCES AND PRINT IT. AND IT TOOK SUCH CARE, SUCH ATTENTION. AND I'M ALWAYS AMAZED THAT THIS IS WHAT PEOPLE USED TO HAVE TO DO TO PRINT THINGS. THEY PUT TOGETHER WHOLE BOOKS AND WHOLE NEWSPAPERS THIS WAY. I LIKE TO THINK OF THE TIME SPENT, THE COMMITMENT TO REPRODUCING WORDS, AND HOW THE PROCESS OF IT WAS GENERALLY NOT SPENT IN ISOLATION.

ON TOUR OUR PRIORITIES WERE; EAT ENOUGH FOOD, GET ENOUGH SLEEP, PLAY AS HARD AS POSSIBLE, HANG OUT WITH OLD FRIENDS AND MAKE NEW ONES. — PRETTY DIFFERENT FROM MY PREVIOUS TOURS WHERE NO MATTER WHAT MY INTENTIONS WERE, I USUALLY JUST ENDED UP GETTING DRUNK AND FREAKING OUT AND RUNNING AROUND TRYING TO HAVE ADVENTURES WITH STRANGERS.

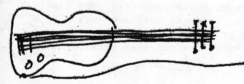

In Pittsburgh me and Miguel went back to the east side after the show so me and Geoff could take apart my guitar and try to solder it back together. Already, only 4 hours from home, the guitar amp had broken and my guitar was shorting out.

A couple houses up from Geoff's house was the Landslide squat. "They call us the retirement home" said Geoff. We were standing around the kitchen eating spagetti and talking about local politics. I'm not totally sure how Landslide works exactly. Our friend Emily lived there for years and I should probably call her up and ask her, but it's late and I can't find her number. I do know that basically, a few years ago, some folks bought a few acres of abandon lot, and they started farming it and squatting the empty house at the edge of the land.

They took me on a tour of the house once, and I remember a beautiful woodstove room with acoustic instruments. Banjo. Fiddle. Guitar. Accordian. The day before our show the cops had come and kicked everyone out of the squat and boarded up the windows and door. In the end there was enough community outcry that the mayor or someone like that told the cops or whoever that they had to let the kids back in, but the day we were there, no one knew what was going to happen.

Miguel went to go hang out with Emily and the other Landsliders while me and Geoff tried to fix my guitar. When he came back he said, "They call this the retirement house but they were doing exactly the same thing over there. Stading around the kitchen, eating spaghetti, talking about local politics."

We slept curled up in a perfect little shack. I like to call that shack "my Pittsburgh home," even though that's the only time I've slept there.

TOUR. AT THE RATE THIS IS GOING, IT'S GOING TO
TAKE YOU A WEEK TO READ ABOUT OUR ONE WEEK TOUR SO I'LL
HAVE TO START CUTTING TO THE CHASE.

IN BALTIMORE WE HAD A LOT OF DUMPSTERED APPLES SO
I WAS SHOWING EVERYONE MY FAVORITE SNACK — APPLE BOATS.
YOU CUT THE APPLE IN HALF AND HOLLOW OUT
THE SEED PART AND THEN FILL IT UP WITH
PEANUTBUTTER AND THEN YOU CAN EAT IT WITH
ONE HAND WHILE YOU DO OTHER STUFF.
MICHAEL WAS TALKING ABOUT ANARCHISM AND HOW MAYBE IT
WOULD BE A GOOD IDEA IF HALF THE ANARCHISTS WORKED ON
POLITICAL ORGANIZING AND HALF THE ANARCHISTS STARTED
PRACTICING CHAOS MAGICK AND THEN WE COULD ATTACK THE
POWERS THAT BE FROM ALL DIFFERENT ANGLES. I DON'T KNOW
WHAT INSPIRED ME TO ASK MICHAEL FOR HIS DEFINITION OF
CHAOS MAGIC. I'VE HEARD PEOPLE TALK ABOUT IT BEFORE AND
IT ALWAYS SEEMS SELF-IMPORTANT AND LIKE A REAL COP-OUT,
BUT I LOVE MICHAEL AND I WANT TO KNOW WHAT HE CARES
ABOUT AND HOW HE THINKS AND WHAT HE WANTS. AND I
ALWAYS THINK IT'S IMPORTANT TO REEVALUATE OUR ASSUMPTIONS,
SO I SAID "WHAT EXACTLY DO CHAOS MAGICIANS DO?" AND
MICHAEL GOT THE GLEEM IN HIS EYES AND HE STOOD UP AND
SAID "FIRST, YOU DRAW A PENTAGRAM IN THE MIDDLE OF
THE ROOM, THEN YOU GRAB YOUR CHERRY VODKA AND YOU OPEN
IT UP AND YOU SPIN AROUND REALLY REALLY FAST!"
I COULDN'T STOP LAUGHING.

IN NEW YORK I EXPLAINED MY DRIVING STRATEGY. "WHENEVER
SOMEONE HONKS I PRETEND THEY ARE SAYING 'I LOVE YOU'."
WE WALKED BEHIND THE MUSEUM AND VISITED THE SCULPTURE
INTERNMENT, WHERE BROKEN OR UNWANTED SCULPTURES ARE
LINED UP AND CAGED IN BEHIND A FENCE AT THE GRAVEL,
OVERGROWN EDGE OF THE PARKINGLOT. I VISITED MY OLD
BEST OF BEST FRIENDS. WE'D HAD AN EIGHT YEAR FRIENDSHIP
BREAKUP, BUT AWHILE AGO HAD A REUNION THAT'S STICKING.
SOMETIMES IT'S WORTH IT TO LET PEOPLE BACK IN. AT LEAST
PART WAY BACK IN.

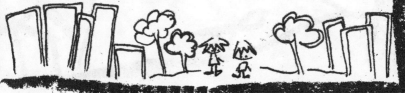

BOSTON HAS THE SWEETEST LITTLE ZINE LIBRARY. MY OLD
FRIEND DAVE TABOR VOLUNTEERS THERE. THE TABOR BROTHERS
CAME TO ASHEVILLE A MILLION
YEARS AGO, WHEN NOT MANY PUNKS OR
WEIRDOS LIVED THERE, JUST A HANDFUL
OF US LIVING IN A BIG PINK TWO STORY
BUILDING NEAR DOWNTOWN. THERE WAS A
BLACK FLAG HANGING WHERE THE AMERICAN FLAG
WAS SUPPOSED TO BE, AND WHEN THE TABORS WERE TRAVELING
THROUGH THEY SAW THE FLAG AND KNOCKED ON THE DOOR AND
SAID "WE SAW THE FLAG AND WERE WONDERING IF ANARCHISTS
LIVED HERE."   THEY STAYED.   I REMEMBER TEACHING
DAVE TO CHAINSAW. HE WRITES A ZINE I'VE ALWAYS LOVED.
HE WANTED TO BE IN A BAND AND I SAID "EVERYONE SHOULD
BE IN A BAND. ANYONE CAN DO IT." AND HE SAID "MAY BE
EVERYONE EXCEPT ME." UNTIL NOW. HE'S FINALLY IN ONE.
THEY PLAYED WITH US AT THE ZINE LIBRARY. AND HE LOOKED
SHY AND NOT SHY, HAPPY, AND I WAS PROUD. EVERYONE
SHOULD BE IN A BAND, IT'S TRUE. THERE'S SOMETHING
UNEXPLAINABLY GOOD ABOUT IT.

dave's zine =
day of recogning
bands + frogs! everywhere!

WE STAYED WITH CATY'S FRIEND JOSH WHO I'D ALWAYS
WANTED TO MEET. HE USED TO DO CONSENT WORKSHOPS + organized THE
SCHOOL OF THE AMERICA'S PROTESTS (THE SCHOOL OF THE
AMERICAS IS WHERE THE U.S. TRAINS RIGHT-WING INSURGENTS
OR THE MILITARIES OF OTHER COUNTRIES TO KEEP THOSE
COUNTRIES SAFE FOR U.S. INVESTMENTS. THIS USUALLY MEANS
BRUTALLY VIOLENT REGRESSION OF ANY TYPE OF FREEDOM
MOVEMENTS. IT INCLUDES ASSASINATING DEMOCRATICALLY
ELECTED LEADERS. IT INCLUDES THE GENOCIDE OF INDIGENOUS
PEOPLE. IT IS AN INTENSE AND SYSTEMATIC VIOLENCE THAT
IS HARD TO DEAL WITH, BUT SO IMPORTANT THAT WE KNOW
THIS HISTORY — THIS CURRENT REALITY.

reading recomendations
THE SCHOOL OF THE AMERICAS - leslie gill
GUNS, GREED + GLOBALIZATION - jack nelson-pallmeyer

SOAW.ORG
KAMARIKUN.BLOGSPOT.COM
NARCONEWS.COM

I REMEMBER TALKING TO JOSH ON THE PHONE BACK WHEN ANDREA
AND I WERE TRYING TO FIGURE OUT HOW TO DO A CONSENT
WORKSHOP. I REMEMBER HIM TELLING ME ABOUT AN EXERCISE
HE DID MOSTLY WITH GUYS. HE'D HAVE THEM PAIR UP, AND
ONE OF THEM WOULD STAND A LITTLE WAYS AWAY, AND THEN
START SLOWLY WALKING, GETTING CLOSER AND CLOSER TO
THEIR PARTNER. THE PERSON STANDING STILL WAS SUPPOSED
TO SAY 'STOP' WHEN THEY STARTED TO GET UNCOMFORTABLE,
BUT ALMOST NO ONE SAID IT WHEN THEY FIRST STARTED TO
FEEL THEIR BOUNDRIES BEING CROSSED. THEY WAITED UNTIL
IT WAS UNBEARABLE. AND THIS FEELING. IT HELPED THEM
TO UNDERSTAND WHY GIRLS AND PEOPLE CAN'T ALWAYS SAY
'STOP' IF THEY DON'T WANT TO BE DOING SOMETHING. THAT
FEELING IN YOUR BODY LIKE YOU SHOULDN'T SAY IT, YOU
MIGHT LOOK STUPID, MAYBE YOU CAN TAKE IT, WHAT IF YOU
SAY IT AND THEY KEEP GOING. ALL THE MESSAGES THAT GET
IN THE WAY AND THE FROZEN FEELING, THE UNBELIEVING
FEELING. A LOT OF US CAN NOT SAY 'STOP' AT ALL.

JOSH AND HIS SISTER BOUGHT A HOUSE IN A KIND OF
FUCKED UP PART OF BOSTON AND FIXED IT UP REALLY NICE
AND BOTH ENTERED LAW SCHOOL. A LOT OF THE PEOPLE IN
THE AREA AROUND THEM WERE GETTING THEIR HOUSES
FORECLOSED ON, AND JOSH AND HIS SISTER AND SOME OF
THEIR FRIENDS THOUGHT 'WE HAVE THIS PRIVLEDGE, WHAT
CAN WE DO WITH IT'. SO THEY FORMED A GROUP, AND THEY
WENT DOOR TO DOOR FINDING OUT WHO WAS GETTING FORCLOSED
ON AND EXPAINING TO THEM THEIR LEGAL RIGHTS AND HELPING
PEOPLE FIGHT.   I LIKED HOW HE TALKED ABOUT IT —
SO MATTER OF FACT, SO DAILY LIFE, NO BLOWING IT OUT
OF PROPORTAON, NO REVOLUTIONARY PATTING ON THE BACK.
JUST — 'WE HAVE THIS PRIVELEDGE, WHAT DO WE DO WITH IT,
HERE'S ONE OF THE THINGS WE DID THAT WAS USEFUL.'

I USED TO WORRY A LOT ABOUT GETTING OLDER — ABOUT PUNKS GETTING OLDER. LIKE WHAT WOULD WE ALL DO? WE HAD BEEN TAUGHT THAT TO BE SUCCESSFUL IN LIFE YOU HAD TO GO TO SCHOOL, GET A JOB, STICK WITH THAT JOB NO MATTER HOW MUCH IT SUCKED. YOU NEEDED HEALTH INSURANCE, YOUR OWN LITTLE APARTMENT, YOU OWN LITTLE GIRLFRIEND, YOU NEEDED TO GO OUT TO DINNER, GO OUT TO THE MOVIES, BUY THINGS TO MAKE YOU AND YOUR LIFE PRETTIER. AS PUNKS WE SAID 'FUCK THAT'. WE WERE

UGLY, WE WERE SLUTTY, WE LIVED ALL TOGETHER OR NOWHERE AT ALL. WE CREATED OUR OWN AESTHETICS. WE GOT EVERYTHING WE NEEDED FROM WHAT THE REST OF THE WORLD THREW AWAY. INCLUDING EACHOTHER. WE WERE THROW OUTS. WE FOUND EACHOTHER IN THE TRASH.

BUT THERE WAS A TIME WHEN MY FRIENDS STARTED DIEING, AND THERE WAS A TIME WHEN MY FRIENDS STARTED STANDING IN THE BACK OF THE ROOM DURING THE SHOWS AND THEN LEAVING. AND I RETREATED SOMEWHAT TOO, BECAUSE THERE WAS A PART OF MYSELF I HAD TO RESCUE. AND NOW THAT IT WAS RESCUED, NOW THAT IT WAS FLOURISHING, I WONDERED WHAT IT WOULD BE LIKE, OUT THERE.

ONCE UPON A TIME, PUNK CYNICISM WAS REBELLION AGAINST A WORLD OPTIMISTIC WITH THE PROMISES OF CAPITALISM; WHEN RONALD REGAN SAID HE'D GIVE MONEY TO THE RICH AND IT WOULD TRICKLE DOWN TO THE POOR, AND WE WERE TOLD THE WORLD'S RESOURCES WERE ENDLESS AND TECHNOLOGY WOULD SAVE US, AND THE MERGER BETWEEN CORPORATIONS AND THE MEDIA WAS GETTING MORE BRILLIANT AND INSIDIOUS. CYNICISM ITSELF WAS A FORM OF REBELLION. BUT NOW EVERYONE'S A CYNIC, DESPITE THE NEW SELLING POINT OF HOPE.

SO HOW DO WE FORGE RESISTANCE? WE FORGE IT WITH VISION, AND BELIEVING IN OURSELVES AND OUR COMMUNITIES, AND LIVING LIVES OF INTEGRITY. and fighting for our beliefs A COUPLE OF MY FRIENDS WHO I THOUGHT WEREN'T GOING TO MAKE IT OUT ALIVE ARE STILL ALIVE. THEY'RE ELECTRICIANS. ONE OF THEM EVEN BOUGHT A HOUSE FOR TWO OF OUR CRAZY AND UNEMPLOYABLE FRIENDS TO LIVE IN. SOME OF MY FRIENDS ARE TEACHERS NOW, SOME ARE WRITING FOR THE WEEKLY NEWSPAPERS, SOME ARE WRITING BOOKS, SOME HAVE UNION JOBS, ONE HAS A RECORDING STUDIO, ONE RUNS A RESTAURANT,

A COUPLE OF THEM WORK AT AN ANIMAL SHELTER, ONE HELPS OLD PEOPLE GROW OLD AND DIE WITH DIGNITY, ONE WORKS AT A RAPE CRISIS CENTER. ONE IS A THERAPIST, ONE IS A DOCTOR, ONE WORKS FOR THE FOREST SERVICE, ONE DOES RESTORATION CONSTRUCTION. SOME HAVE BABIES AND FAMILIES, SOME HAVE GONE BACK TO SCHOOL. SOME LIVE ALONE, SOME STILL LIVE ALL TOGETHER.   FOR THE MOST PART, THOSE OF US WHO LIVED, MADE IT THROUGH WITHOUT AS MUCH GIVING UP AS I'D EXPECTED.

A BUNCH OF THEM STILL PLAY MUSIC. MOST OF THEM ARE STILL INVOLVED, IN ONE WAY OR ANOTHER, IN CREATING OR MAINTAINING CULTURES OF RESISTANCE, OR WORKING TO BUILD MORE EMPOWERED COMMUNITIES.

IN PROVIDENCE, MERIDITH GIVES ME HER ZINE. IT'S A ONE SHEET WITH A DRAWING OF TWO CATS, TWO WITCHY CATS STANDING OVER A CAULDRON, STIRRING. IT'S KIND OF CRYPTIC, WITH A SENTANCE HERE AND THERE, LIKE A MAP OF SOMETHINGS IN HER HEART OR LIKE AN INSIDE JOKE SHE'S PARTIALLY LETTING ME IN ON. AND IT SAYS TO ME, "I AM FINALLY HAPPY. I AM TRUELY IN LOVE." AT LEAST THAT'S WHAT IT SEEMS TO SAY.

IN VERMONT, PAULA COMES TO SEE US. SHE WAS MY IDOL WHEN I WAS 15. SHE KNEW EVERYTHING AND MORE THAN I EVER THOUGHT I WOULD. SHE KNEW HISTORY AND PLANTS AND PHILOSOPHY AND PROTEST TACTICS AND COULD IDENTIFY ANIMALS IN THE WOODS BY THE NOISES THAT THEY MADE. SHE SHOWS UP IN BRATTLEBORO AS ELEGANT AS EVER AND I LOVE HER JUST AS I ALWAYS HAVE. WE'RE MORE LIKE EQUALS NOW. AND EVEN THOUGH WE'VE PROBABLY ONLY SEEN EACHOTHER 3 TIMES IN THE PAST TEN YEARS, THE FRIENDSHIP STILL FEELS NATURAL AND STRONG.

WE PLAY WITH ANTOINE'S BAND, MY OLD FRIEND FROM ASHEVILLE. HE'S JUST BOUGHT A MILK COW WITH A GROUP OF PEOPLE WHO ALL TAKE TURNS TAKING CARE OF IT, LEARNING HOW. WE PLAY WITH UKE OF PHILLIPS, CORNERS, DAN USED TO INTERN ON MY SISTERS FARM AND HAS BEEN OUR FRIEND NOW FOREVER, AND AMY IS ONE OF MY FAVORITE ARTISTS AND THEIR VOICES SOUND SO STRANGE AND PERFECT. EVERYONE SITS AROUND THEM AND REQUESTS SONGS AND I THINK "HOW DOES EVERYONE KNOW THE TITLES?" IT'S LIKE A DREAM COME TRUE. WE STAY WITH DALIA AND SATURN, MY NEW FRIENDS WHO I LIKE SO MUCH I WOULD ALMOST THINK OF MOVING TO VERMONT JUST TO BE NEAR

THEM, EXCEPT I LIVE IN OHIO NOW. I HAVE A HOME.
IN THE MORNING, SATURN BUILDS UP THE FIRE AND DALIA

GOES OFF TO THE BAKERY AND WE GO TO HELP BUILD A YURT,
EXCEPT WE'RE LATE AND IT'S PRETTY MUCH ALREADY BUILT
AND THERE'S A STORM COMING EVERYONE SAYS WE'LL NEVER
MAKE IT OUT. THEY TELL US ALL KINDS OF WEIRD BACK
ROAD ROUTES, BUT WE JUST HEAD SOUTH, TAKE THE FREEWAYS
AND WE MAKE IT. HOME. SWEET HOME.

you'll never make it.
you could try taking
county road 2 to 127 to
county road L - that ones
dirt but it's pretty good
all the way to mass

WE'RE JUST
GOING SOUTH
TO THE FREEWAY

SNARLAS 7" RECORD
available for $5
from me
CINDY
POB 29
athens oh 45701

or dorisdorisdoris.com/music distro

315

W is for

Why Haven't You Known

The other day someone I know said "It's not really capitalism that's the problem. We just need to create ecological accountability for corporations." and a few months earlier, someone else I knew had said "If only we could convince everyone to turn off their lights more!"

I was so surprised in both cases and didn't even know where to begin, but I remember when I thought those ways too. and I remember reading the article "Why Haven't You Known" which was about the atomic bomb tests the U.S. did on the Bikini islands. The fallout poisoned people. The women gave birth to what they called "jellyfish babies;" babies that had a heartbeat but no form and died within an hour. The women of the islands wrote this essay to U.S. feminists and activists, saying - these are the horrors that you have turned a blind eye to - Why Haven't You Known?

These days I am surprised when people think reform is still possible. It just seems like we're inundated by the horrors every day - war and racism and poverty and prisons, gender hatred and rape and enviornmental destruction, the inability of electoral politics to fill anyone's real needs. but I suppose the inundation with no radical analysis leaves people floundering. In which case, I really recommend the book <u>A Culture of Make Believe</u>, by Derek Jensen.

TONI WESCHLER author of TAKING CHARGE OF YOUR FERTILITY

THIS IS THE GREATEST BOOK IF YOU WANT TO UNDERSTAND MORE ABOUT YOUR MENSTRUAL CYCLE, ANATOMY, IF YOU'RE INTERESTED IN USING FERTILITY AWARENESS AS A FORM OF BIRTH CONTROL (or for trying to get pregnant). WESCHLER is really thorough, funny, + pissed off at the medical world's treatment of women.

Winona La Duke

author and activist

totally changed my life!

♡

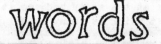

words

I can't believe how the fuck it keeps happening; people
waking up to someone they know touching them. How the
hell can anyone think it is ok to initiate sex with
someone who is sleeping?

Do they think about our abuse histories? Or the fact
that we can't say "no" when we're asleep? Do they understand our complex defense systems and how vulnerable and
terrified we might feel waking up to this assault? Do
they know that even if we go along with it all, once we
wake up, it doesn't necessarily mean we wanted it? We
have complex ways of protecting ourselves. Do they think
about this?

The truth is, I used to crawl in people's beds too.
I thought it was ok. I thought of course all guys wanted
it. I never considered the fact that I might be capable of
assault. But of course, I am. A lot of us are.

Are you seeing this? Will you promise to take steps
to never do it again?(like don't get in bed with someone
when you're wasted or unsure about your intentions. Stop
making excuses for yourself. Look at your life for real.)

I am sick of how it all keeps happening. I can't
stand how often people tell me something like this: "I told
him, early in the night, that just because we were getting
drunk together didn't mean I wanted to fuck him. I
specifically said fI don't want to have sex with you" and
then later, he was just on me. Do we call this rape?"

Or how many times I've heard "I didn't say no outright,
but I tried to make it clear." And then there are all the
times we try to comfort someone or find comfort in their
arms, and they think it's an invitation to do what they
want. We trust people and they don't understand (or care?)
about the difference between emotional openness and sexual
desire. Or how it happens; if we're slutty or flirty
people think we're open game. If we're shy, they think it's
a form of flirt and really they just need to be persistent
in pressuring us. This game is not always a fun game for
all of us.

Yesterday, a tough girl friend of mine said "I have
not had consensual sex all year." The day before I heard
friends laughing about two people we knew who had been
wrestling and one of them had just thought it was comraderie
until the other person ...

and everyone is laughing at the story because it is a boy - boy story, which I don't think is funny at all.

The day before that I was reading a zine where she's calling someone out. She says "That was assault, asshole!" but at the end of the page it says "I should have fought."

I am sick of people saying, "well, if you didn't want it, why didn't you say something. I never would have had sex (or whatever(with you if I'd known."

I am sick of the blame and self blame. We have had practically everything taken away from us and can not always speak. And what kind of world are we building? If it's still seen as our responsibility to say something? Why isn't it their responsibility to ask and watch for signs and signals, and ask again?

You know how there are supposedly two instinctual responses — fight or flight? Well, there's also freeze. you can see it everywhere in nature, especially in animals that are under constant attack.

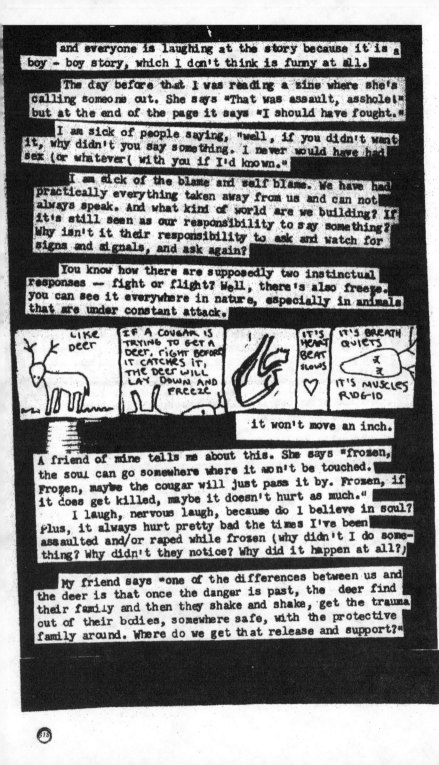

it won't move an inch.

A friend of mine tells me about this. She says "frozen, the soul can go somewhere where it won't be touched. Frozen, maybe the cougar will just pass it by. Frozen, if it does get killed, maybe it doesn't hurt as much."

I laugh, nervous laugh, because do I believe in soul? Plus, it always hurt pretty bad the times I've been assaulted and/or raped while frozen (why didn't I do something? Why didn't they notice? Why did it happen at all?)

My friend says "one of the differences between us and the deer is that once the danger is past, the deer find their family and then they shake and shake, get the trauma out of their bodies, somewhere safe, with the protective family around. Where do we get that release and support?"

"At the punk show?" I say.

"Come on now, really." She says, and of course, it is true. It is not the same. She says "we don't get support and release. We are almost never in a place of safty. The trauma builds in us. We freeze our voices, our bodies. We become frozen inside."

She thinks it is instinct and culture. I think it is systematic oppression and patriarchy. But sometimes now, alone in my room, I shake and I shake and I scream.

more words

Maybe we need 100 new words for when our friends or acquaintances or partners assault or rape us. One word to describe, "I let you because I was half asleep and too tired to do anything else." One that's "I was to sick of arguing about it." One for "It's fucked up and scary the way you talk to me. One for "I told you I didn't want to do that." One for, "why didn't you notice I wasn't present anymore." One for, "we had an agreement you would use protection." One for, "you said if I didn't do it you'd leave me. What choice did I have?"

Maybe we need 100 new words to talk about rape and sexual assault and sexual manipulation: words that speak clear about the seriousness of what is being done to our bodies. Or maybe our friends and acquaintances and partners need to have the courage to hear "You raped me, ore "that was assault" (I still barely ever use these words because I know the backlash consequences. I know that no no one has the courage to hear their actions defined that way. They don't want to admit they are capable of rape or assault. They don't want to admit that patriarchy exists and that it gives them the God and State granted rights to do these things. They don't want to look at the physical and political nature of their actions. They want to blow it all off. They have a million different reasons for what they did.)

Every time I've tried to talk to someone about sexual stuff that they did to me that I didn't want, their first reaction is to (usually frantically) try to explain it away. They want the story to different than the one I'm telling. They want me to see it through their eyes and absolve them. They say "But I thought," they say, "I never would have," even "No, that's not what happened" (as if their experience was the only one). They try to make me out as crazy. They say I am blaming them for things that are really just stored up from my past.

I am not crazy. I am aware that capitalism and patriarchy and all systems of control depend on the denial of both the oppressor and the oppressed. I know that patriarchy values logic over emotion, and that "too much" emotion, too strong of a response, will label you crazy, and that women especially are considered crazy lot of the time. We are not crazy. What happens to us is real. All the attempts to silence us won't change this reality.

I carry with me a whole history of sexual abuse, and so do most of us. Each sexual act does not exist in a vacuum and I'm sick of people treating it as if it does. I never want to hear the fucking words, "Well, why didn't you stop me?" again. I want to hear, "oh my god, I'm so sorry" and then I want them to ask for my story. I want them to be able to take it instead of asking for pity. If I tell them to fuck off and leave me alone, then I want them to respect that. If it's someone I love, I might want them to hold me so I can cry. If it's someone I hate, I want to be able to punch them without the community saying "dude, that's so fucked up! She hit him!"

I want all of them to say, I believe you. I'm taking this seriously. I hate what I've done and I'm going to change. I'm going to commit myself (or recommit myself) to looking deep inside of myself and changing my behavior and looking at this world and what it's made me into, and it's my responsibility. I'm going to take this seriously. Thank you for having the courage to tell me. I'm going to work as hard as possible to make sure I never do that to anyone ever again."

I want them to say that and feel it and mean it and follow through.

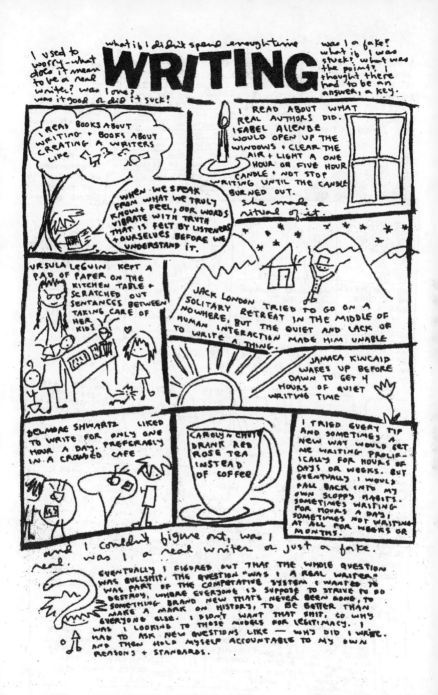

I WRITE IN MY JOURNAL BECAUSE IT HELPS ME TO LEARN TO BE PRESENT AND TO PROCESS WHAT I SEE + FEEL + THINK

dear diary

I am here in Arizona. My Grandma is dieing, maybe. outside is the weird green of the watered lawn here in the desert that I wish could return to desert. when do we stop trying to make things what we want them? should I tell her to fight to stay alive or should I let her go?

I WRITE BECAUSE IT HELPS ME TO SEE THE WORLD IN NEW WAYS + FIGHT THE BRAINWASH OF BLACK WHITE, FAT THIN, BLOND BROWN.

WRITING HELPS ME TO LOOK MORE + SEE MORE

he leans forward when he walks. Her face has strong expressions.

she looks like she wants to say something but she doesn't.

she rubs her thumb under her chin. He has the longest eye lashes hidden.

I WRITE DORIS BECAUSE I BELIEVE THAT IN ORDER TO CHANGE THE WORLD FUNDAMENTALLY, WE HAVE TO CHALLENGE OURSELVES AND EACHOTHER TO BE BRAVE AND ALIVE

LETS JUST JUMP ON THE BED

OK

AND WE HAVE TO TAKE OUR EXPERIENCES + FIND THE LESSONS IN THEM AND PASS ON THESE LESSONS IN A WAY THAT DOESN'T ALIENATE

and zines are a perfect place for me to work on becoming a better writer + to work at articulating + editing + learning to spell a little bit better + learning to draw. I write it all down in my journal + then look at it and think "what is the essence of this - what is the important part?" Sometimes it is just one sentance worth saving. I write from there + edit + write + edit. I believe in care but not a stifling fear or ego driven perfection.

HOWS IT GOING?

PRETTY GOOD. I'VE BEEN THINKING ABOUT THE SLOGAN "GROWING UP = GIVING UP" and HOW I LOVE GROWING UP

IT HELPS ME THINK OF NEW SUBJECTS TO TALK TO PEOPLE ABOUT SO LIFE STAYS GOOD + NOT BORING GOSSIP.

here, I made this

IT HELPS ME TO HAVE A PROJECT I CAN FINISH + PUT OUT THERE TO FEEL CONNECTED + NOT SO ALONE.

X marks the

Pe X andSassy   just   in t
ate   in the   es a   I ca
those minihorse: neig   le gr

hey run towards me the crook of an arm my head in the
oulder warm under the blankets in a stick fort sleepi
stone boulders back in the woods the field that is no
a pine forest walking down the street with my raccoo
nywhere the building rooftop mural alley the whisperi
basement shows the landfill my dumpstered writing des
at night where it crosses the river pensacola beach
tourists the recycling center late at night when you
the bottles you want grandma bessie bell's pine tree
e under the stairs where I painted rainbows on the wa
in the stacks of books at the library hiding in the
deep bathtubs with gretchen the cat lapping water u
on the tree limb in the back field watching the dogs
expressions of a new friends face the way they walk
hide the nook behind the building on telegraph where
ry to eachother grandmas basement with the orange ca
ayed cards like 52 pick up and i was all alone playi
f the road up to jenny house the park at the end of
oorway at 6th and market on the train the last trai
the community garden the middle of the mississippi
ry waters with the minks playing like i wish i coul
ep into a novel that I can't put down screaming wit
show singing along with all my friends pressed clos
e van going from one place to another in courtneys
ng on the counter top real Finish saunas iceskating
ts the back of the van the great sand dune national
there are buffalo not caged in inside the donut sho
e the wash where the coyotees breed behind the libra
d up boat in cape cod alleys doorsteps to abandon ho
where we slept under the sidewalk inside museums suck
any place to call home the chair at robin and pauls
the back shack in pitsburgh the top of the hill when
he miniture hot air balloons in the middle of the ni
powered by candles and went up and up and up so pret
sisters crib go fish through the laundry shoot erin
yard when she let me set up my tent back there and l
he week of escape telling stories of kimba the smell
ds study the floor of the station wagon on long road
ad lands the railroad tracks by gilman railroad trac
under the loading dock at the box factory on the lo
e candle factory the voidvot spot or however you spe
eachers of the unused baseball field at night with t
back and forth my bed when its raining out curled u

There were times when I wanted adventure. My friends hopped trains and came back filthy, covered in dirt and eachother. full of escape stories, fighting the cops stories, and the random encounters with strangers - normal people,- who reached out and gave them something, a ride, some food, some part of their lives.

in a world that made people so empty and shut of off and judgemental and alone, it was these random small things that sometimes gave us hope.

i felt kind of like a poseur. but I watched everything around me and I learned everything I could.
When the rain came through the roof, I learned to patch it. When the sink wouldn't stop dripping, I took it apart. When the van broke down, i looked under the hood. I read the manuel. I bought tools, a worthy investment, and lost them. When my garden wouldn't grow I asked my sister

WHAT AM I DOING WRONG?

THERE'S NOT A SCRAP OF SUN BACK HERE

I hadn't noticed.

and it's funny because it never felt like it was adding up that much, but now we bought a house and I tear out the walls and ceiling, rewire the lights, hang up the drywall, redo the plumbing. There's a lot I don't knowm My friends come and help me. But I know enough that I know this is possible. to make a home livable.

Sometimes I look in the mirror and there are ways my face is changing. some wrinkles. I try not to look in the mirror too often. I think "how ugly." and then I look at women my age or older and their wrinkles which I think are totally beautiful

there are things we're not supposed to look at or think about. there are things we're not supposed to be curious about. there are things we're not supposed to learn.

I say learn them, look, think, be curious. don't give away your power if you can help it.

when I moved here, I couldn't stop crying. Sometimes the crying would come so suddenly and strongly I would fall to the floor. It seemed extremely dramatic, but I had no control over it. and I wasn't depressed exactly. there was a big part of me that was happy.

I read "burnout is caused by a failure to mourn" I tried to let the sorrow pass through me.

I thought that since I didn't have any friends here and couldn't remember how to make friends it would be the perfect time to write a few books. I was going to write my political autobiography - more about the politics and less about my life. I got a library card at the college library and a whole stack of books about Ronald Regan and about the wars and U.S. intervention in Central America in the 80's. I layed in bed and read a lot and took a lot of notes and felt really isolated - like 'I'm ok, but where is the joy in life?'-   I decided maybe I better work harder at making some friends first.

I told Caty

"I've got a new full time job."

what is it?

"trying to make friends"

Every day I'd be busily doing stuff around the
house - we were renting a sweet house in the country
with a pond and acres of woods on a dirt road. Every
day I'd sigh and say "I guess it's time to go to
work", and I pack up my backpack and head in to
town. Since I didn't feel very outgoing, making
friends mostly consisted of just sitting around one
of the two places I felt sort of comfortable, the
coffee shop or the collective resturant/bar. I'd
bring my normal paying work with me, and I'd sit
at the booth tieing knots in the ends of scarves
I'd woven. I'd write out invoices or whatever it is
I had to do.

I figured if I was just around long
enough, may be the people would find me. I also
tried to talk enthusiastically to anyone who I had
even vaguely met before. I waved at people who I
thought should be friendly to me. Some of them
looked like I was crazy. some of them said hi. Johnny
invited me to the Make Believes show. Finally! A
show to go to! There are a lot of bars and shitty
college bar shows and I hadn't figured out how to
find the shows that weren't just misogynist jockrock.

The MakeBelieves were incredable. if they come
to your town, go see them.

I got obsessed with Mikey, the one visibly
queer boy in town. "Do you think he's queer or
just a hipster" I asked Caty. She said "the
hipsters here don't look very gay yet."   well,
now that I think about it, she probably didn't
say that. I was probably just talking to myself.

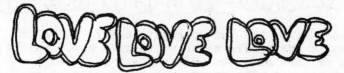

Mikey had a shirt that said "Love Love Love" in
bubble letters. His hair was kind of curly with
one patch dyed blue or green. The color hadn't
taken very well. He had those kind of sad or tired
or hungover eyes. I wrote him a note and tied it
up with string. I made him a fortune cookie with
the fortune saying 'a new friend would bring you
much happiness.'
If I ran into him at night when he
was drunk he'd call me his straight wife and I'd
loudly claim that I was not straight! I was like 80%
gay. His eyes weren't tracking. We never did become
proper friends. I gave him my Doris Anti-Depression
Guide and he told me he really liked it, it had
some real LOL moments. When I got home I asked Caty,
"do you know what LOL means?" She said "oh, I just

read an article in the New Yorker about text
messaging. I think it means 'laugh out loud'.

The New Yorker. boy oh boy.

I came up with a brand-new tactic for making friends.
Usually before I would just try to be unobtrusive,

Like, if I found people I wanted to be friends with,
I just tried to hang around them and not get in
their way. I tried to watch them and anticipate
their needs and fulfill their needs before they
even realized them. I took care of them when they
were sick or brokenhearted. I pulled secrets out

of them. I tried to make myself indispensable.

My new friendship approach was really different.
I figured I would try and do the thing that was
hardest for me to do - ask people for help.
It was something I was trying to practice. And I
knew that generally people really like to help other
people when they can and it's sort of flattering to
be asked for help with something, as long as the
something is a useful thing and not too boring or
sucky.

Like I asked the two toughest looking girls in
town if they would teach me to ride a motorcycle.
One of them said she would except she didn't
know how yet. The other girl had road rash on
her shoulder. she laughed her perfect laugh and
said if I wanted to learn from her, she'd teach
me. I asked the grad-school writer girls I met
if they'd read something I wrote and tell me if
it made sense. We ended up starting a writing
group. I asked Johnny for direction. I asked
White Horse if I could borrow their shop-vac.
I asked Sarah if there were any punk or notsopunk
houses where people did stuff together not just
couples and she said 'sure. Tocmanistan. I'll
go down there with you.' There were people on

the front porch, bikes in the bushes, a practice
space in the garage. I said "can I come over and
cook in your kitchen when I'm in town? Can I
set up an office in the back? Do you want to start
a band? Do you want to go on a friendship date?'

I like how people can be shy and not shy at the
same time. Lizzy had the prettiest sparkly sweater.
the nicest blush. she asked me thoughtful questions
about things that mattered in my life and hers.
Indigo wanted advice about relationships and
collective organizing. Miguel was quiet sometimes,
and stood on chairs and slept in his freebox and
held my hand when I couldn't stop crying.

and I know it has been said a million times in
zines - the list of things that make friends
be friends. and I know it has been said a million
times - how we need to make sure there are always
houses people can come to, places we can gather.
how we need to make sure to welcome. to not
isolate. to keep taking risks. to keep seeing
beauty. to keep alive and alive in the world.
and to remember to thank our friends for the things
they have given. and to remember to give. reach
out. risk. love.

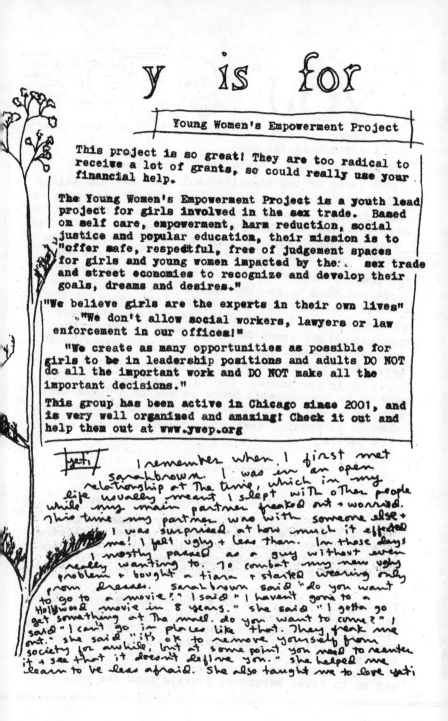

y is for

Young Women's Empowerment Project

This project is so great! They are too radical to receive a lot of grants, so could really use your financial help.

The Young Women's Empowerment Project is a youth lead project for girls involved in the sex trade. Based on self care, empowerment, harm reduction, social justice and popular education, their mission is to "offer safe, respectful, free of judgement spaces for girls and young women impacted by the sex trade and street economies to recognize and develop their goals, dreams and desires."

"We believe girls are the experts in their own lives"
"We don't allow social workers, lawyers or law enforcement in our offices!"

"We create as many opportunities as possible for girls to be in leadership positions and adults DO NOT do all the important work and DO NOT make all the important decisions."

This group has been active in Chicago since 2001, and is very well organized and amazing! Check it out and help them out at www.ywep.org

I remember when I first met sarahbrown. I was in an open relationship at the time, which in my life usually meant I slept with other people while my main partner freaked out + worried. This time my partner was with someone else + I was surprised at how much it effected me! I felt ugly + less than. In those days I mostly passed as a guy without even really wanting to. To combat my new ugly problem + bought a tiara + started wearing only dresses. sarahbrown said "do you want to go to a movie?" I said "I haven't gone to a Hollywood movie in 8 years." she said "I gotta go get something at the mall. do you want to come?" I said "I can't go in places like that. They freak me out." she said "it's ok to remove yourself from society for awhile, but at some point you need to reenter it + see that it doesn't define you." she helped me learn to be less afraid. She also taught me to love yeti

YOU

I wrote this for you:
You who needs city, needs land/ trees/sea.

You whose mother committed suicide. You who thinks
your feelings get out of control. You who has only one
real friend, or none. who feels like a visitor in the
city you live and like you're the only person who is
ever uncomfortable. You in the "Year of Magic" you
created. you brave and alive. so excited to see what
you could do if you really wanted to and set your
heart and mind to do. You trying to get out of an
abusive relationship. You who has lost track of the
person you want to be and is searching under every
rock and around every corner. afraid to cry or that
you cry too much. You who wants to make everything
new. makes art of the small things you find in the
street or in the fields. You in isolation, behind the
bars or in your parents house or out in a world that
refuses to see or value you. wanting to feel the
comfort of knowing that other people have felt like
you before.

---

and for me.
when I read your letter that says

"The only place I have ever felt safe and ok is in
the sunflower fields of Kansas, with the sunflowers
turning slowly with each minute; always turning their
yellow faces to face the yellow sun. And always in
the sunflower fields, I'm reminded of you."

I read this letter and am so immediately overwhelmed.
and I wonder how much love will I have to receive
before I allow myself to actually receive it -- Allow
myself to let it in through the barriers that are
bracing against loves eventual removal.
I do not know where these barriers live inside of me,
and so to these barriers, I write this for you.

Z is for

ZORA NEALE HURSTON

When I was a teenager, there were not many women being published, and a lot of the really great works of literature by women had been allowed to go out of print. Thankfully, the feminist + womanist movements of the 70s were dedicated to rediscovering forgotten artists. Zora Neale Hurston was one of the greatest writers of the mid 1900's.

She wrote the amazing novel <u>Their Eyes Were Watching God</u>, which Alice Walker describes by saying "There is enough self-love in that one book — love of community, culture, traditions — to restore a world. Or create a new one." (from the dedication in the book <u>I LOVE MYSELF when I'm laughing... And Then Again when I'm looking Mean + Impressive</u>, which is another great one.)

zebras

Zapatistas

Oh, I was so happy when the Zapatistas came to be known! It was January 1, 1994, the first morning that the North American Free Trade Agreement went into effect. In Southern Mexico, in the state of Chiapas, an indigenous led guerrilla army took over 4 cities and declared war on the Mexican Government. They demanded "work, land, shelter, bread, health, education education, democracy, liberty, peace, independence and justice." They fought against the genocide of indigenous Mexicans by the Mexican government and against the total war of corporate rule over the whole world. I love the Zapatistas. They were the first revolutionary group in my time that didn't seem mired down in old socialist dogma or defensive anarchist philosophies or nationalism, but instead just made sense - a kind of humble, extremely smart and visionary sense.

read: <u>Beyond Resistance: Everything</u>

zines

to write a zine you need paper + pen, scissors and glue stick. a photo-copier somewhere. some courage. maybe the zine is something you do, you + your friends together. a project to work on to bring you some joy + some focus. maybe you've learned something + you want to share it. maybe you've been told to keep quiet + you need to break it. maybe your rage is so huge you need a starting space to begin to express it. or your love for this world makes you want to change it.

you do not need permission you write + reflect + try + find the truth of what you want to say + write again and send your imperfect words out into the world. imperfect but done with care. you are worth it.

here